Patrick Netter's
high-tech
fitness

Patrick Netter's
high-tech fitness

By Patrick Netter
and the High-Tech
Fitness Team

Principal Photography by
Ken Merfeld

Workman Publishing, New York

Library of Congress Cataloging in Publication Data
Netter, Patrick.
Patrick Netter's High-tech fitness.
1. Physical fitness.
2. Exercise.
3. Exercise—Equipment and supplies. I. Title.
II. Title: High-tech fitness.
GV481.N44 1985   613.7′028   84-40317
ISBN 0-89480-771-4

Technical adviser on photography: S. Richard Gunter
Cover photography: Ken Merfeld
Cover design: Tedd Arnold
Art Direction: Paul Hanson
Book design: Judith A. Doud

High-Tech Fitness™ is a trademark of High-Tech Fitness,
Inc., 617 N. La Cienega Blvd., Los Angeles, CA 90069.
Application is pending for registration in the U.S. Patent
and Trademark Office.

Workman Publishing Company, Inc.
1 West 39 Street
New York, New York 10018
Manufactured in the United States of America
First printing October 1984
10 9 8 7 6 5 4 3 2 1

Wende Chinchilla West, my partner in this book, assisted me in every aspect that needed attention—from discussing and originating concepts, to stylizing the photography, to tracking down needed details.

Without her professionalism, inspiration, dedication and love, this book would never have come together.

HIGH-TECH FITNESS TEAM
BOARD OF ADVISERS

LEROY PERRY, JR., D.C.

Chiropractic orthopedist. President of International Sports Medicine Institute. Co-Founder, with Wilt Chamberlain, of the Foundation for Athletic Research and Education.

WILLIAM R. PRIHODA, M.S.

Bio-mechanist and exercise specialist.

SUKI RAPPAPORT, Ph.D.

Movement educator, author of publications on body transformation and gravity inversion.

BILL RODGERS

World renowned fitness and running expert. Four-time New York and four-time Boston Marathon winner. Author of *Marathoning*.

AM ROSEN, N.D.

Nutritional consultant.

JACK L. ROSENBERG, D.D.S., Ph.D.

Director for the Rosenberg Institute of Integrative Body Psycho-Therapy.

MYRON S. SHAPERO, M.D., F.A.A.F.P.

Member of the American College of Sports Medicine. Physician Specialist for the 1984 Olympic Games. Diplomate, American Board of Family Practice.

HARRY AND SARAH SNEIDER

Personal trainers to numerous Olympic athletes. Fitness directors at Ambassador College, Pasadena, California.

JACKSON SOUSA

Founder/President of Jackson Sousa Professional Fitness Training Group.

CHAMPION K. TEUTSCH, Ph.D.

Clinical psychologist. Published author on motivation and psycho-geneticism.

TRAINING GROUP, INC.

Los Angeles-based personal training company.

MARJORIE TYSON, B.S.

Clinical nutritionist. President of Integrated Health, Inc.

DARRELL L. WHITE, I.S.I.D.

National Interior Design Award recipient. Expert in designing home and corporate gym interiors.

ACKNOWLEDGMENTS

I cannot list all the people who've helped put High-Tech Fitness on the map and this book together. But I'd like to at least single out my following friends and business associates who have put up, cajoled, influenced and inspired me to finish this monumentally healthy project!

Annie Brody, my literary agent, for coming to me with the idea and keeping me on track; Syd Field and John Manning for helping me to put the original proposal together; Peter Workman, Sally Kovalchick, Paul Hanson, Mary Wilkinson and Judy Doud, at Workman Publishing, for continuously believing in and finishing this project with style; Annette Annechild for helping to structure the book and supplying great energy; Ken Merfeld and associates for an excellent photo job; Darrell White for always coming up with creative design ideas; Ben Pesta for his speedy and jocular way of writing; Joy Grau for her great attitude and technical help; Drew Mearns, my capable business adviser, for his sagacious marketing help; the High-Tech Fitness retail staff—Carol Whitt, Bobby Omatsu, Andrew Schatz, Jerry Matt, Rosemary Meyer, Monett Schwartz, Don Parker, Fred Flynn. And the following special humans: my mother, father and sister, Holly and Tommy Harp, Steven Eisen, Richard Leivenberg, Carreiro's Gymnastics Classes, Rick Nathan, Mark Reisman and Al Yesk.

I'd like to thank the following model workout people:

Annette Annechild, Carmel the Cat, Belinda Lee Gunter, Marie Landwirth, Ken Marts, Bess Motta (cover), Don Parker, Eric Parkinson, Bill Prihoda, Karen Rushmore, Zetta Whitlow, Carl Wilson (make-up), Delane Vaughn, Richard Gunter.

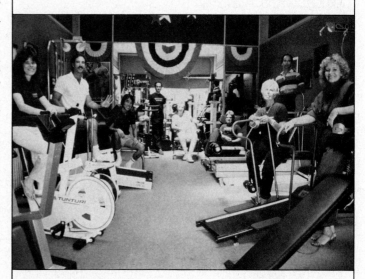

Patrick Netter and his staff, shown in his flagship High-Tech Fitness store in Los Angeles.

The following companies were generous with their cooperation, helping to make this the first and best compendium of quality fitness equipment in the world.

Amerec Corporation

AMF American Athletic Equipment Division

BackSaver Co.

Bally Fitness Products Corporation

Better Living Designs

Biosig Instruments, Inc.

Bio-Technology, Inc.

California Gym Equipment Co.

Cemco Physical Fitness Products

Computer Instruments Corp.

Computerized Biomechanical Analysis, Inc.

The Dance Center

Excel, The Exercise Company

Fitness Master, Inc.

Fitness Equipment Co., Inc.

Fitness Equipment of California

Fitness Products

Gravity Guidance, Inc.

Gym Equipment International, Inc.

Gym-Mobile Corporation

Gyro Jump

Haden Industries Inc.

Hemokinetics

Heartmate, Inc.

Hoggan Health Equipment Mfg.

H.W.E., Inc.

Ivanko Barbell Co.

Jacuzzi Whirlpool Bath

Kyga Stick Co.

J. Oglaend, Inc.

Libin & Associates

MacLevy Products Corporation

Marcy Gym Equipment Co.

Maxisports Inc.

M & R Industries Inc.

Nautilus For The Home

New Balance® Athletic Shoe, Inc.*

Nordic Fitness Equipment

Norelco

Nu-Barres Co.

Oasis Tank Co., Inc.

Paramount Fitness Equipment Corporation

Polder, Inc.

Precor, Inc.

PaVage Fitness Innovations

Pro Form, Inc.

Quality Gym Sales, Inc.

Queststar

Samadhi Tank Co.

Spenco Medical Corp.

Swim Gym

Total Gym By West Bend

Training Group, Inc.

Trampolking Sporting Goods

Triangle Mfg. Corp.

Trileen Inc.

Trotter Treadmills

Universal Gym Equipment Co.

West Bend Company

Zemco, Inc.

Zestron, Inc.

CONTENTS

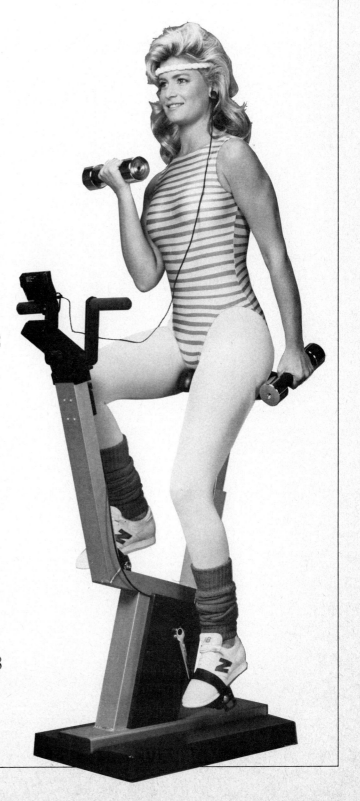

FOREWORD

Exercise, until the twentieth century, has been almost exclusively an outdoor activity. The ancient Olympic Games, for example, began in a sacred valley in Greece in 776 B.C.

These games were actually religious festivals held in honor of the Olympian god Zeus, and had little to do with health or fitness, except for preventing death by war. Every four years, the Greek nation and its warring tribes laid down their arms and came together in peaceful competition.

The first of the "modern" Olympic Games was held in Athens, Greece, in 1896. Since that time, world-wide interest in athletic events and physical fitness has steadily increased. Today, more than a third of the American population 16 and over engage in a regular exercise program and, it is estimated, over 30 million of us are involved in running alone.

Why are we so interested in physical fitness today? One of the major reasons is that medicine has made so many advances in the fitness industry that the benefits of exercise are now apparent: increased feeling of well-being; decreased pain; decreased psychological stress; weight loss; strengthening of heart and lungs; lowered risk of heart disease; lowered high blood pressure; and improvement in diabetes condition.

In addition to these advantages, people who exercise are better able to stop smoking, and it is said that regular exercise may help thicken the supporting structures of the skin and delay wrinkling.

As I indicated earlier, exercise was almost always an outdoor activity. However, with the invention of indoor sports such as racquetball and the movement of basketball courts and swimming pools into sheltered areas, exercisers were able to become fit without having to battle the elements.

The emergence of commercial health clubs and the recent aerobic-dance interest attracted even more fitness buffs indoors. The problem, though, is oftentimes these facilities are either inconvenient, crowded or time-consuming.

Since *regular* exercise is so vitally important to health and well-being, the more convenient it is to do, the better your motivation to do it.

That's where Patrick Netter's *High-Tech Fitness* comes in. For the first time since the ancient Olympic Games, fitness can become the "domain of your domain." In other words, now you can equip your home with the proper equipment and exercise in privacy, at your own pace.

This book is unique, because it tells you literally everything you need to know to stay in shape at home. Its advice on fitness and nutrition is medically sound. Its expert tips on setting up your own home gym equipment and their proper use are carefully thought out and researched by professionals.

I believe in what Patrick Netter has to say. I've referred people to him, and they've benefitted from his expertise in fitness and his knowledge of home gym equipment. I've incorporated the ideas related in this book into my own home fitness system. I believe in fact that the information presented here is of value to all of us. I recommend this book without hesitation.

Irving Dardik, M.D., F.A.C.S.

Chairman, U.S. Olympic Committee's Sports Medicine Council
Co-author, *Quantum Fitness*

INTRODUCTION

As a boy, I was always interested in sports and fitness. I played tennis on various school teams. After leaving school, I belonged to several gyms. I managed to keep my body in pretty decent shape.

But I know now that physical fitness was essentially a hit-or-miss proposition for me. I was always finding reasons why I couldn't work out on a given day or night. It was too cold outside. It was too hot. There was a smog alert. There was a chance of rain. I was worried about America's balance of payments deficit. My cat was having an anxiety attack. You know the excuses. Chances are, you've used them yourself.

Today, my home gym is an integral part of my life. I'm proud to own it, and to use it. It *works* for me. These past several months I've gone from bench pressing about a hundred pounds to almost 200 on my weight machine. I started out running two miles in the hills in 24 minutes, and since working out on my aerobic equipment, I can now run that same course in 17. I can do 55 push-ups in one minute and, with a 10-pound weight on my chest, can do 50 sit-ups in 52 seconds. My resting pulse is in the low 60's. My home gym has clearly made me fitter, healthier, and happier.

Of course, in the same way that a highly knowledgeable clothing designer knows what fabrics, styles, and cuts work well, I have the advantage of knowing how best to equip a home fitness center for my family and friends. You've probably seen those T-shirts that say, "Show business is my life." Well, the home gym business is mine.

I graduated Phi Beta Kappa from San Diego State University with a B.A. in psychology. I'd originally planned to go on and take a Ph.D., but I decided to take some time off to see how the world worked. I realized I was going to have to find some sort of job. Then as now, the world wasn't beating down the doors of brand-new psych grads.

So I answered a classified ad. Somebody had an "exciting new home fitness product," and was looking for salesmen. I called the phone number in the ad, and a very nice fellow assured me, "You won't have to worry, Patrick. This product practically sells itself!" It sounded like a good deal to me, especially if I could get the product to make house calls.

The item in question turned out to be a rebounder. It didn't *exactly* sell itself, but I couldn't help noticing that more and more people were becoming receptive to the idea of staying in shape at home. I invested $300 in stock, stacked the rebounders in the living room of my apartment, and went to work.

As I worked (and worked out) in my home, I received a lot of customers' inquiries about other types of home fitness equipment. I began to diversify my line. Eventually, I rented a store and displayed my wares on the floor for everyone to see. After all, you can only store so many multi-station weight machines in your living room.

At about this time, the Hollywood community became fitness-conscious. My staff and I found ourselves consulting with and selling equipment to such celebrities as Robert De-Niro, Gary Collins and Mary Ann Mobley, Jon Voight, Burt Bacharach and Carole Bayer Sager, Barbara Carrera, Pierce Brosnan, Robert Redford and dozens more. All these people were looking for our advice on how to set up fitness centers in their own homes, and what equipment might be right for them.

Today, my High-Tech Fitness, Inc. store in Los Angeles carries over 500 different items. My customers range in age from the teens to the nineties. They are workers, professionals, athletes, and entertainers. Besides my celebrity clients, there've been over 25,000 others you *haven't* heard of. Although *The Guinness Book of World Records* has no such category, I'm reasonably confident that my High-Tech Fitness Team and I have put together more home gyms than anyone else in the world.

I've watched my business grow from the living room of my apartment into a profitable and self-sustaining retail enterprise. It's grown so rapidly because today fitness is the "in" thing. And the home is now the "in" place to work out. Why? It's more convenient. It saves time. We have entertainment areas in our homes, so keeping fit is less boring.

And a home gym is ultimately a better investment than continuing to pay the rising costs of health club membership. In the '80s, a home gym is one of the new status symbols. And it's a *functional* status symbol, one that keeps you healthy and happy.

Obviously, I'm far from the only person to have figured all this out. That's why the market is flooded with fitness devices. It seems like there are a dozen new ones every time you turn around, each equipped with LED displays, warning lights, whistles, and bells. If you're like most consumers, you know what to look for when you're buying a food processor, a microwave oven, or a new car. But the home fitness boom has happened almost overnight. How do you determine which exercise bike, rower, or weight machine is best for you?

I believe you'll find the answers here. We're going to take the mystery out of buying, setting up, and using home gym equipment so you can build the body you've always wanted.

What's in store for home fitness in the future? I can see four trends at work that will make home gym equipment even better and more useful tomorrow:

1. It's becoming more beautiful, so it can fit in any room without making that room look like, well, a gym.

2. It's becoming more versatile. The trend is toward one unit performing more and more functions.

3. It's becoming more compact. More of us are living in smaller houses and apartments these days, and equipment manufacturers are responding to this fact.

4. It's becoming more electronic. The same computer chips that are enriching California's Silicon Valley are letting us exercise more scientifically and efficiently. They're even helping us to stay motivated!

Ten years ago, I started out with a $300 investment and a cluttered apartment living room. Today, I think I have the best staff, the best minds, and the best equipment in the home fitness field. I've put these resources to work—overtime—in producing this book. So get ready to enter the fascinating world of High-Tech Fitness. Your mind and body will thank you for it.

To your fitness,

Patrick

Patrick Netter
October 1984

INTRODUCING HIGH-TECH FITNESS

High-tech fitness is the application of modern technology to the fitness requirements of today's lifestyles. It is a product of the convergence of two modern trends that we've all seen at work: the growth of science and technology and our increasing preoccupation with health and appearance. Specifically, high-tech fitness is the kind of fitness you can achieve by working out with equipment designed to help you get in shape, such as rowing machines, stationary bicycles, treadmills, rebounders, and multi-station weight machines.

So what's the difference between building muscles by pumping iron and building muscles by using a Nautilus machine? Why isn't fitness just ... well, plain old *fitness?* Is all that equipment really necessary for good health?

Strictly speaking, no. It's not necessary to use a 747 to get from New York to Los Angeles, either. Our ancestors managed the trip in Conestoga wagons. Of course, a 747 takes only a few hours, instead of a few months, and reduces your likelihood of getting lost or dying of thirst en route. But you don't *have* to fly to get from one coast to the other. It's only faster and safer and cheaper and more convenient and more fun to do it that way.

Technology has created a similar revolution in fitness. The *kind* of fitness you achieve the high-tech way is exactly the same as if you were sufficiently diligent about doing your push-ups and chin-ups and presses and aerobics and. ... A healthy body is a healthy body, and I'm not going to try to fool you into thinking there's a magic formula that will let you build one with no effort.

High-tech fitness is anything but magic. It's just faster and more convenient and more fun than doing things the old-fashioned way.

High-tech fitness is *faster* because today's high-tech equipment is designed to achieve specific results. It takes advantage of our increased knowledge about mechanics and human physiology, and it lets you put that increased knowledge to work.

It's *more convenient* because fitting out your own home gym with high-tech equipment enables you to work out at home on your own schedule, regardless of weather or other conditions. And, because it's more convenient, you're more likely to stick to your own personal fitness program.

It's *more fun* because working out on a rebounder or stationary bike while monitoring your own progress or even watching TV is an enjoyable thing to do.

High-tech fitness has some other advantages going for it, too. It's safer than previous methods of exercise, because today's home gym equipment is designed and constructed with safety in mind. It saves time, because you can walk down the hall to your home gym instead of driving to your health club or local "Y." It's aesthetic, because much of the home fitness equipment on the market these days is beautifully designed. It's less boring than your dad's Fort Benning boot camp physical training routine, because the versatility of modern home gym equipment lets you vary your exercises. And most important of all, it keeps you motivated, because you can use your own equipment to design a personal fitness program that's fun and effective for *you*.

I've described high-tech fitness as a revolution, a revolution that's changed the lives of ordinary people. The wheel, the plough, the printing press, the automobile, and the computer brought about technological revolutions. They changed the way people lived. High-tech fitness will change your life as well. Your health is the foundation of everything good in life, and this new approach to exercise will help you develop the potential for greatness that lies locked within you. High-tech fitness will change the way you look, the way you feel, and the way you have fun. And I guarantee that you'll like the changes.

THREE ASPECTS OF FITNESS

The human body is a miraculously complicated machine that operates most harmoniously when each component functions in a precise and delicate balance. In order to evaluate the efficiency of this organism, three separate aspects must be considered—physical, nutritional, and mental.

Physical Fitness

The components of physical fitness can be further broken down into five categories: aerobic fitness; strength; flexibility; balance and coordination; and the capability to relax and reduce stress.

Aerobics—The heart is your most important muscle. Its function is to keep every cell of your body supplied with oxygen and nutrients. It does this by pumping blood through your body 40 to 200 times a minute, each and every minute of your life. Your *cardiovascular fitness* is a measure of your heart and circulatory system's ability to do this work. As your cardiovascular fitness increases, your heart can pump more blood with each stroke, allowing it to rest longer between strokes.

Another sign of improved cardiovascular fitness is a lower resting heart rate (normal pulse), and a faster recovery rate after exertion. This is known as the training effect and is evidence that your cardio-respiratory system is working more efficiently. Improved circulation of blood to your brain and heart results in increased mental clarity and a decreased risk of cardiovascular problems. Circulation to every organ and body tissue is also improved, contributing to better overall health and a slowing down of the aging process.

The best way to improve your cardiovascular health is by *aerobic conditioning*. Aerobic simply means "with oxygen." Exercise routines that increase your body's ability to take in and use oxygen are called aerobics. To facilitate aerobic conditioning, you must push the heart rate into the target heart rate range and hold it there for at least 15 minutes. And you must do this at least three times a week.

Fitness activities that require repetition of very few movements such as jogging, swimming, cycling, and brisk walking are aerobic—provided you do them at your target heart rate three times a week, for at least 15 minutes per workout. Golf, bowling, softball, and power lifting are not aerobic, because the actual exertion

YOUR TARGET HEART RATE

AGE	YOUR MAXIMUM HEART RATE (BEATS PER MINUTE)	YOUR TARGET HEART RATE RANGE (BETWEEN 70% AND 85% OF MAXIMUM BEATS PER MINUTE)	YOUR TARGET HEART RATE (75% OF MAXIMUM BEATS PER MINUTE)
20	200	140-170	150
25	195	137-166	146
30	190	133-162	142
35	185	130-157	139
40	180	126-153	135
45	175	123-149	131
50	170	119-145	127
55	165	116-140	124
60	160	112-136	120
65	155	109-132	116
70	150	105-128	112

involved in these activities is performed in short spurts. All aerobic activities include an element of endurance.

Your target heart rate equals 70 to 85 percent of your maximum pulse rate and is easily calculated by the following formula. Subtract your age from 220 to find your maximum pulse rate. Then multiply that number by .70 and .85 to determine the range of your target heart rate.

For example, suppose you are 35 years old. Your maximum pulse rate is 185 beats per minute, that is, 220 minus 35. Your target heart rate (.70 to .85 × 185) is 130 to 157 beats per minute. You need to raise your pulse rate to these figures three times a week, for at least 15 to 20 minutes per workout, to benefit from aerobic exercise.

You can use this formula to figure your own target heart rate, or you can find your approximate values from the table in the illustration.

If you haven't been exercising regularly, choose a target heart rate near the bottom of your range. In our example, you'd aim for 130, or 70 percent of your maximum pulse rate.

If you exercise regularly and have a low resting pulse, you'll need a tougher workout to maximize your benefits. You should train in the 75 to 85 percent range of your maximum pulse. In our example, you'd strive for 139 to 157 beats per minute.

In addition to helping to prevent heart disease in the healthy, controlled aerobic exercise can even be good for those recovering from heart conditions. However, you should only undertake a *rehabilitative* aerobics program under the supervision of a physician.

You've probably already figured out that to exercise the aerobic way, you have to be able to take your pulse. The easiest and most accurate way is to use one of the digital-readout electronic monitoring devices discussed on pages 88–97. But you can also do it the old-fashioned way, by hand. Place the fingers of your right hand over your left wrist. Count the number of pulse beats you feel during a 15-second interval. Multiply by four to get the number of pulse beats per minute.

With a little practice, you'll be able to take your pulse quickly and accurately. Speed is important, because of the training effect mentioned earlier. As your cardiovascular fitness improves, your pulse rate will quickly drop to your resting pulse when you stop exercising. So if you wait too long to take your pulse, your reading will be inaccurate, and your workout won't maintain your target heart rate. With electronic monitors, you won't have this problem. They display your pulse while you're exercising.

Pulse rate monitor systems are now being developed that not only allow you the sophistication of accurate monitoring, but also will give you a complete computer print-out, in graph form, illustrating your entire workout.

EXERCISE: THE BEST WAY TO GET RID OF BODY FAT

The best way—in fact, the *only* way—to take off weight and keep it off is by a combination of exercise and proper nutrition. A diet is a short-term solution to the problem of food intake. Proper nutrition means a change in your eating habits *for life.* You need to eat enough to keep hunger pangs away, while getting the vital nutrients your body requires.

Getting enough exercise is at least as important as eating right. The proper amount of regular exercise will burn the fat right off your body. And it will stay off—your weight won't go up and down, as it does on the diet roller coaster.

Best of all, a program of regular exercise will "teach" your body to burn more calories. As you replace fat with muscle, your caloric needs increase because lean muscle tissue burns more calories than fat. That's why regular exercisers weigh 20 percent less than average Americans, even though they actually eat *more.* In fact, some exercisers manage to stay thin in spite of some pretty serious overeating.

When it comes to exercise and weight loss, there are two myths you should be aware of. The first is the idea that you can exercise until you lose a certain, desired amount of weight. Certainly exercise will burn fat from your body. But if you stop working out, the fat will come back. That's what happens to most people as they grow older. They become less active than they were as children and they begin to add pounds of fat to their bodies.

The second myth is that we can measure the weight-reducing value of an exercise by looking only at the number of calories burned during that exercise. All of us make this mistake at one time or another. It's especially prevalent among dieters. They look at the amount of calories in a given piece of food, then calculate the amount of exercise needed to burn that many calories. This sort of reasoning can make working out seem hopeless. After all, it might take an hour of pumping iron just to burn off the calories in a small dessert!

We can certainly be suspicious of such logic because of the many active people who eat more than average, yet remain quite thin. In fact, your body burns calories at an accelerated rate not only during exercise, but for hours *after* your workout is over! Your body doesn't slow down all at once. While it's cooling off, it's still burning calories at a faster rate than when it was at rest.

In addition, the good effects of exercise accumulate in your body. The way you eat now probably isn't "off" by too many calories, or you'd be gaining lots of weight, year after year. You're probably only consuming one or two hundred calories a day more than you should. By exercising three or four times a week, you can change this surplus into a daily deficit. Your metabolic rate increases gradually with exercise. As your body becomes leaner, gets into high gear, and "learns" to burn more calories (instead of getting along on fewer, as happens when you diet), you'll burn extra calories every hour of the day—even while you sleep. Eventually, you may have to start eating more just to keep from getting too thin!

Don't take your pulse until you've worked hard enough to get it up into your target range. With a little experience, you'll be able to gauge it, approximately, by your breathing.

When your pulse hits your target rate, keep exercising at about the same level of intensity for 15 to 30 minutes. If you slack off, your pulse will drop below the target rate, and you'll lose your aerobic benefits.

You should also beware of overtraining. If you step up your level of activity too much, you can put unnecessary strain on your bones and joints as well as your heart. So when you are ready to increase your exercise workload, proceed gradually and do not do so until your heart rate and your physical tolerance feedback tell you it is okay.

Remember, to benefit from aerobic conditioning you must repeat your workout at least three times (better four or five) a week. Any fewer repeats will start to cost you the positive results you've achieved. After about 12 weeks of inactivity, you'll be back to where you started before you began your program.

Strength—Amazingly enough, between one-fourth and one-half of your body weight is muscle. You have three basic types of muscles: your heart, the smooth muscles that force food down through your digestive tract, and your skeletal muscles. There are over 400 of these skeletal muscles attached to your bones by tendons. They control all body movement and allow you to lift and carry, push and pull.

Muscular strength depends on three main elements: muscle mass (the amount of muscle tissue you have), muscular coordination (the ability of the various muscles to interact smoothly), and the amount of energy stored in the muscle cells (in small structures called mitochondria). Strength improves control of your movements and the amount of force you can generate. With adequate strength you can carry out all your daily activities with greater ease, reduced fatigue, less physical strain, and a lower risk of injury.

When you're strengthening your skeletal muscles (just as when you strengthen your heart muscle), you use the overload principle. A muscle becomes stronger when you work it harder than it's accustomed to and then allow it to rest. As it rests, it resets itself at a slightly higher level of performance. When work that was difficult becomes easy, it's time to increase your workload. This is called the adaption principle.

There are three basic types of strength training: isometric, isokinetic, and isotonic. Isometric exercise works your muscles against static resistance, such as by pushing against an immovable object (body parts have no visible movement). It builds a muscle's strength for a limited range of motion. This training is less than ideal, because for almost all activity, you need strength through some range of motion. Isokinetic exercise is activity in which the movement is controlled by a machine. The problem here is that isokinetic machines are too expensive and impractical for most people. And it has not yet been shown that they produce strength any better or any faster than isotonic work.

Isotonic exercise moves your muscles through their entire range of motion against gravity or gravity plus resistance. For most people, this is the most efficient way to develop strength and muscle tone. Weight machines and free weights work your muscles isotonically.

All strength training works by the exertion of your muscles against resistance. Resistance is provided either by gravity or a mechanical device. When you're lifting your own body weight (as in push-ups or chin-ups), working with free weights (as in bench presses or curls), or using a weight-stack machine, you're working against gravity.

If you want to improve your performance in most sports, training for muscle tone and strength will be an important part of your fitness program.

MUSCLES OF THE HUMAN FEMALE

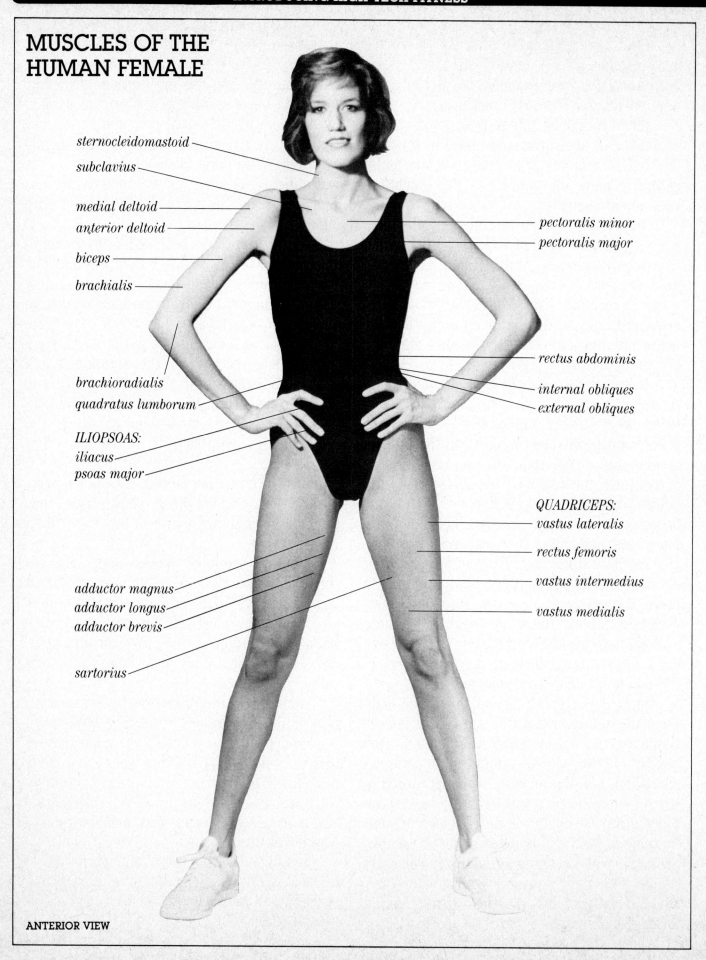

sternocleidomastoid

subclavius

medial deltoid

anterior deltoid

biceps

brachialis

brachioradialis

quadratus lumborum

ILIOPSOAS:
iliacus
psoas major

adductor magnus
adductor longus
adductor brevis

sartorius

pectoralis minor
pectoralis major

rectus abdominis

internal obliques
external obliques

QUADRICEPS:
vastus lateralis

rectus femoris

vastus intermedius

vastus medialis

ANTERIOR VIEW

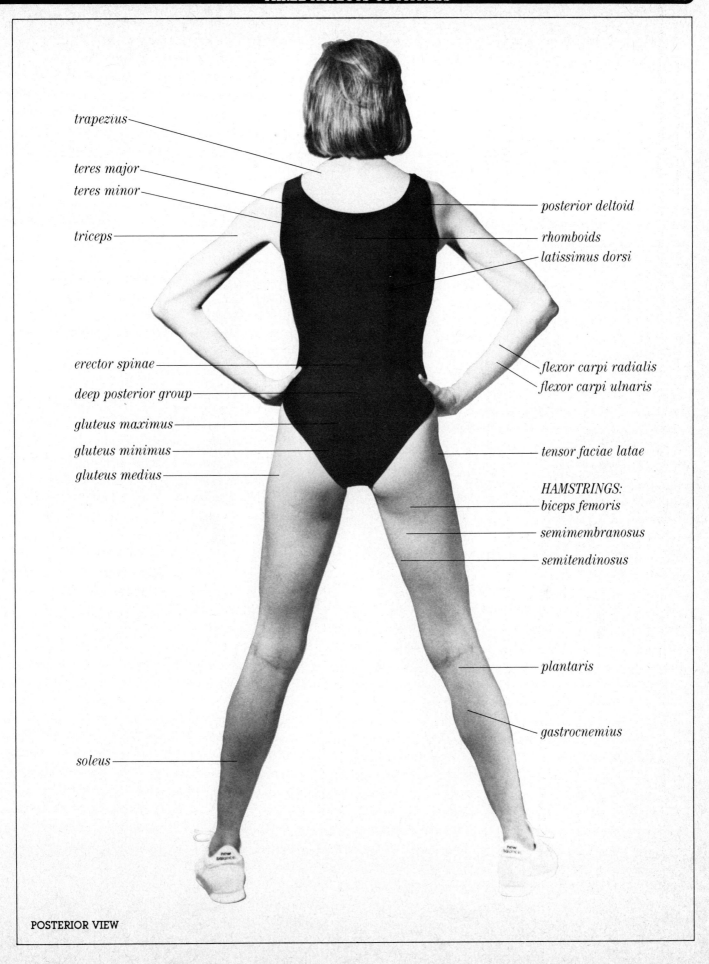

trapezius

teres major

teres minor

triceps

posterior deltoid

rhomboids

latissimus dorsi

erector spinae

deep posterior group

gluteus maximus

gluteus minimus

gluteus medius

flexor carpi radialis

flexor carpi ulnaris

tensor faciae latae

HAMSTRINGS:
biceps femoris

semimembranosus

semitendinosus

plantaris

gastrocnemius

soleus

POSTERIOR VIEW

MUSCLES OF THE HUMAN MALE

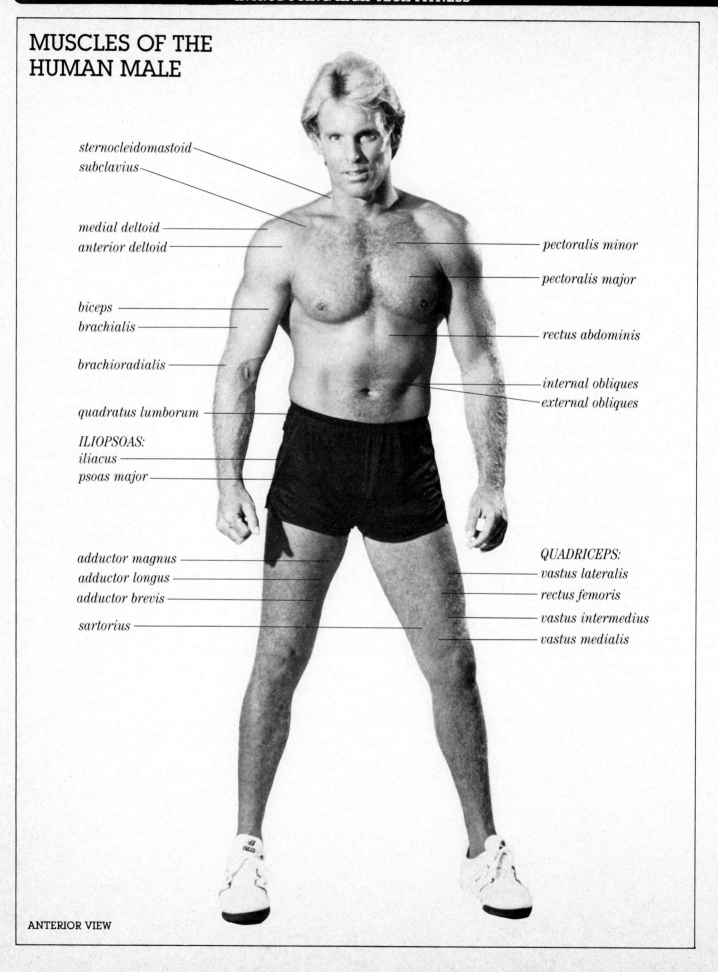

sternocleidomastoid
subclavius

medial deltoid
anterior deltoid

biceps
brachialis

brachioradialis

quadratus lumborum

ILIOPSOAS:
iliacus
psoas major

adductor magnus
adductor longus
adductor brevis

sartorius

pectoralis minor

pectoralis major

rectus abdominis

internal obliques
external obliques

QUADRICEPS:
vastus lateralis
rectus femoris
vastus intermedius
vastus medialis

ANTERIOR VIEW

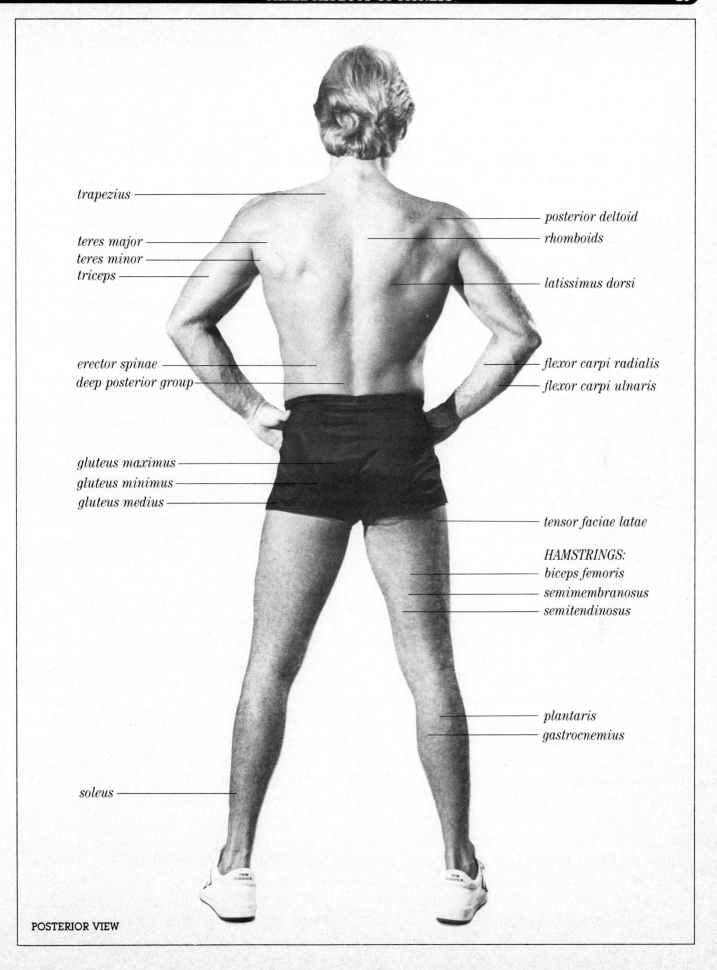

trapezius

posterior deltoid

rhomboids

teres major

teres minor

triceps

latissimus dorsi

erector spinae

deep posterior group

flexor carpi radialis

flexor carpi ulnaris

gluteus maximus

gluteus minimus

gluteus medius

tensor faciae latae

HAMSTRINGS:

biceps femoris

semimembranosus

semitendinosus

plantaris

gastrocnemius

soleus

POSTERIOR VIEW

Flexibility—Although flexibility exercises are usually the simplest part of any fitness program, they are frequently overlooked or hurried. This is understandable. The stretches we do for flexibility are typically slow, small, subtle movements, not at all as exhilarating as aerobics or as dramatic as lifting weights.

But we can't overstate the importance of stretching your body regularly and properly. The process of repeatedly moving our bodies, whether in sport, exercise, or ordinary daily activities, overworks some muscle groups and overlooks others. Stretching the tight, overworked muscles brings our bodies into balance and comfort and reduces physical and mental stress.

Long, pliable, flexible muscles enable joints to move freely and smoothly. Stretching works on the connective tissues that encase muscles and the large "plates" of fasciae into which many of your limb muscles are inserted. Connective tissue and fasciae can be underused (because we do not exercise properly or at all), or overused (because we are tense, or because muscles are weak and tire easily). When this happens, they become shorter and less pliable. They restrict the length of our muscles, limit the movement of our joints, and generally make us feel painful and stiff.

Gently stretching the fasciae and connective tissues makes them longer and more supple, and gives you a greater freedom of movement. You can alleviate muscle cramps and help injured muscles to recover by stretching. You can also eliminate muscle tightness caused by fatigue and emotional tension.

Flexibility is an important part of fitness because it prepares your muscles for exercise and relaxes your entire body.

Balance and Coordination—Balance and coordination are a more subtle aspect of fitness. They allow your body to move with grace and fluidity. Trampolines, balance beams, rings, and uneven parallel bars are all designed to improve your balance and coordination.

Recent studies show a correlation between good balance and coordination and higher self-esteem, increased mathematical skills, and heightened ability to develop athletic skills. That's why educators are beginning to incorporate the development of balance and coordination into their curricula. It's best to begin this development at an early age, but a fitness program including balance and coordination training can be beneficial regardless of your age or fitness level.

Government statistics indicate that the higher incidence of domestic accidents among older people occurs due to a deterioration of balance skills. It's never too late to incorporate balance and coordination exercises into your personal fitness program.

Relaxation and Stress Reduction—"Stress" is one of those words that's in the air these days. You can hardly pick up a magazine without finding an article about it. We all suffer from it in some degree, and it's one of the most dangerous elements of modern life. Stress wears down the body and greatly accelerates the aging process. It's been linked to many diseases, including heart disease and cancer.

It seems obvious, then, that one of the most useful things we can teach ourselves is how to relax. Yet few of us have this skill.

Your ancestors 50,000 years ago led a *very* active life. A typical day at the office consisted of hunting down an aurochs (a prehistoric ox with 10-foot horns and hooves the size of meat platters) and trying to kill him with stone knives. Other activities included running from wolves, cave bears, and each other. It was a stressful existence, but the stress was short-term. Your thousand-times-great-granddad either ran from his problems, or they ate him.

Things are different today for most of us—let's hope. We don't do much physical work. We've traded our clubs and stone knives for swivel chairs.

Stress is different, too. There's more of it, and our stress levels almost never return to what our ancestors would have considered normal. Our bodies, built to handle the short bursts of stress our progenitors experienced, now must adapt to high levels of stress that are nearly constant from cradle to grave. The effects of that stress are absorbed in our bodies.

Most of us thus get a fraction of the exercise we were designed for, and many times the stress. Yet our bodies are basically the same as those of the prehistoric hunters who once roamed the plains. Technology has inflicted these physical problems on us as a sort of flip side to its benefits. Now technology can help us cope with these problems.

That's what fitness, particularly high-tech fitness, is all about.

Learning to stretch and breathe correctly aids tremendously in stress reduction. Inversion devices, hot tubs, flotation tanks, saunas, foot massagers, table and chair massagers, and manual massagers all help the body to relax into a calmer state. Biofeedback devices, such as pulse monitors, can help you identify your level of stress and reduce it. But the best-known and most effective way of alleviating stress is a regular exercise program.

After assessing your current state of health (and consulting a physician if in any doubt) and carefully digesting the five components of physical fitness, you can begin to formulate your own personal fitness program. You may choose to work on all five areas at once, or to concentrate on a particular area. By achieving fitness in all five areas, you'll look and feel your best. A fit body is one that's adapted to its environment, that's competent and becoming, worthy and prepared, in as good physical condition as the body of an athlete or a racehorse, and in good health.

Nutritional Fitness

Just as you cannot run a car without fuel, you cannot run the body without adequate nutrition. "Adequate" must be emphasized—not just any food substance you shovel into your mouth will work. If you put the wrong quality of gas and oil in your car, it will not only impair performance, but may also lead to an eventual breakdown. The same is true of the physiology of our human machinery.

Just as there are different makes and models of cars, so there are different body types. And if you think about it, the kind of body you have goes a long way to determine what activities interest you, and the way you spend your time. For example, a big-boned, heavily muscled body might be drawn towards exercise that involves heavy body contact (such as wrestling or football). A thinner, more highly strung type of body might be drawn to exercises that involve more refined flexibility and balance (such as dance or yoga). These are but very general examples. There are no hard and fast rules. But whatever forms of exercise you choose, how well your metabolism functions will go a long way to determine your performance level.

Our bodies change in order to adapt to the kinds of demands our daily activities place upon them. In primitive times, we needed thick, heavy muscles for strength to survive. There were times when, due to the uncertainty of food production, people would bulk up by retaining excess fat on their bodies. But today—with refrigeration, mass transportation, and push buttons—a new kind of demand is being placed on our bodies. We need stamina and endurance, so we must have efficient aerobic metabolisms—pumping the blood, oxygen, and essential fluids throughout the body-brain unit—to feel sharper, clearer, and more able to take advantage of our modern technology. In order to achieve this most desirable state of functioning, it is necessary to both exercise the body and to feed it the proper kinds of nutrients.

If you prefer eating three meals a day, breakfast should be the second heaviest meal. The kinds of foods you eat should depend on the season of the year and the inclination of your body. Don't just eat something because you think you're supposed to. Know what's beneficial and listen to your body. Your state of mind, energy level, and your environment continuously recombine to place different demands on your system. For instance, in hot weather the body may crave lighter foods and fluids (you will perspire). Most of the more delectable fruits are summer fruits. They're enzymatic and will start your body cleansing. In cold weather months you may desire more butter and cheese for extra body warmth and slow-burning energy storage. As you learn to combine a knowledge of what these foods do for your metabolism with a sense of what the body needs for any given level of activity, you will begin to gain more control over the workings of your metabolism. Then you can safely mold your system to the level of performance you desire.

If you feel like staying light and having some quick energy, then you might choose a luscious fresh fruit salad for breakfast. If you need a boost of energy for the mind and muscles, you might want to have eggs (soft cooked) along with some lightly steamed vegetables and/or grain.

If you're really ravenous, feel low in body warmth, or face a strenuous task and your energy must be constant for a while, you should start thinking of whole grains. If you choose to eat three meals, try to keep them proportionately light and uncomplicated.

To ensure good digestion, there are several important considerations to keep in mind. The first is food combinations. The less complicated the combinations of food, the easier they are to digest. Some foods will combine easily with each other (grains with vegetables; meat with vegetables). Some foods will actually enhance the available energy to be derived (beans and rice). Some foods challenge each other and have to battle it out for digestive enzymes (raw vegetable versus raw fruits; complex carbohydrates versus proteins from animal flesh). Sugars (in the form of sweetened desserts and very sweet, ripe fruits) cause the fastest secretion of enzymes necessary for their assimilation. If eaten too close to more complex foods, especially the meat proteins, sugars may usurp the digestive system, preventing secretion of the proper enzymes for digesting the other foods. Melons should be eaten separately from other foods. For instance, watermelon is a natural diuretic that can be very cleansing to the kidneys. But because of its unique enzymatic activities, it makes digestion of other foods difficult.

If you digest better, then you assimilate more of the nutrients in food. In turn, you can burn the calories easier, and your system will stay lighter and more energized. For instance, the heavier the meat you consume, the more time and energy you have to expend digesting it. Of the flesh foods, fish and chicken are the easiest to digest, and lowest in saturated fat–forming cholesterol. Lamb comes next, followed by the beefy red meats. Pork takes the most time to digest in the stomach.

Each person's ability to digest varies with his circumstances and the state of his metabolism. But once you understand how your system operates, you have a means of gauging and adjusting your body's needs to the level of performance you desire.

Just as important as how you combine foods is the quality of the foods you eat. Re-

WHAT HAPPENS WHEN YOU DIET?

- Much of the weight you lose won't be fat. Instead, you'll lose fluids, muscle, and organ tissue, possibly exposing yourself to health risks. Losing muscle will change your body composition, so you may wind up with a higher percentage of fat, even though you weigh less. And every pound you gain back will make you look even worse.
- You risk poor nutrition. It's hard enough to eat properly with normal amounts of food. It's almost impossible with low-calorie diets.
- The more you diet, the harder it gets. If you teach your body to get by on less food, it will adapt, making it harder to lose more weight. And when you go off the diet you'll gain weight, if you eat sensibly.
- Dieting is inconvenient, especially over the long run. Eating is a social activity, and it's pretty hard to diet in a restaurant or at a party.
- Your energy level will be lower. You may become less active, and that will make you fatter. You'll feel "down" much of the time. Depriving your body of the food and pleasure it's accustomed to can make you moody and irritable.
- Dieting is no fun! It's unpleasant, and difficult to keep up.

WHAT HAPPENS WHEN YOU EXERCISE?

- You lose fat, not muscle. Your body becomes not only thinner, but more attractively shaped.

- You won't jeopardize your nutrition.

- Losing weight will grow easier with time. As you become more fit, you'll become more active, making it even easier to lose excess pounds.

- You'll find more things to do with your family and friends, because exercise is a great social activity. You may even find yourself meeting new people.
- Your body will become more stable, strong, and flexible—and thus, less prone to injury. Back pain and other symptoms of muscular imbalance may be relieved. Your other physical processes, such as sleep and elimination, will become easier and more regular.
- You'll have fun! As you grow stronger and fitter, you'll enjoy exercising more and more.

fined, devitalized, chemically processed foods are often not only nutritionally worthless, they can even impair the functioning of your metabolism. Our bodies haven't changed much in the past fifty thousand years. When operating in a state of nature, our food choices were limited to locality and seasonal availability. Combinations were simple, if not singular. Today we have an overabundance of edible choices, too many of which have never touched the soil of earth or seen the light of day. Remember, the quality of food you put in your body goes a long way to determine how well you function.

Your state of mind also affects your metabolism. Our bodies still carry the same functional designs they had when we were primitive. In the state of nature, reactions to life-threatening situations were the main causes of stress, and during such moments you wouldn't stop to eat. Today, much of our stress is generated by our thinking, but our bodies can't tell the difference. All too often, we drag our anxieties with us to the dinner table and shovel anything down. If such is the case—especially if you don't give it notice by chewing well and savoring the tastes—the body may fail to secrete the necessary digestive enzymes. Learn to relax and enjoy your meal. No matter how busy you are, find some way to slow yourself down before the meal (walk in the garden, meditate, hug somebody you like, or lie back and listen to music). Once in a receptive and more sensitive frame of mind, the body knows it should be digesting and will take care of business.

If you eat three meals a day, lunch should be your most potent. By then your metabolism is going full throttle and is ready to digest. The average metabolism usually slows down around 3:00 p.m. If functioning healthfully, it should by then have converted the bulk of the fuel necessary to handle its needs for the rest of the day. Therefore, heavier foods should be eaten by 3:00 p.m.—for both energy and weight control. As the metabolism slows down, it lowers the rate of calorie consumption. The later you eat and the heavier the foods, the harder it is to burn calories and keep your weight gain in balance.

Try to drink about eight glasses of purified or distilled water throughout the day. When it comes to meal time, drink as little as possible with the meal. Too much fluid will water down the digestive enzymes.

Dinner should be light and simple, more a pick-me-up than a full-blown meal. Many very physically active people find it more advantageous to consume two moderate major meals, and to snack lightly throughout the day. Instead of eating first thing in the morning, earn your breakfast (so to speak). Get up, be active, drink lots of water, and eat around 11:00 a.m., when you're really hungry. Snack lightly every two hours on small amounts of simple, easy to digest foods (an apple with a few raw almonds, a couple of bites of yesterday's casserole, cottage cheese and sprouts, or a small sliver of whole-grain sprouted bread). Have your dinner by about 4:00 p.m.; after that, snack lightly. If you can do some exercising sometime between your last meal and bedtime, you'll fire up your metabolism and wake up feeling lighter.

Whether you choose three meals spaced evenly throughout the day, two meals with snacks, or another alternative, listen to the needs of your body. If you don't know how, contact a knowledgeable health expert. Have your body professionally evaluated. This is especially important if you've been out of shape for a while, or if there are any medical complications. Then let yourself be guided to excellent health. You'll soon be over the hurdles and able to consciously take control of your own progress.

Mental Fitness

The effects of a person's mental attitude on the success or failure of any fitness program cannot be overestimated. You must motivate yourself not to become a fitness dropout, and the best way to do that is to make your exercise program something you look forward to, a time to work hard but also have fun. If you develop a regimen that's interesting, challenging, and convenient, you won't *want* to stop.

Choose a program that fits your schedule, with routines you enjoy. Set realistic short-term and long-term goals—but don't bite off more than you can chew.

Do everything you can to replace any negative feelings with positive feedback. Associate with other high-tech users and learn from and encourage each other. Concentrate on your successes, not on your aches and pains.

Build your confidence by becoming more informed. Subscribe to fitness periodicals, ask health professionals for advice and information—one little tip or minor adjustment can make the difference between floundering and real progress.

Motivate yourself by a technique called "imaging." First, relax. Imagine yourself working out, and repeat the image until it becomes familiar. Then, imagine yourself as you want to look. Making this mental connection between exercise and your goal of an ideal body will help you achieve that goal.

You can even reprogram your subconscious by repeating certain "affirmations" to yourself while you exercise:

- "I am now building my ideal body."
- "Every cell, fiber, muscle, and organ of my body functions perfectly."
- "Every day, in every respect, I get better and better."
- "My equipment and I cooperate perfectly with one another."
- "I'm doing better, feeling better, and looking better than ever before."
- "I always win, because I am a winner."

Use any technique that works for you to guarantee the success of your fitness program. Remember, exercise is not just a temporary get-in-shape measure, it's a lifetime commitment to yourself and your health.

EQUIPMENT AND HOW TO USE IT

There are two things that every piece of home gym equipment has in common with every other piece. They're all designed to get you in shape, and they all cost money. Unless you have absolutely no regard for the latter, you'll naturally want the best stuff you can afford, i.e., the best *value*. That's what this section is about.

There's no doubt that the fitness equipment industry is going through a major growth cycle. We're now even seeing some of the larger conglomerates entering this once mainly "Mom and Pop" business.

The industry's current expansion phase could affect you, the consumer, in several ways:

• To capture larger market segments, companies are manufacturing in greater volume. This usually results in lower prices.

• As in the auto industry, the trend in fitness equipment is toward one-upmanship. We're seeing more equipment that can be used in a multiplicity of ways, and units are being built with more and more features, such as the many varieties of electronic feedback. Furthermore, consumers are more quality-conscious than ever. This "investment mentality" is forcing some manufacturers to upgrade their products. They're now using better materials and paying more attention to quality control.

• The fitness industry is a competitive market, and as with any competitive market, prices will go up and down. We've tried to list the approximate average selling price of each piece of equipment we show. Bear in mind that the price you pay *may* vary significantly from the price listed in this book. And remember: The integrity of the company from which you buy could be an important factor if you have problems with your equipment later on.

Every piece of equipment rated on the following pages has been investigated by the High-Tech Fitness Team. We've found that all these units are effective at doing what their manufacturers say they'll do. No two pieces have exactly the same features. This doesn't mean that some are good and some are bad—we've left the bad ones out. What it does mean is that you should decide what you want a given unit to do and what you can afford to pay, then read the evaluations carefully and come to a conclusion about which unit best fits your goals and budget. We've evaluated all units for compatibility and modularity; that is, you can buy a piece at a time, and most will complement each other. We've also tried, whenever possible, to present equipment with the best monitoring and feedback systems. Exercise is a repetitive business, and it helps break the monotony when you can see how fast you're going, how hard you're working, and how far you've traveled. Our feeling is, the more feedback, the better.

When you're looking at home gym equipment, beware of look-alikes. The equipment industry is seeing more and more knock-off designs. Just because two items *look* alike doesn't mean they have the same functions, or that their components are of comparable quality. I've seen more "flywheel"-type bikes that rattle, and more "heavy-duty" rebounders that don't hold up, than I care to see.

What criteria did we use to evaluate home gym equipment? We asked the following eight questions about each unit we tested:

1. Is it a quality product?

2. Is it manufactured by a reputable company? If you have questions or problems with the product, will the manufacturer likely still be in business?

3. Is it a low-maintenance product? (Unfortunately, all lemons don't come from trees or Detroit.)

4. Is it attractive (relatively speaking)? If you leave it set up in your living room or your bedroom, will your friends point at you and laugh?

5. Is it portable? (Again, everything's relative. Obviously, a multi-station weight machine isn't going to be as portable as even the most awkward jump rope.)

6. Is it reliable? Does it perform over the long haul, and does it come with a manufacturer's warranty? (These warranties are usually good for a year.)

7. Does the product come with an owner's manual, giving specific instructions for care and use?

8. Is it a good dollar value?

Although we have used and tested most of the following units, we can't guarantee that they'll do everything in the world you expect them to. *Properly used,* all the equipment in this chapter is safe for most people and will perform satisfactorily. But *you* have to use it. Regularly. And correctly. Improperly used, each item carries its inherent risks. Even the humble dumbbell won't contribute to your fitness if you drop it on your foot.

We've tried our best to present the most current technical specifications and price data. Due to the changing nature of manufactured product lines and designs, some maybe slightly inaccurate.

STATIONARY BICYCLES

A stationary bicycle is a device that lets you simulate the movements of bicycle riding in the comfort and convenience of your own home. Out of over a hundred models on the market today, we have selected twelve. They range from simple, portable bikes to the most sophisticated computerized models. By examining the wide range of features, you can see which one best fits your needs.

When shopping for an exercise bike, you will want to carefully consider its flywheel mechanism, for this is the key to insuring smooth pedaling action. Generally, the heavier the flywheel the better. But technically, it's the flywheel mass *and* flywheel rotational ratio that will determine the fluid motion. A light flywheel, or a bike that uses a bicycle wheel with no counterweight, will make the pedaling action jerky. And this can get rather annoying.

Other things to look for are a comfortable seat (wide padded ones seem to be best for home cardiovascular use); a secure seat-locking mechanism (some either constantly slide downward with use or wiggle from side to side during pedaling); the ability to vary tension or resistance (in a way that is easy and repeatable from workout to workout); easily adjustable foot straps (or at least pedals with a slip-resistant surface); a sturdy frame (that will not constantly need tightening or bend with use); movable and adjustable handlebars (to accommodate the height of the user as well as various exercise positions); and whatever feed-back features you desire—such as an odometer for distance ridden, a timer for duration of ride, a speedometer for miles per hour, a caloric expenditure meter for calories burned, a pulse monitor for tracking your heartbeat, or an ergometer for calibration of work load.

An ergometer gives you an exact readout of the amount of work you're doing at any given time. These devices used to be found only on bicycles utilized for testing, but now they are included on more commercially priced models. The High-Tech Fitness Team feels the ergometer can be an important feature. The only way to calibrate your fitness progress is by maintaining a constant, repeatable work load and seeing how your pulse rate improves at that level—and then increasing the work demand accordingly. If your bike does not have an ergometer, it is difficult to accurately control the work load and increase your program when it is appropriate.

Stationary bicycles come equipped with almost every accessory except a horn and lights. Diversionary devices, such as a rack to hold a book so you can read while you pedal, are popular. One bike we've seen even comes with a TV monitor and a collection of videocassettes that simulate a cycling tour of Germany. It only costs about six times what you'd pay to fly yourself and your bike to Germany and ride on your own.

As always with aerobic training equipment, we recommend a pulse monitor. Padded seat covers and foot straps make the ride more pleasurable and comfortable. We usually don't recommend those bicycle machines that combine the action of pedaling with the action of rowing—they seem to compromise the effectiveness of both activities. Better to buy a bike and a rowing machine. If you cannot afford two pieces of equipment of that magnitude and want to work the upper body while you are cycling, a set of HeavyHands or small dumbbells will do the job.

ANATOMY OF A STATIONARY BICYCLE

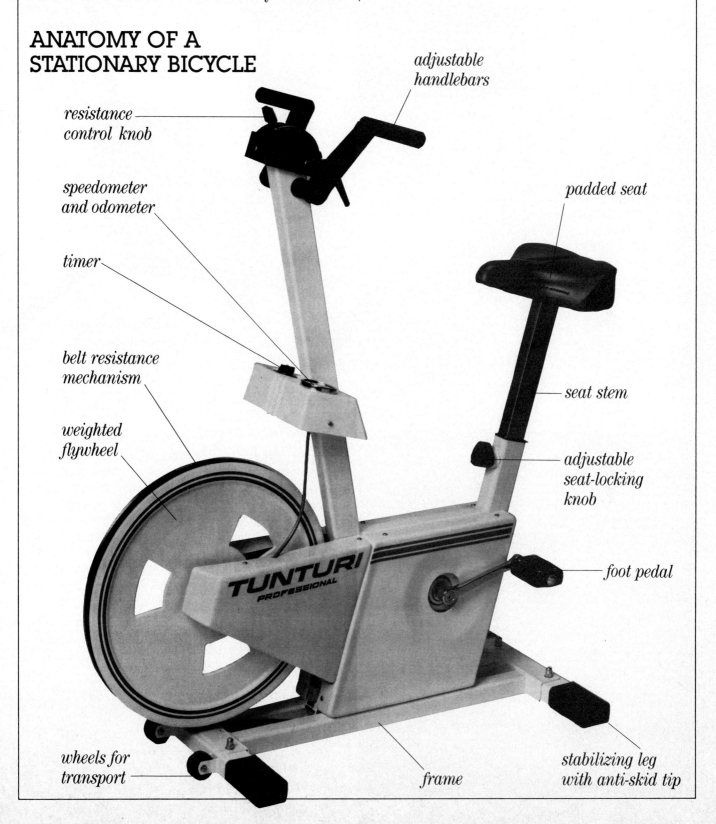

resistance control knob

adjustable handlebars

speedometer and odometer

timer

belt resistance mechanism

weighted flywheel

padded seat

seat stem

adjustable seat-locking knob

foot pedal

wheels for transport

frame

stabilizing leg with anti-skid tip

HIGH-TECH TRIMBIKE™

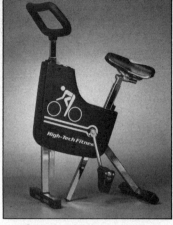

This West German-made bike comes completely assembled. It folds down to the size of several shoe-boxes and can easily be stored in a small closet. It has a nice, clean appearance (black and chrome). Families with children will appreciate the fact that its flywheel is completely enclosed, leaving no chance for little fingers to get caught.

The TrimBike has push-button controls for twelve seat and handlebar adjustments. It has an easy tension adjustment, pedal straps, and a medium-heavy flywheel—features not usually found on the less expensive bikes. But its ride is significantly smoother at the lower tension settings than at the higher resistance levels.

WEIGHT: 44 lbs.
SIZE: 16″ × 32″ × 44″ h (noncollapsed)
APPROXIMATE COST: $200

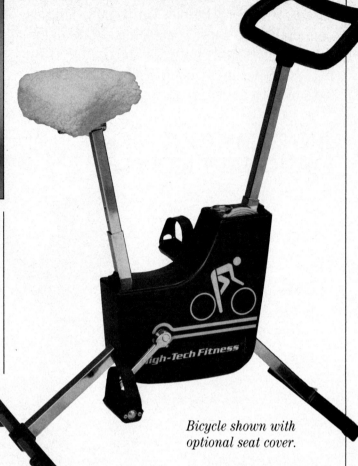

Bicycle shown with optional seat cover.

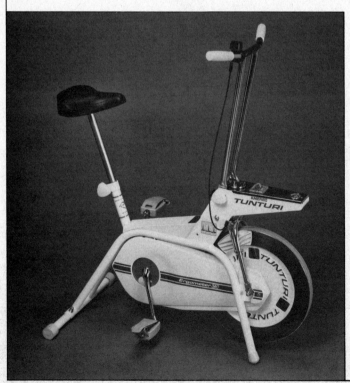

TUNTURI ERGOMETER

Probably the most widely recognized stationary bike around today, the Tunturi Ergometer is well built and sturdy. Its 40-pound flywheel gives it a smooth ride. Disc brakes make it a relatively quiet machine and allow for infinite tension adjustments, from freewheeling (no resistance) to heavy resistance.

The Ergometer's precision controls let you measure rpm, distance, levels of resistance, and elapsed time. The bike's colors are white with green and chrome trim. It can be moved by rolling it on its flywheel, but it doesn't collapse for storage.

Over the years, the Tunturi Ergometer has proved to be relatively maintenance-free.

WEIGHT: 73 lbs.
SIZE: 20″ × 37½″ × 42½″h
APPROXIMATE COST: $450

PRECOR® 820e

This stationary bike is made of anodized aircraft aluminum. Power is transferred to the precision-balanced 26-pound flywheel through a unique V-belt drive system. This design eliminates chain and flywheel "chatter," not to mention the need for lubrication common on chain-driven bikes.

The 820e's electronic module is conveniently located (along with the micro-adjust tension knob) near the padded handle grips. The electronics display is powered by a 9-volt battery and shows your total time, pedal rpm, and distance. The micro-adjust tension knob has "click" stops to enable you to set your work load precisely. You can set the handgrips in any one of four riding positions. It is black with anodized aluminum.

WEIGHT: 55 lbs.
SIZE: 16″ × 25½″ × 42″ h
APPROXIMATE COST: $450

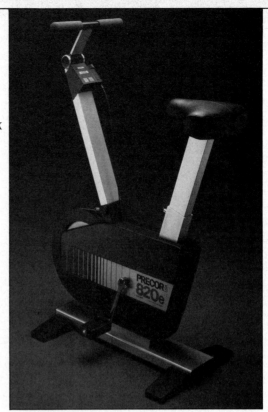

M & R INDUSTRIES, INC. AVITA 450

The American-made 450 has a 45-pound flywheel, very heavy for its class. High-density felt disc brakes provide quiet, even resistance. Its handlebars are immovable, and the frame is welded for stability. The colors are black and chrome.

The 450's instruments include an ergometer calibrated in watts, a pedal rpm indicator, an odometer, and a 60-minute timer.

WEIGHT: 78 lbs.
SIZE: 15½″ × 39″ × 42″ h
APPROXIMATE COST: $475

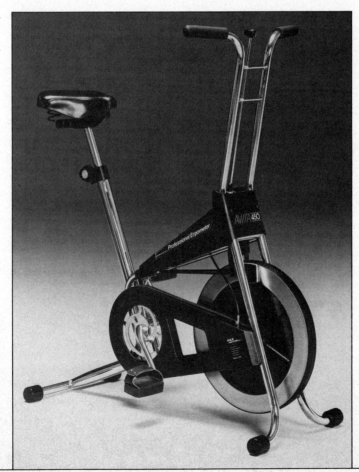

MONARK 867

This Swedish bike is built on the same frame, flywheel, and chain guard as Monark's 865, 868, and 869 models. It features a finely tuned belt resistance mechanism, with a tension control that can be adjusted to 20 different settings. Other features include quick-release, infinitely adjustable handlebars; an adjustable pin-through seat stem; sound-absorbing rubber feet; a large, heavy, and well-balanced flywheel; a speedometer and odometer; wide pedals for extra foot comfort; and wheels for easy transportation. The Monark 867 has a white lacquer finish with blue trim.

WEIGHT: 56 lbs.
SIZE: $23'' \times 44'' \times 39''$ to $42''$h
APPROXIMATE COST: $550

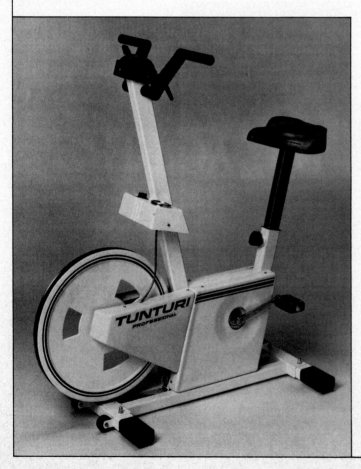

TUNTURI PRO TRAINER

The Finnish-made Tunturi Pro is a Harley Davidson among stationary bicycles. It's sturdy, heavy, and built to withstand lots of punishment. That's why you'll find it in many gyms and health clubs. If you're heavy, or if you just like the feel of a sturdy piece of equipment, the Pro might be the bike for you.

This no-frills machine has a very comfortable seat, handlebars that rotate 360°, 11 resistance levels, a tachometer that measures up to 200 rpm, and a timer. Its 50-pound flywheel is about the heaviest on the market, and its durable belt brake provides smooth and strong pedaling resistance.

The Tunturi Pro is white with green trim, and can be rolled from place to place. It does not collapse for storage.

WEIGHT: 125 lbs.
SIZE: $19\frac{1}{2}'' \times 43'' \times 47''$ h
APPROXIMATE COST: $575

BODYGUARD® 990

This machine is well constructed, yet portable. It comes with foot straps, an easy-to-adjust resistance regulator, and level adjusters to help maintain your balance on uneven floors.

The 990 has probably the most accurately balanced ergometer of any stationary bike. Its precision accuracy makes it especially suitable for cardiac and orthopedic rehabilitation patients. The Bodyguard comes in a combination of ivory, white, and chrome.

WEIGHT: 115 lbs.
SIZE: 20″ × 36″ × 44″ h
APPROXIMATE COST: $750

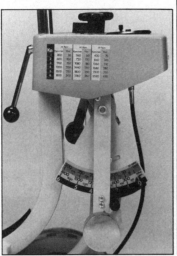

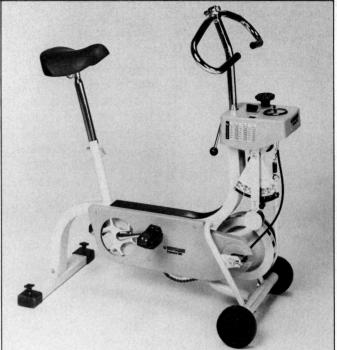

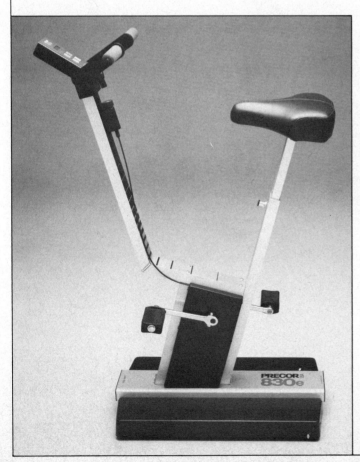

PRECOR® 830e

The 830e's precision-balanced 25-pound steel flywheel is horizontally placed and enclosed. It rotates faster than the flywheel on any other stationary bike we've used. The quicker the rotation, the smoother the ride. Thus, the 830e's ride is unusually fluid and virtually noiseless.

This model comes equipped with rollers on the bottom for easy transportation. However, because of its unique flywheel position, don't ride it on long shag carpeting, as the shag tends to catch. The 830e's high-tech design is clean and sleek; the colors are black and anodized aluminum. The handgrips rotate a full 360°, and the seat is hand-adjustable and comfortable.

The 830e's touch controls are simple to use. Its display reads out elapsed time, rpm, distance (accurate to ± 2%), calories burned per minute, and total calories burned.

WEIGHT: 60 lbs.
SIZE: 16″ × 26″ × 42″ h
APPROXIMATE COST: $800

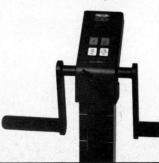

EXERCYCLE®

The best known of all stationary bikes, the Exercycle has been around for over forty years. It looks it, too. This machine's sturdy, strictly functional design marks it as a no-nonsense piece of gym equipment.

The Exercycle's ½-horsepower motor is driven through a gearbox, instead of by chains or pulleys. The motor permits only two speeds, 60- and 90-pedal rpm (30 and 45 on the Senior model). The basic machine comes with *no* monitoring equipment. A Personal Exercise Planner (shown), including ergometer, timer, intensity adjustment, warm-up/cooldown light, and condition-ing seconds adjustment, is an extra-cost option.

The Exercycle's seat, pedals, and handlebar move simultaneously. They're powered by the motor, but you can accelerate the movements by pushing, pulling, and pedaling. This feature allows you to combine cycling with rowing and other movements.

The machine comes in two color choices: metallic gray, and ivory/coppertone. If you have a back problem, you may want to check with your physician before using the Exercycle.

WEIGHT: 160 lbs.
SIZE: 14″ × 58″ × 41″ h
APPROXIMATE COST: $1,600; up to $2,100 with options

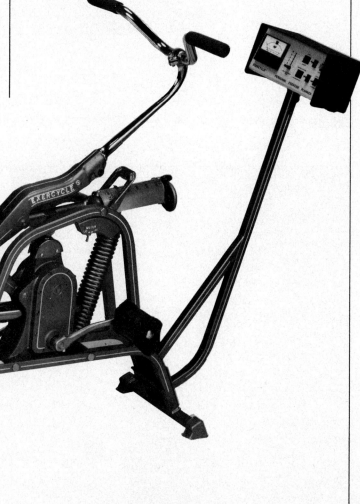

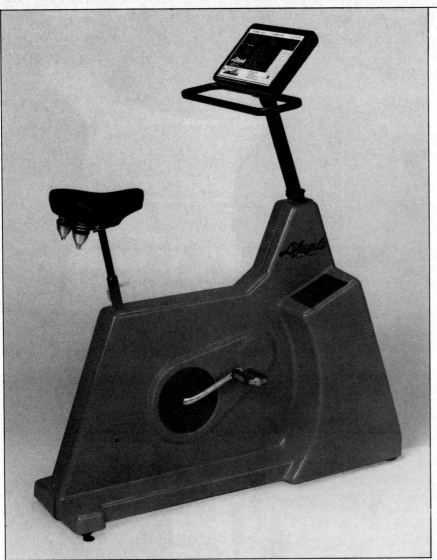

BALLY LIFECYCLE™

If you're a member of a gym or health club, you may have seen or used the Lifecycle. This bike has as many high-tech features as some cars.

The Lifecycle's on-board computer is about as snazzy as you could wish for. You can set it for any of 12 levels of difficulty and for any of 3 different exercise programs. The manual program gives you a preselected fixed work load, the same as with most stationary bikes. The standard and random programs include a "hill profile"– a series of varying resistance levels that simulate a warm-up, a group of hills of different heights and grades, and a cool-down period.

The Lifecycle displays calories burned per hour (although this fluctuates greatly), pedal speed, elapsed time, the program and resistance level being ridden, and upcoming resistance levels. The Maximum Oxygen Uptake readout, when used with a heart-rate monitor, lets you know how much your cardiovascular system is improving. You generate power to run

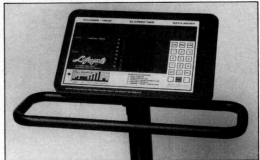

the computer by pedaling.

The Lifecycle comes in red, blue, white, orange, or yellow. Its seat is comfortable. Older or out-of-condition people should be careful not to exceed recommended heart rates. Even at the first level of difficulty, the workout can be a strenuous one.

WEIGHT: 100 lbs.
SIZE: 20″ × 46″ × 46″ h
APPROXIMATE COST: $1,995

DYNAVIT® 30

Developed in West Germany for cardiovascular rehabilitation, the Dynavit 30 is the most sophisticated electronic/computerized bike on the market. There's no drag on its perfectly balanced copper flywheel, which is enclosed. Resistance is created by a magnetic field, so nothing touches the flywheel itself. This arrangement makes for an exceptionally smooth and quiet ride.

The Dynavit's computer monitors your heart rate (with its own pulse monitor), pedal speed, work load, oxygen uptake, distance, and calories burned. It's recommended for older people, people in stressful situations, and those who are very serious about their cardiovascular conditioning. It comes in black, black and white, or black and orange. For high-tech, this bike looks and functions in a class by itself.

WEIGHT: 116 lbs.
SIZE: 14″ × 30″ × 28″ to 35″h
APPROXIMATE COST: $3,500

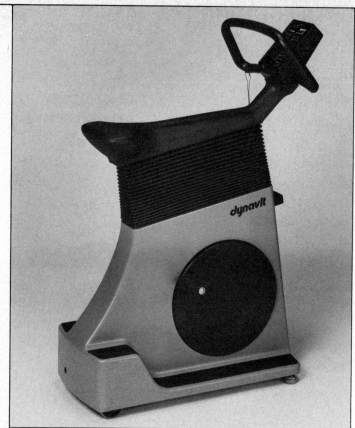

HEART MATE

Like the Lifecycle, the Heart Mate is a mechanical marvel.

The Heart Mate's computer gives you readouts on pulse rate, calories burned per hour, calories burned per workout, and how quickly your fitness level is improving. There are 20 fitness levels, plus a computerized heart-rate recovery test.

This machine comes in red, beige, blue, or black. Built-in AM/FM radio and black-and-white TV are standard; color TV is an extra-cost option. If you want entertaining distractions, this bike has them.

WEIGHT: 200 lbs.
SIZE: 26¼″ × 40″ × 53″ h
APPROXIMATE COST: $3,995 (color TV extra)

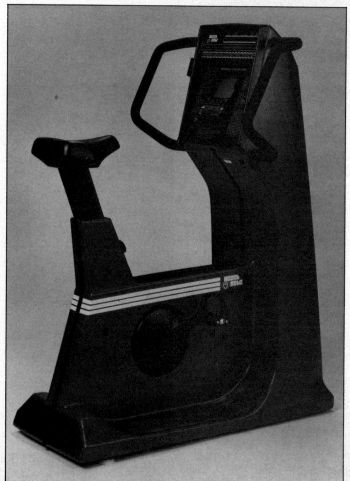

How to Use a
STATIONARY BICYCLE
S

Stationary bicycles are a wonderful adjunct to an exercise program. Any exerciser will find them easy to use. You'll develop a stronger heart, you'll use oxygen more efficiently, and there will never be a fear of falling, skinned knees, or speed demons in sports cars or on skate boards. Because using a stationary bike does not require bearing the body weight on your feet, ankles, knees, or hips, they may enable you to exercise even though you may have chronic medical problems or injuries in these areas.

Before you mount your bike for the first time, read over our list of suggestions and observations. It will make the experience as positive and productive as possible.

- Check that the seat is fastened securely and adjusted to the height which is correct for your leg length. The seat should be situated so that when one leg has depressed the pedal as far down as possible, the knee of that leg is just slightly bent.

- Check the handlebar positioning if it is adjustable. For most long-duration endurance work, the handlebars should be raised so that the arms, shoulders, and neck are very relaxed. If they are tense they will rob your legs of energy you could be using to pedal. If you are training for racing, you may want to rotate the handlebars downward to mimic the racing position. (If this is important to you, make sure you ask for this feature when purchasing a bike—not all have the option.)

- Start at a slow speed and at the lowest resistance. This gives cyclists at all levels the needed period of warm-up and time to get acclimated to the bike itself.

- Wear lightweight rubber-soled shoes to enhance the friction of the foot on the pedal. This will keep your feet from slipping off while pedaling. Foot straps obviously hold the foot securely on the pedal also and are recommended.

- Be conscious of your body movement while pedaling. If you find that your hips are moving from side to side, or your torso is getting a lot of movement, your seat may be adjusted too high or you may be trying to pedal against too great a resistance.

- Try to feel the evenness of each leg stroke as you pedal. The flywheel should be turning in a continuous fashion, not a jerky one. Usually the "hum" of the flywheel is irregular or changes pitch if you are pedaling with unequal force on one leg or the other.

- Get up to the speed and resistance you desire slowly. This allows the muscles to get used to the increasing work load and cadence.

- Remember that going faster or pedaling against more resistance will affect your pulse rate. You will reach your training zone more quickly. This means you should be monitoring your pulse to make sure you are not doing too much, too soon, too fast.

- After getting used to your bicycle, you may want to enhance the scope of your workout by adding hand weights to increase the work load. Working your arms as well as your legs has been shown to give better cardiovascular results. It has also been suggested that the same amount of work feels less taxing when it is spread out over all four limbs. And adding hand weights to your cycling program also improves the shape and tone of your upper body.

Begin with 1-pound weights. Since you will be diligently monitoring your pulse rate as we have advised, you will know when it is time to increase your work load by adding weight.

• When adding to your overall work load, increase only one parameter at a time. In other words, add speed or resistance to your pedaling *or* pedal for a longer period of time *or* add weight to your hand weights. By all means don't do all of them at once.

• Cycling is an aerobic activity and should be done at least three times a week for a minimum of 15 to 20 minutes.

• Don't forget to pay attention to how your muscles and joints feel in your feet, ankles, knees, hips, and lower back. These areas, in addition to your heart, get a good workout on the bicycle. It is very possible for your cardiovascular system (as indicated by your pulse rate) to tell you it is time to increase your work load while your skeletal system (as indicated by muscle or joint stiffness and soreness) is telling you *not* to increase it. Remember the old adage "the squeaky wheel gets the grease," and listen to your muscles and joints. They will adapt, and then you can move onward and upward injury-free.

BASIC BIKE RIDING

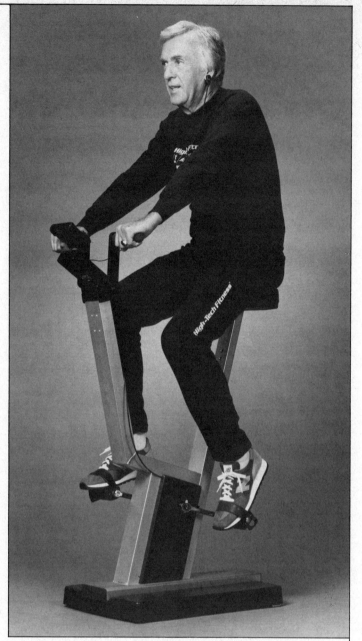

STARTING POSITION: Sit on your bicycle with the seat's height adjusted so that your knee is slightly bent when your foot reaches the bottom of the pedal rotation. Secure your feet to the pedals with the toe straps (if your bike has them), keep your torso upright, and place your hands comfortably on the handlebars.

MOTION: Keeping your upper body upright and stable, pedal the bike normally in a smooth and continuous motion. Adjust the wheel resistance and pedaling frequency to your own requirements. Remember to warm up below your target heart rate for 2 to 5 minutes, then increase speed and resistance until you're within your zone.

PRECAUTIONS: As with any aerobic exercise, start slowly and increase resistance over time. Some people may experience tenderness in the knees from bicycling. If this happens, reduce your work load and/or time on the bike.

AREAS STRENGTHENED: Cardiovascular and respiratory systems, thighs, calves.

MUSCLES STRENGTHENED: Quadriceps, gastrocnemius, soleus, hamstrings, gluteals.

BIKE RIDING WITH TRICEPS FLYS

STARTING POSITION: Sit in the basic riding position. Grasp a weight in each hand, and raise your elbows to shoulder height, so that elbows and shoulders are aligned. Let your lower arms hang straight down.

MOTION: As you pedal, straighten your arms so that they are fully extended from the shoulder, palms down. Then slowly lower the weights back to the starting position. Do this rhythmically, in conjunction with your pedaling motion.

PRECAUTIONS: This exercise may seem awkward at first. Concentrate on maintaining your balance and keeping your torso straight. Start with light weights, 1 to 3 pounds, and increase at a comfortable yet challenging pace.

AREAS STRENGTHENED: Cardiovascular and respiratory systems, thighs, calves, shoulders, back of upper arms.

MUSCLES STRENGTHENED: Quadriceps, gastrocnemius, soleus, deltoids, triceps, hamstrings, gluteals.

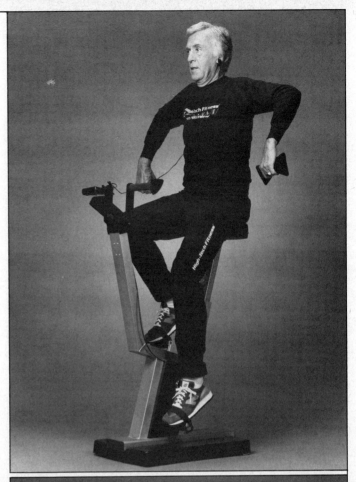

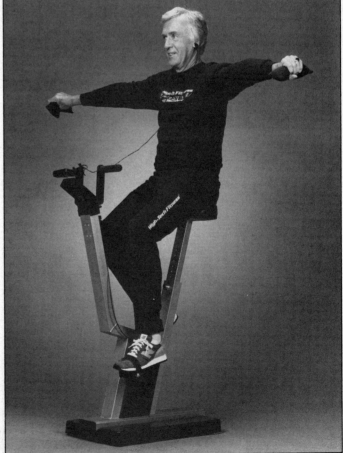

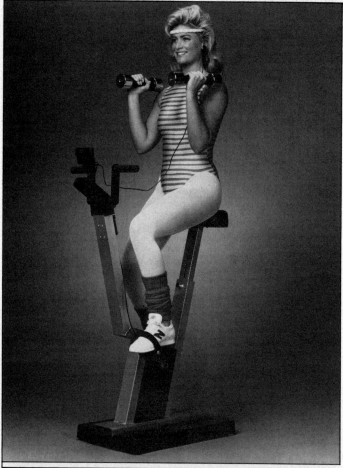

BIKE RIDING WITH BICEPS FLYS

STARTING POSITION: Sit in the basic riding position. Grasp a weight in each hand, and let your arms hang straight down at your sides.

MOTION: As you pedal, bend your elbows, bringing the weights up to your shoulders, palms facing each other. Then extend your arms straight out to the sides, palms down. Bring the weights back in to your shoulders, then back down to your sides to complete the motion. This should be done rhythmically, in conjunction with your pedaling.

PRECAUTIONS: This exercise may also seem awkward at first. Concentrate on maintaining your balance and keeping your torso straight. Start with relatively light weights, 2 to 4 pounds, and increase as desired.

AREAS STRENGTHENED: Cardiovascular and respiratory systems, calves, front of upper arms and shoulders.

MUSCLES STRENGTHENED: Quadriceps, gastrocnemius, soleus, biceps, deltoids, hamstrings, gluteals.

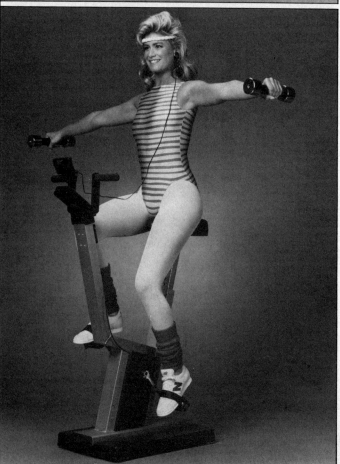

BIKE RIDING WITH BICEPS CURLS

STARTING POSITION: Sit in the basic riding position. Grasp a weight in each hand, and let your arms hang straight down at your sides.

MOTION: As you pedal, bend one elbow and bring the weight up to your shoulder, palm facing the shoulder. Then straighten your arm and lower the weight back to the starting position. Alternate arms to maintain your balance. Do this movement rhythmically, in conjunction with your pedaling motion.

PRECAUTIONS: Concentrate on maintaining your balance and keeping your torso straight. Start with light weights, 2 to 5 pounds, and increase according to your goals.

AREAS STRENGTHENED: Cardiovascular and respiratory systems, thighs, calves, upper arms.

MUSCLES STRENGTHENED: Quadriceps, gastrocnemius, soleus, biceps, hamstrings, gluteals.

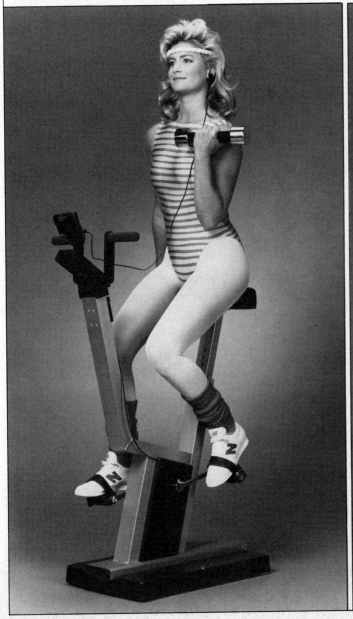
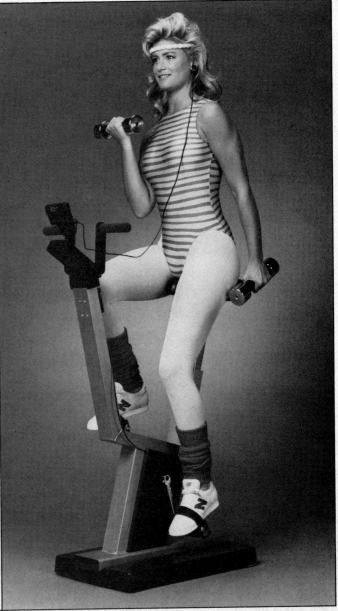

TREADMILLS

The revolving belt of a treadmill provides a surface on which you can walk, run, or jog without going anywhere—and without the risks of being rained on, mugged, or hit by a moving vehicle.

Both motorized and manual treadmills are available on the market. The motorized variety has two advantages. First, they help you maintain a steady pace, thereby controlling your heart rate and giving you a better, more predictable workout. Second, since you're actually moving to keep up with the movement of the belt instead of propelling your body forward with each stride, the skeletal stress from "heel-strike shock" is minimized. This may lessen the tendency toward shin splint injuries as well as other common runners' ailments. A treadmill is not a cure-all in this sense, though, for if you have basic gait or posture abnormalities, any repetitive movement like running can aggravate the problem. When shopping for a motorized treadmill look for a reliable, quiet, heavy-duty motor, variable speed capability that is easy to adjust, an emergency on-off switch, a speed indicator, front and/or side handrails, and a starting speed that is slow enough to allow walking. Most motorized treadmills operate on house current.

The major advantage of manual (nonmotorized) treadmills is that they are considerably less expensive. Walking or running on a manual treadmill is quite different from normal walking or running. In order to keep the belt moving smoothly, you have to push it behind you with each stride. The normal movement is more a process of falling and catching oneself with each stride. On a motorized treadmill, the movement is closer to the normal one. The manual treadmill, therefore, uses more of the muscles on the back of the hip and thigh than the motorized type, although involvement of these muscles can be enhanced on any treadmill by adjusting the surface incline. In choosing a manual treadmill, the mechanical features (usually rollers) that cause the belt to rotate freely and frictionlessly should be scrutinized. The more freely they move, the less you will notice the need to push backward with your feet. It is not a bad idea to inquire about keeping these rollers lubricated. Other features to look for in a manual treadmill are quietness, a comfortable belt surface from the standpoint of padding and traction, and a generally smooth running belt which remains centered on the machine during use. Side and front handrails are usually needed at first for balance, and a timer and odometer are nice to help quantify your workout.

Some treadmills, both motorized and nonmotorized, have an adjustable elevation feature which enables you to run up hills of varying steepness. This way, you can emphasize different muscle groups if you like, make your workout more strenuous without running faster or longer, and have the option to train for numerous sports that require uphill locomotion (hiking, rock-climbing, skiing). This feature becomes less useful if making the elevation adjustment requires too much time and too many tools. For the average recreational fitness buff, adequate levels of fitness can be achieved by running on level surfaces.

If you cannot, for medical reasons, do any running and must just walk, the elevation adjustment will give you some work-load versatility that you would not otherwise have. The inclined surface will let you work hard enough to build and increase your cardiovascular fitness without having to increase your pace (or the trauma on your joints) by moving from a walk to a run.

Along with the treadmills, we've included a cross-country ski simulator in this section. This is a specific treadmill-like device that mimics the exact motions of the sport for training purposes. For general fitness purposes this device has the advantage of giving your upper-body musculature (chest, shoulders, arms, and back) a workout in addition to your lower body (feet, ankles, calves, thighs, and hips), with virtually no skeletal shock. The biggest drawback to these devices is the relative coordination needed to condition effectively. However, once you get the hang of it, you'll get a terrific workout.

We recommend that you use a pulse meter with your treadmill. As with other home gym equipment, it's a good idea to buy whatever monitoring devices you can afford. They provide valuable safety controls and motivational tools for the exerciser.

ANATOMY OF A TREADMILL

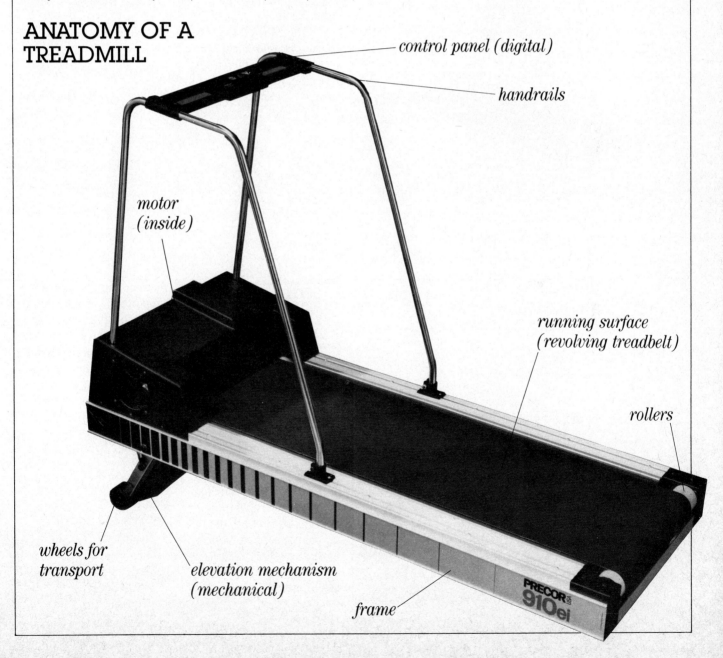

control panel (digital)

handrails

motor (inside)

running surface (revolving treadbelt)

rollers

wheels for transport

elevation mechanism (mechanical)

frame

PRECOR 910ei

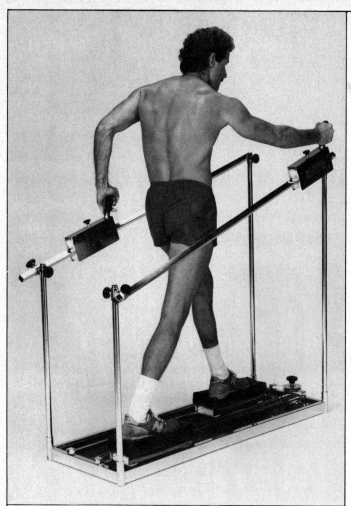

FITNESS MASTER XC-1

The XC-1 is a cross-country ski simulator. These devices, originally designed to help cross-country skiers train when there is no snow, are also excellent rehabilitative tools, especially for people who suffer from back and neck pain. Instead of running, you slide back and forth on footpads mounted on roller tracks. With sliding there's no heel shock and less strain on the lower back.

The XC-1 allows you to exercise your arms by means of a variable-tension pulley arrangement. You can set the tension for your arms and legs separately. The runway remains level, but the angle of the side rails is adjustable. The XC-1 comes with a 2-year warranty and a free 30-day home trial period.

WEIGHT:	68 lbs.
SIZE:	20″ × 58″ × 48″ h
APPROXIMATE COST:	$550

PORTABLE MODEL-35 (not shown)

APPROXIMATE COST:	$379

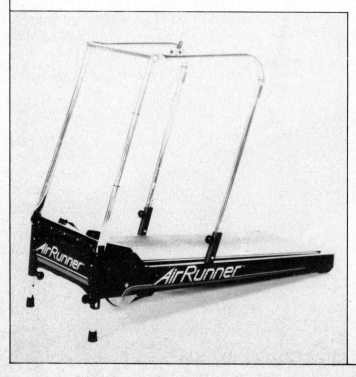

GRAVITY GUIDANCE® SYSTEM AIRRUNNER™

This nonmotorized unit is a prototype from Gravity Guidance, the inversion people. It has three outstanding features to minimize the effects of running or jogging on your spine and joints: the belt's cushioned surface is made of copolymer rubber and features rows of tubular air channels; the platform beneath the belt is designed to bow slightly downward during use; and the belt and platform are supported by eight rubber shock absorbers.

The AirRunner has a very smooth operation, adjustable elevation, speedometer, odometer, timer, and a two-position handrail. It comes in black, with chromed rails. The AirRunner folds flat for storage.

WEIGHT:	94 lbs.
SIZE:	18″ × 48″ × 39″ h
APPROXIMATE COST:	$595

TUNTURI JOGGING MACHINE

The Tunturi is a sturdy, well-built, nonmotorized treadmill. The low friction between the running surface and the treadbelt is the secret of its quiet action. An instant load adjustment accommodates a wide range of body weights and exertion levels. A convenient tracking adjustment keeps the mat centered. The side handrails and elevation are adjustable. It also has solid rubber caps which reduce noise and prevent slipping. The Tunturi's speedometer/odometer is easy to read and reports your progress at a glance. Its colors are the familiar Tunturi white and green.

WEIGHT: 91 lbs.
SIZE: $13\frac{1}{2}'' \times 55'' \times 36''$ to 48" h
APPROXIMATE COST: $700

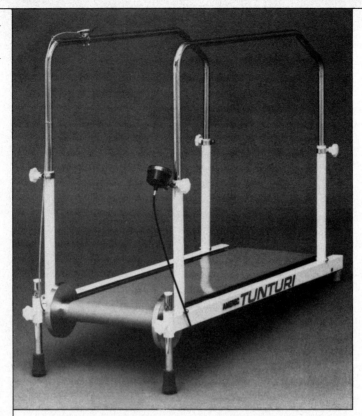

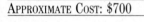

FITNESS EQUIPMENT CO., INC., MARATHON 1500

The 1500 is a quality low-cost machine, complete with elevation. It has a wooden base, with sturdy side and front handrails for safety. The ¾-horsepower motor allows you to adjust your speed from 0 to 4 mph. The hand-cranked elevation mechanism adjusts the grade from 5 to 15 percent. The speed control knob is easy to reach while you're exercising.

WEIGHT: 105 lbs.
SIZE: $20'' \times 66\frac{1}{2}'' \times 54''$ h
APPROXIMATE COST: $900

M & R INDUSTRIES, INC., AVITA 350 AEROBIC JOGGER

The 350 is powered by a 1½-horsepower heavy-duty motor. The speed is adjustable from 0 to 10 mph. It has a smooth surface, a 60-minute timer, a light aluminum frame, and rubber-coated, tapered end rollers with permanently sealed ball bearings. Although it has no elevation capabilities, it is a good value.

WEIGHT: 112 lbs.
SIZE: 22″ × 61″ × 51″ h
APPROXIMATE COST: $1,200

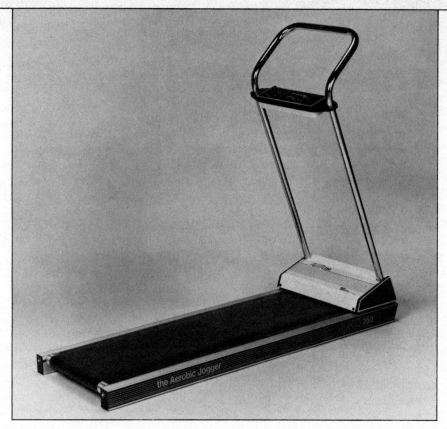

PRECOR® 910ei

This contemporary-looking machine features cushioned handrails, reasonably quiet and smooth running action, a graded elevation unit (0 to 15 percent grade) that operates with a gas-assisted spring arm, and an emergency stop mechanism that cuts off the motor when you press any two keys on the control panel. Its color scheme is black, polished stainless steel, and anodized aluminum.

The 910ei's easy-to-use fingertip computer key pad gives you digital readouts on time, mph (calibrated in tenths), and distance covered (in hundredths of a mile). You can adjust your speed from 1 to 8 mph.

WEIGHT: 155 lbs.
SIZE: 26″ × 72″ × 43″ h
APPROXIMATE COST: $2,300; without elevation, $2,100

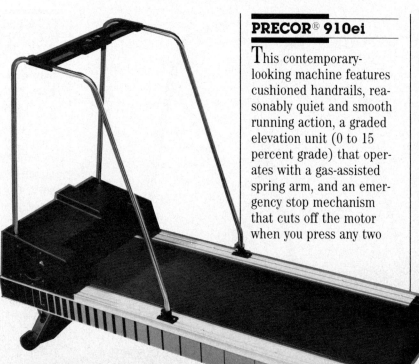

PRECOR® 935e ELECTRONIC TREADMILL

The 935e's frame is made of anodized aluminum and welded for strength and durability. It has a padded handrail and simple fingertip controls. This unit's top speed is 10 mph.

The running surface is a specially formulated elastomer (plastic), and it travels on a low-friction bed, making each step solid and accurate, whether you're running or walking.

The 935e's microprocessor gives this treadmill a sexy electronics package. The display tells you speed, distance, time, calories per minute, and total caloric expenditure. No other treadmill in this price range gives the calorie information. The machine divides each "footplant" (step) into segments. The microprocessor "reads" each segment and adjusts the belt speed to minimize sticking and jerking.

WEIGHT: 165 lbs.
SIZE: 28¼" × 75" × 46½" h
APPROXIMATE COST: $2,695

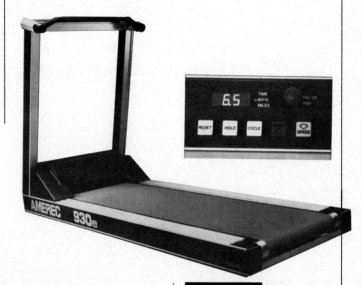

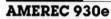

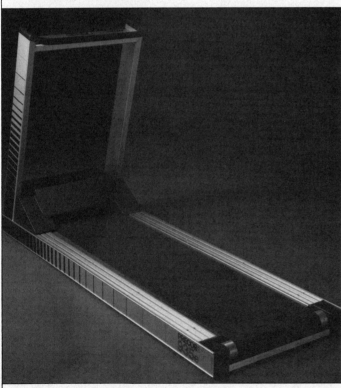

AMEREC 930e

The 930e is probably the sleekest-looking treadmill on the market. The black and anodized aluminum unit features a foam-handled front support, an easy-to-use red emergency stop button, and probably the longest running surface available today. However, it does not have an elevation capability.

The highly visible touch-control computer panel is 9 inches wide. It tells you your speed (adjustable from 0 to 10 mph), calibrated in tenths of a mile; distance traveled, in hundredths of a mile; and time in seconds, up to 59 minutes and 59 seconds.

WEIGHT: 200 lbs.
SIZE: 28" × 75" × 45" h
APPROXIMATE COST: $3,000

TROTTER UNITROT 330

Trotter, the manufacturer of the 330, has helped set an industry standard for quality and reliability.

The Unitrot 330 is a heavy-duty motorized unit. It features front and side handrails, easy-access controls, *motorized* elevation adjustable from 0 to 25 percent grade, safety footpads, and wide decks for ease in getting on and off. The 330's Data-Pak tells you elevation, speed in miles per hour or minutes per mile, and time in minutes and hundredths. You can adjust the speed from 2.5 to 10 mph or order it with an alternate range of 1.4 to 6 mph. The machine is off-white with chrome rails.

Trotter also manufactures its own Pritikin Institute–model treadmill.

WEIGHT: 300 lbs.
SIZE: 31" × 62" × 56" h
APPROXIMATE COST: $3,500

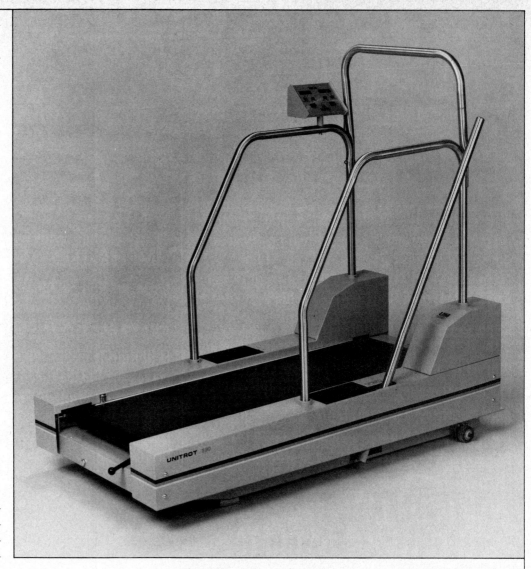

How to Use a
TREADMILL

For all practical purposes, using a treadmill is merely walking or running. However, these familiar movements do occur in a context that initially makes them feel awkward and perhaps more difficult than the normal activity. Having the ground move underneath you (as on a motorized treadmill), or having to push the ground backward with each step (as on a manual treadmill), may temporarily make you feel unstable and make your movements erratic or uncertain. However, after one or two practice sessions you won't know the difference. Once you are able to move with the momentum of the particular machine, there is no perceptible difference from walking down the street. The following suggestions and observations should get you started safely and help you to proceed successfully.

• Turn the unit on, if it is motorized, and check that it is operating smoothly. The treadbelt should be taut and centered on the machine. If the unit is adjusted to an incline position, check the adjustments to see that they are secure.

• Once you have inspected your treadmill, stand with your feet on the outside deck, straddling the treadbelt. Start the treadmill at the lowest speed and then hop on. (Starting it when you are standing on it puts a lot of stress on the motor and may eventually burn it out.)

• Start at a slow speed and then work up to a faster one. This gives all runners at all levels a needed period of warm-up and a time to get acclimated to the treadmill itself.

• It is a good idea to utilize the hand or front railings for stability and balance at first.

• Wear well-cushioned footwear and per-haps an additional insole for foot and ankle stability. Because many treadmills utilize rollers underneath the belt surface, one of the most common treadmill-caused ailments is plantar metatarsalgia—a bruising of the bones on the bottom of the forefoot.

• Be conscious of your posture. It is possible to overaccentuate forward lean and/or back arch when running on a treadmill. It helps tremendously to have a mirror at the side if it is convenient for your gym setup.

• Pay attention to your right and left footfalls as you walk or run. The movement and force of your steps should feel and sound even. On a manual treadmill unevenness may interrupt the gliding of the belt enough to make it jerky or actually cause it to stop.

• Remember to land first on the heel and allow the weight to be transferred along the outside border of the foot to the ball of the foot, from which you will push off and land on the opposite heel. On a motorized treadmill there may be a tendency to overstride to keep up with the belt, forcing you to land on the forefoot first. On a manual type, you may lean forward and run on the balls of the feet if you are having difficulty keeping the belt moving smoothly.

• Always work up slowly to the speed you desire. This will allow you to develop the necessary changes in cadence and stride length needed at the higher speed.

• Always elevate the running incline gradually. It is important to realize that increasing the incline increases your work load. Your pulse rate will reach training levels faster when you are going up a hill. This means you could work your heart too fast too soon by increasing the incline too rapidly or in too large an increment.

• Once familiar with your treadmill, you may want to enhance the scope of your workout by adding hand weights. Doing this has several advantages. It will increase your work load and decrease the time it takes to get your pulse rate up to training level, just like running on an incline, but it does not require the postural adjustments that running uphill requires. Working all four limbs under load has been shown to have a better aerobic training effect than just working two limbs. It has been said that the same amount of work feels like less when using all four limbs because the aerobic demands are being spread over more body musculature. And it also gives your upper body attractive shape and tone. For best results make sure each leg movement is done in a "duet" with one arm movement. Remember to begin with a small 1-pound weight. If you are monitoring your pulse rate, you will know when you need to work harder and add more weight. Remember, running with too heavy a weight can have negative effects on joints and other body parts.

• Walking and running are aerobic activities and should be done a minimum of three times a week for at least 15 to 20 minutes.

• Don't forget to pay attention to the effect of your exercise on the muscles and joints of the feet, ankles, knees, hips, and lower back. These areas, in addition to your heart, get a good workout on the treadmill. It is not uncommon for your cardiovascular system (as indicated by your pulse rate) to adapt more rapidly than your skeletal system (as indicated by muscle or joint soreness and stiffness). To remain injury-free, you should be monitoring the feedback from both systems.

• Finally, don't forget to cool down by slowly walking one to five minutes.

TREADMILL WALKING

STARTING POSITION: Set the treadbelt at a slow walking pace (1 to 3 mph). Hold on to the handrails and straddle the moving treadbelt with your feet. Put one, then the other, foot on the moving treadbelt, while supporting yourself with the handrails.

MOTION: At first, walking on a treadmill may feel awkward, but you should become accustomed to it quickly. Just walk normally, taking long strides instead of short, choppy steps. Look forward, not down at the moving treadbelt. Once you get used to it, you'll find it easier and more natural to let your arms swing at your sides instead of holding on to the handrails.

PRECAUTIONS: As with any aerobic exercise, start slowly and increase your work load over time. Adjust speed, elevation, and time on the treadmill to your own requirements. Warm up (2 to 5 minutes) before you start working within your target heart rate. Remember that walking on an incline (as in the photo) is more strenuous than walking on a level surface.

AREAS STRENGTHENED: Cardiovascular and respiratory systems, thighs, calves.

MUSCLES STRENGTHENED: Quadriceps, gastrocnemius, soleus.

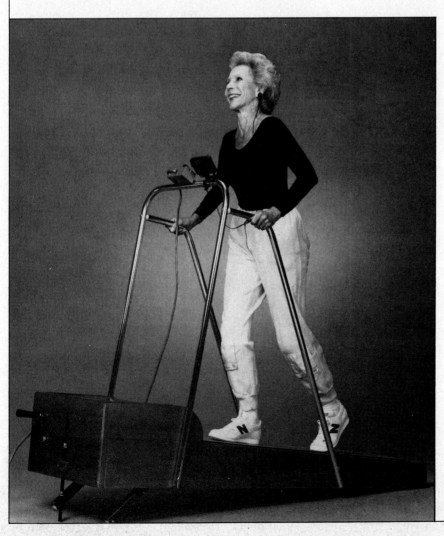

TREADMILL RUNNING

STARTING POSITION: Start slowly, using the same procedure as with walking.

MOTION: There's a transitional stage between a fast walk and a slow jog. *Slowly* increase the treadmill's speed as you increase your own speed. Eventually the treadmill should be moving fast enough for you to run at a pace that challenges you within safe, comfortable limits.

PRECAUTIONS: Never run out of control, or past the point of slight discomfort. If you feel dizzy, dehydrated, or nauseated, slow down, then stop. Running on an incline (not shown) is significantly more challenging than on a level surface.

AREAS STRENGTHENED: Cardiovascular and respiratory systems, thighs, calves.

MUSCLES STRENGTHENED: Quadriceps, gastrocnemius, soleus.

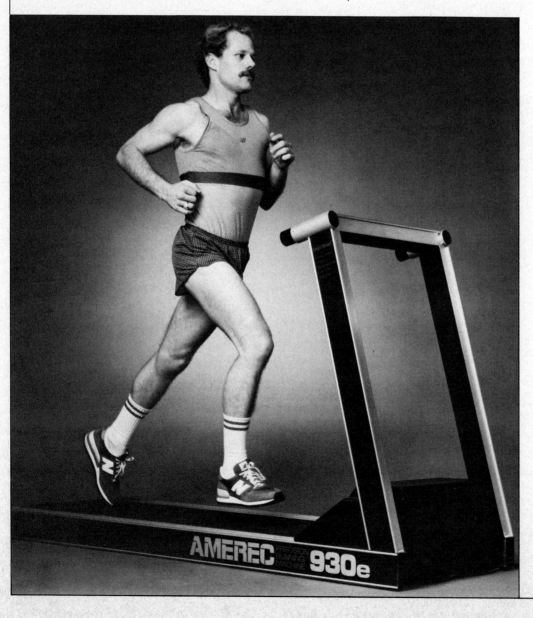

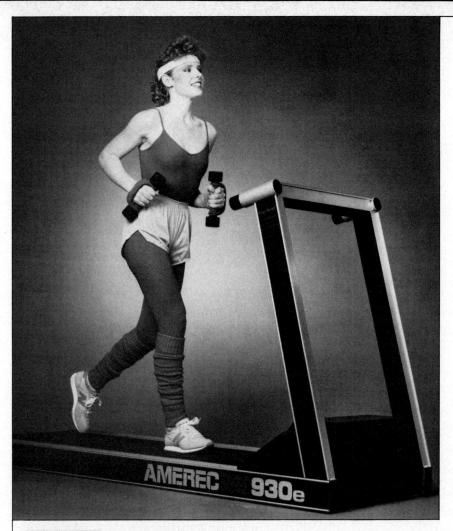

TREADMILL RUNNING WITH WEIGHTS

STARTING POSITION: Grasp a weight in each hand, and start slowly, using the same procedure as with basic running.

MOTION: Walk or jog normally on the treadmill while holding the weights. Swing your arms at your sides, as you would when walking or jogging on the ground.

PRECAUTIONS: Start with very light weights (1 to 2 lbs.). There's a much greater difference between jogging with and without weights than you might expect, and you'll be surprised at how heavy the weights feel at first. You'll probably hit your target heart rate much faster than usual. Bear in mind that the motion of walking or running with weights is slightly different from ordinary walking or running, so it's especially important to start slowly. Weight work is definitely an advanced treadmill exercise.

AREAS STRENGTHENED: Cardiovascular and respiratory systems, thighs, calves, front of upper arms and shoulders.

MUSCLES STRENGTHENED: Quadriceps, gastrocnemius, soleus, biceps, deltoids.

ROWING MACHINES

A rowing machine is possibly the single most cost-effective piece of home exercise equipment you can own. Rowing is a strenuous aerobic activity that builds cardiovascular and respiratory fitness. It burns calories like a '68 Eldorado burns gasoline. It provides weight and strength training for all major muscle groups by allowing you to do a variety of exercises. And rowing makes your entire body more flexible. For all these reasons, if you can afford only one piece of equipment for your home gym, we recommend that you consider making it a rowing machine.

A rowing machine lets you simulate the action of rowing a boat while pushing against mechanical resistance instead of water. There are two basic types. Sculling machines require your arms to move in an arc, and the more popular shock-absorbing resistance machines move your arms forward and back in a more or less horizontal plane.

Because rowing is an aerobic exercise, you should work out at least three times a week for at least 15 to 20 minutes per session at your target heart rate. All the rowers illustrated here, except the scull-type, can easily be placed upright for storage in a small closet.

When shopping for a rowing machine, look for smooth seat action, a comfortable seat, dual shock absorbers, a solid stabilizing frame, swiveling footplates, and a timer or stroke counter. If you're buying a sculling machine, make sure that the resistance joint is well constructed. Try out machines to see that the length of stroke is proportionate to your height. This can be a problem if you're over 6'2".

The resistance you're working against in a rowing machine is provided by shock absorbers—usually one shock per rowing arm. In all rowing machines now available, the cylinders of these shocks are filled with oil, which is the resistance medium. When you stroke the rowing arm, your stroke pulls a quantity of oil through a small opening. Some rowing machines have gas-assisted shocks. In these, a small bag containing either Freon or nitrogen is attached to the cylinder. The gas in the bag helps keep air out of the oil in the cylinder. Air bubbles in the oil reduce resistance and prevent you from getting the kind of workout you want.

The fact is that not much air gets into a rowing machine's shock absorbers in the first place. It's a different story with the shocks on your car—a car bounces around a lot at 60 miles per hour, and that causes plenty of air bubbles. Your rowing machine sits on the floor and bounces hardly at all. So gas-assisted shocks are perhaps a needless extravagance.

The size of the shocks, however, can make a difference in your rower's durability. Generally speaking, the larger the diameter of the shock absorbers, the better. A larger cylinder will dissipate heat better than a small one, and larger components usually don't wear out as quickly as small ones.

All rowing machines allow you to adjust the resistance you're rowing against, so you can give yourself either an easy or a severe workout. Most have an adjustment knob or T-knob on each rowing arm. To increase the work load, you loosen the knob and move the adjustment clamps up the arm. To decrease resistance, loosen the knobs and lower the clamps. There are usually dots, lines, or other reference markings around the adjustment clamps, so you can be sure you have equal tension on both rowing arms. All rowers come with instructions that tell you how to adjust them.

We recommend that you use a pulse monitor with your rowing machine. Chest-mounted monitors work best for this purpose. Because of the arm movements, the ones you wear on your finger don't work very well at all.

There are over two dozen rowing machines on the market. We've selected those that offer smooth action, good value, and reliability.

Rower shown in upright storage position.

ANATOMY OF A ROWING MACHINE

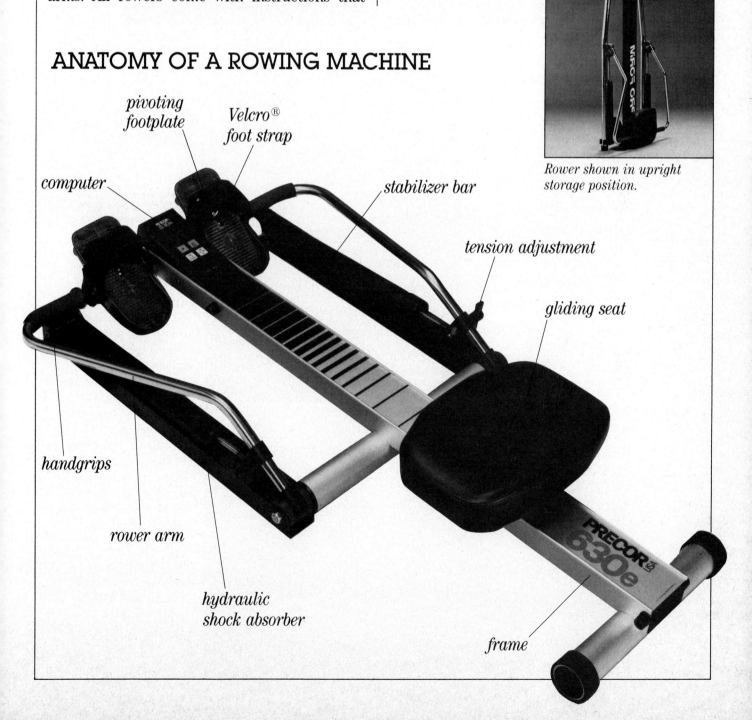

pivoting footplate

Velcro® foot strap

computer

stabilizer bar

tension adjustment

gliding seat

handgrips

rower arm

hydraulic shock absorber

frame

PRECOR® 612

This lightweight but well-built rower of black and anodized aluminum is reasonably priced and features the latest in hydraulic engineering: a new valve system for the oil-filled resistance pistons. The result is that the 612 operates quietly and gives you a smooth, consistent pull throughout each stroke. Swiveling footplates, wide Velcro® foot straps, and a wide, thickly padded seat ensure that your workout is comfortable as well as quiet.

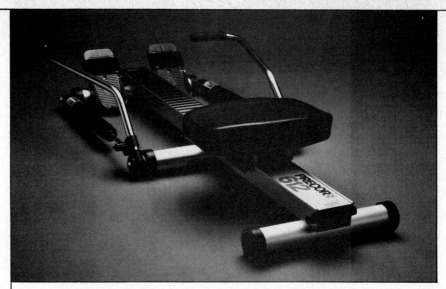

WEIGHT: 30 lbs.
SIZE: 30″ × 52″
APPROXIMATE COST: $280

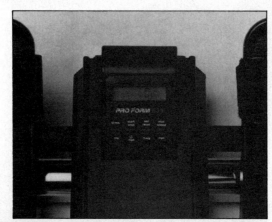

PRO FORM® 935

The 935's unique one-piece chrome tubing frame is one of the sleekest (and most stable) designs available. This black and chrome machine has smooth seat action, swiveling footplates, and rotating handgrips.

The 935 allows the buyer the option of a sophisticated computer, which operates off a 5.6-volt battery. Its LCD reads out stroke rate, maximum rowing speed, average rowing speed, and total miles rowed. There's also a stopwatch display.

WEIGHT: 29 lbs.
SIZE: 30″ × 48″
APPROXIMATE COST: $350;
$400 with computer

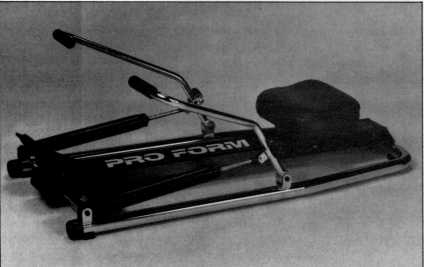

AVITA 950

The Avita 950 is one of the best buys on the market. Its gas-assisted cylinders provide maximum resistance and quiet operation. The rowing arms work smoothly, thanks to ball bearings, and the cushioned seat moves on ball bearings in an internal track. Other features include a 60-minute timer, wide foot straps, and footplates that swivel independently.

The 950's chrome steel tubing frame is sturdy enough to easily handle the kind of workout an athlete will give it. (The frame is guaranteed for five years; all other parts are guaranteed for one year.) The frame's construction makes this the heaviest of all the portable models listed here.

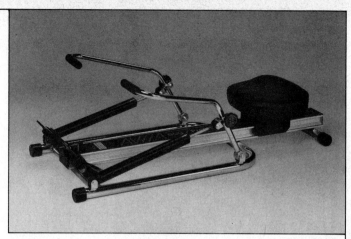

WEIGHT: 40 lbs.
SIZE: 34″ × 49″
APPROXIMATE COST: $350

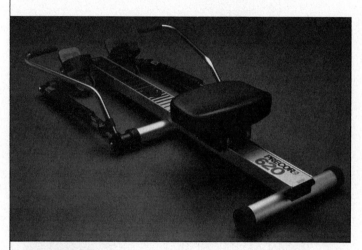

PRECOR® 620

This anodized aluminum rower's box frame is rigid enough for even the most enthusiastic rowers. The upholstered seat is heavily padded for extended workouts. There is a mechanical counter that displays total strokes. The footplates swivel, and your feet are held in place by Velcro® straps.

The 620 was designed to be worked hard, so its two oil-filled shocks are the largest of those on any rower. Precor's new Ventrika™ valving system makes this machine unusually quiet, smooth, and durable. You can set your work load with the micro-adjust knobs on each rowing arm. Fractional settings are easy with the 620's system.

Because of its 53″ frame, the 620 is suitable for people up to 6′7″ tall.

WEIGHT: 35 lbs.
SIZE: 32″ × 53″
APPROXIMATE COST: $395

MAXIMUS™

Gym Equipment International's rower features eight marked tension positions, a four-digit single-cycle stroke counter (non-electronic), and just about the largest seat of any rowing machine we've seen. Maximus is a good bet for tall people.

WEIGHT: 35 lbs.
SIZE: 30″ × 50″
APPROXIMATE COST: $400

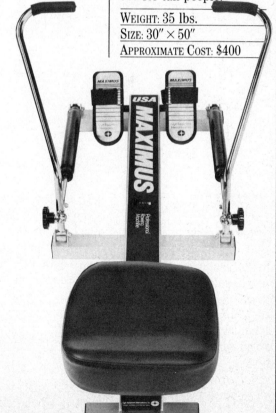

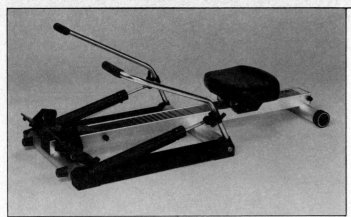

PRECOR® 630e

The black-and-anodized-aluminum 630e was the first true ergometric rower designed for consumer use. This machine requires virtually no assembly and comes with heavy-duty hydraulic shocks, an all-welded frame, a long shaft to accommodate taller users, a wide base for heavier users, and smooth, quiet seat action.

The 630e's sophisticated computer operates off a 9-volt battery. The LCD reads out time, strokes per minute, total

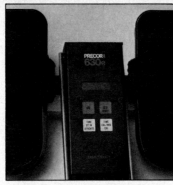

strokes, calories burned per minute, and total calories burned. A state-of-the-art rower from a state-of-the-art manufacturer.

WEIGHT: 33 lbs.
SIZE: 30″ × 51″
APPROXIMATE COST: $550

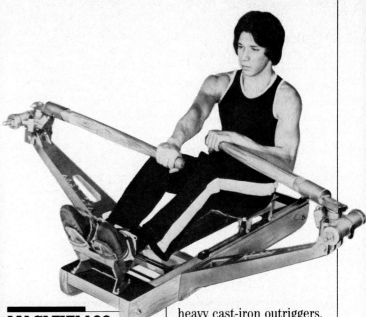

MACLEVY 190

The 190 is the only sculling machine evaluated in this chapter. MacLevy describes it as an "Extra-Heavy-Duty Rowing Machine" designed to hold up under rigorous use by groups of exercisers in a gymnasium setting. As you can imagine, this machine's virtual indestructibility requires that it be fairly large, and not portable at all.

Each hardwood oar has its own adjustable hydraulic unit. The hydraulic cylinders are mounted on heavy cast-iron outriggers. The seat has absorbent shock bumpers both front and rear. The heavy hardwood base is mounted on elevated legs, with non-skid rubber bumpers to prevent creeping and protect floors. The oars are mounted on protective steel collars attached to the hydraulic units. Clearly, this is a machine designed for the serious oarsman.

WEIGHT: 135 lbs.
SIZE: 53″ × 58″
APPROXIMATE COST: $1,200

AMF LIFE STYLER™ 5000

This machine's unique design features a pulley-and-handle system, instead of conventional rowing arms. Its extended aluminum seat guide accommodates long-legged rowers, and front-mounted rollers make it easy to store. The Life Styler 5000's

LED readout displays resistance, time, and calories burned.

This unit will work your legs a little more than most rowing machines.

WEIGHT: 77 lbs.
SIZE: 15″ × 82½″
APPROXIMATE COST: $595

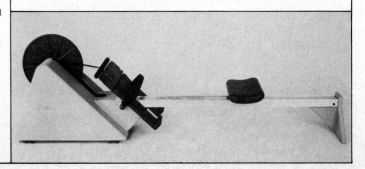

How to Use a
ROWER

As we've said earlier, rowing is just about the best all-around aerobic exercise you can get. It works virtually all your major muscle groups, and there's no problem with shock to your body (as is the case with running).

All rowing machines have footplates, a seat, a sliding base on which the seat rests, and "oars" (which are actually handlebars). The footplates are located at the end of the rower. They should swivel to let your feet move as you row, but they're stationary with respect to the long axis of the machine. You push against them as you row. The seat slides along the machine's long axis toward the end opposite the footplates. When you row, then, you're pushing your body weight back and forth along the length of the rowing machine.

The first step in using a rower is to find one you feel comfortable in. You need to get used to the fit of the foot straps and the footplates. Most rowers are designed to fit people of "average" height. In our review of the individual machines, we've indicated which ones fit people 6'2" and over.

Sit down in your rower in a tuck position and strap your feet into the foot straps. The seat should be as close to the footplates as possible. Grasp the handlebars firmly, using either an overhand or underhand grip. The handlebars will be forward and almost straight down in this position. Sit up as straight as you're able, given the position of your hands and arms.

The first rowing motion is a strong, smooth push of your feet and legs against the footplates. Push until your legs are as fully extended as possible. This push works the quadriceps, gluteals, and hamstrings. At the end of your push, you should be leaning backward from the hips, legs partially extended, arms almost fully extended and grasping the handgrips.

A nearly simultaneous motion with the leg push is a strong, smooth pull of the handlebars toward your chest. Avoid the impulse to lean forward and bend your back into your stroke. Instead, keep leaning back as much as you can, and keep your back straight. This isolates your abdominal, shoulder, arm, and back muscles. Once you've completed this motion, you return to your beginning position by pulling forward with your legs and pushing on the handlebars. This final stage works the muscles that were stretched during the earlier movements.

Rowing is a great calorie-burner, and you should monitor your work load in whatever way you prefer. Depending on your needs and your rower's equipment, you can chart total strokes, strokes per minute, time elapsed rowing, calories burned per minute, and/or total calories burned.

The most common mistake beginning rowers make is to set the oars' resistance too high. Start with a sufficiently low resistance so that you can row for 15 or 20 minutes without exhausting yourself. If it's under 15 minutes, you won't get any aerobic benefits. As your skill and level of conditioning improve, you can increase the resistance to give yourself a tougher workout. But be advised that various rowing motions put some strain on the lower back.

And don't worry about your workout not being tough enough. In fact, you should keep towels near the machine, because you're likely to pump so much sweat you'll think you're rowing on a lake, instead of on your living room floor. Try to set a weekly goal of calories burned, distance rowed, or time spent working out.

With the sleek machines in this book, you won't be able to row your way to Tahiti—or even across the floor of your home gym. What you *will* do is develop a stronger heart, a more efficient cardiovascular system, and a leaner, meaner body. And if you ever do decide to go near the water, you can bet that nobody will kick sand in your face.

ARM PULLS

STARTING POSITION: Sit in the machine with your legs straight out, feet strapped into the footplates. Hold the handles in an overhand grip.

MOTION: While keeping your legs straight, alternately pull each hand toward your torso.

PRECAUTIONS: Adjust the machine's resistance so you can pull the handles as far back as your shoulder joint will let you. Getting a full range of motion gives you better results. Avoid the urge to overly twist your torso or overarch your back. Try to move only your arms.

AREA WORKED: Front of arms, back of shoulders and underarms, upper back.

MUSCLES WORKED: Biceps, posterior deltoids, latissimus dorsi, trapezius, rhomboids.

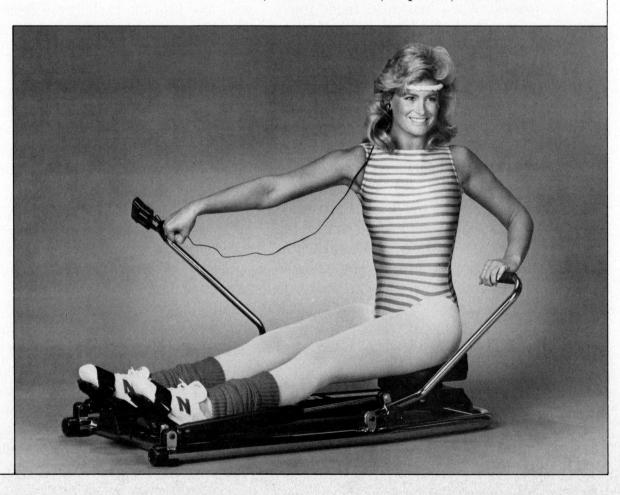

ROWING

STARTING POSITION: Sit forward in the machine, with your feet strapped to the footplates and your knees up to your chest. Hunch your shoulders forward slightly, and hold the handles in either the overhand or underhand grip. (The underhand grip is a bit easier and works your biceps more, because your biceps have a more advantageous angle of pull than in the overhand.)

MOTION: Straighten your legs and bend your arms by pushing on the footplates and pulling the handles toward your chest. Lean your torso slightly backward during this movement. To return to the starting position, reverse the sequence by bending your knees and straightening your arms.

PRECAUTIONS: You'll need practice for your arm and leg actions to occur in a smooth and coordinated fashion. Your speed and style will be yours alone, since they'll depend on your own strength and limb lengths.

AREAS WORKED: Front and back of thighs, hips, entire back, front of arms, back of shoulders and underarms, upper back.

MUSCLES WORKED: Quadriceps, hamstrings, gluteus maximus, erector spinae, biceps, posterior deltoids, latissimus dorsi, rhomboids, trapezius.

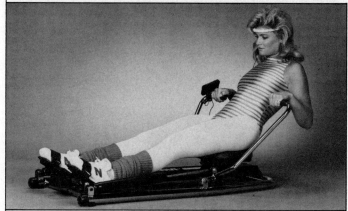

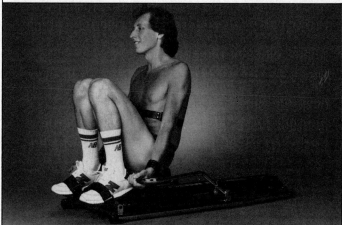

The overhand grip

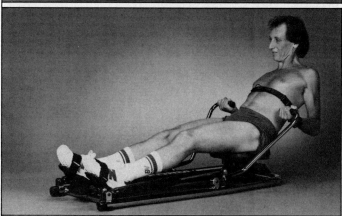

The underhand grip

SIT-UPS

STARTING POSITION: Strap your feet to the footplates and bend your knees slightly. Clasp your hands behind your head.

MOTION: Lower your torso slowly backward and downward, toward the floor. Allow your body to unfold segmentally, lowering first your waist, then your ribs, chest, shoulders, neck, and head. Sit up slowly in reverse segmental order.

PRECAUTIONS: Sit-ups are a must for a healthy back, but they can cause an unhealthy one if you do them incorrectly. Do not arch your lower back at all during this exercise. If you have back problems, bend your knees to form a 90° angle and fold your arms across your chest. Lower your torso backward only as far as you can without strain or pain in the lower back. Sit back up from that point. As you get stronger, you will be able to lower your torso farther.

AREAS WORKED: Front of torso, front of thighs, front of neck.

MUSCLES WORKED: Rectus abdominis, internal and external obliques, quadriceps, sternocleidomastoids.

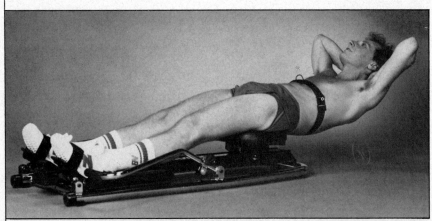

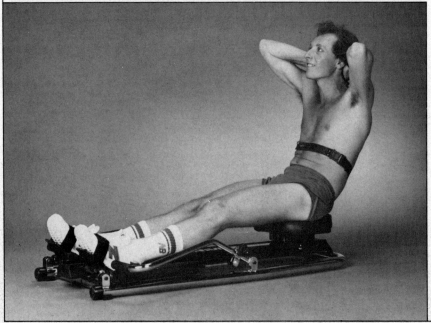

CHEST PRESS

STARTING POSITION: Sit upright in the seat, facing away from the footplates so the rowing handles are close to your chest. Place your feet securely on the floor and grasp the handles. Your elbows are bent.

MOTION: Push the rowing arms forward by the handles until your arms are fully extended and parallel to the floor. Return to the starting position, slowly resisting the force of the machine, until your hands are once again close to your torso.

PRECAUTIONS: For best results, keep your torso upright and motionless during this exercise. It's easy to cheat unconsciously by leaning forward to assist your chest and arm muscles. Remember to keep your shoulders relaxed, that is, lowered, not shrugged up toward your ear lobes. (This will prevent tension in your neck and will focus your energy on the exercise.)

AREAS WORKED: Front of chest and shoulders, back of upper arms, underside of forearms.

MUSCLES WORKED: Pectorals, anterior deltoids, triceps, flexor carpi radialis and ulnaris.

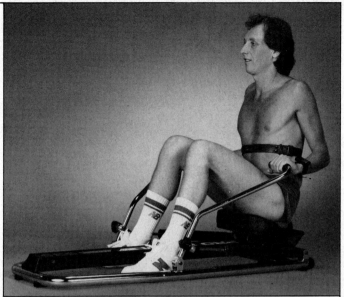

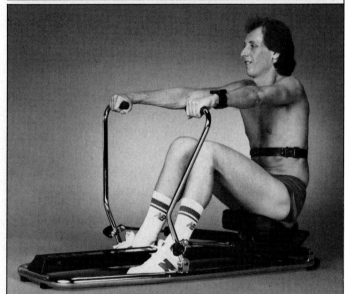

REBOUND EXERCISERS

Most people, when they've heard of rebounders at all, think of them as "those mini-trampolines." They're wrong. Rebounders are members of the trampoline family, but they aren't actually trampolines or mini-tramps. The difference is that the purpose of a full-size trampoline, the kind we're all familiar with—a device consisting of a fabric bed, a metal frame, and comparatively loose 9- to 12-inch springs—is to propel the user into the air, usually to do acrobatics. A mini-trampoline is a smaller version, also with fairly loose springs, that propels the user into the air to do gymnastics and vaulting. You usually see these at gymnastics meets or at the circus. Gymnasts hit the mini-tramp from a running start, and they land somewhere other than on the mini-tramp's fabric bed.

A rebounder is also small, but it has tighter springs than either the full-size or the mini-trampoline. On a rebounder, you don't jump to achieve a certain height. The rebounder's purpose is simply to let you jump up and down while the springs absorb the shock of your body's weight when you land. That's why a standard 8-foot ceiling will accommodate virtually any person who wants to rebound.

Rebounding exercises incorporate aerobics with strength training, balance, and coordination, and they condition the entire body in a way that places very little undue stress on the neurological and skeletal systems. The basic rebounding movement consists of bouncing up and down from a standing or seated position. Eventually, sandbag, wrist, or ankle weights are added to increase the aerobic value. Rebounding with weights or jumping rope on a rebounder is enough of a workout for even the most seasoned athlete.

When you shop for a rebounder, look for square or rectangular models. You will see round rebounders that are less expensive (and less sturdy), but the round shape tends to pronate your feet (turn them inward) too much. They're like firemen's safety nets, where you are drawn toward the middle. Besides giving you better foot support, rectangular units are more stable. But even circular models cushion the shock of jogging or jumping better than any type of stationary surface.

Make sure the springs around the mat are made of music wire, not a cheap bedspring-type. The best material for the mat seems to be polypropylene, a tough nylon weave that yields when you bounce but will stand up to constant use. Stay away from canvaslike material—it tears too easily. Polypropylene is ultraviolet-resistant, so you can leave your rebounder outside. However, like all equipment with metal components, the springs and frame will likely discolor and eventually rust.

You'll also want your rebounder to have spring-loaded or shock-absorbing legs. Shock absorbers reduce the shock trauma to your body, they make the springs around the mat last longer, and they make bouncing more fun.

The more you use your rebounder, the more accessories you'll want. Sandbags provide extra resistance; the Olympic Trainer weight system is an excellent one. You'll see wrist and ankle weights illustrated elsewhere in this book. As with any aerobic exercise, you'll want a pulse monitor. A chest-mounted monitor is currently the only kind that won't be jarred into ineffectiveness as you bounce. As you become more sure of yourself, you'll probably want a jump rope to increase the intensity of your workout.

At press time, there still seems to be only one well-designed rebounder on the market— sturdily built, square or rectangular, and with shock-absorbing legs. However, we understand that several companies have similar units in prototype stages. They should be worth checking out.

ANATOMY OF A REBOUNDER

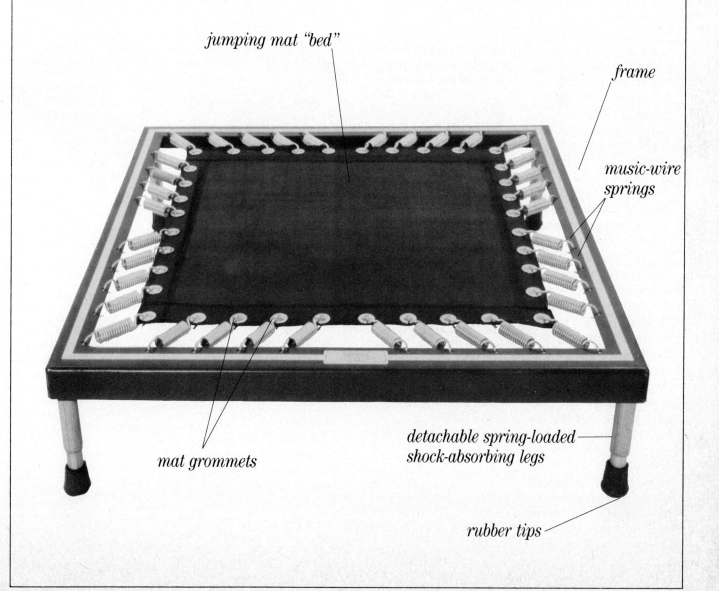

jumping mat "bed"

frame

music-wire springs

mat grommets

detachable spring-loaded shock-absorbing legs

rubber tips

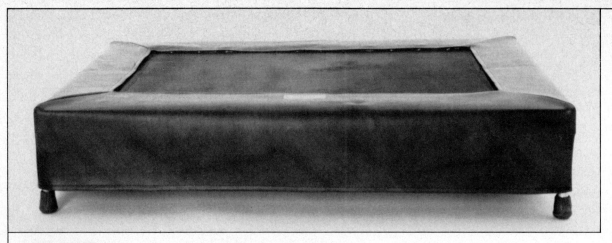

SOFTJOGGER™ REBOUNDERS

Rebounders let you work out aerobically by jumping, jogging, and twisting, all with minimal shock to your entire skeletal system. We chose SoftJoggers because they are the only production-model rebounders that incorporate the three basic components necessary to a good rebounder: square or rectangular design for even bouncing and stability; shock-absorbing legs; and overall high-quality materials and workmanship.

SoftJoggers' mats (jumping surfaces) are made of polypropylene, a tough lining-type material with high tensile strength. The mat's grommets are inserted in such a way that the mat wears well and doesn't tear easily. The springs are made from music wire. And the angle-iron frame also yields when you jump, giving you added shock absorption.

SoftJoggers' two drawbacks are that they are relatively cumbersome to carry around and that they take up a fair amount of space. You can store one by resting it on its side against a wall, or by sliding it under the bed. The legs may eventually start to squeak. If so, apply a little lubricant (such as 3-in-1 Oil or petroleum jelly) to stop the noise.

The larger rebounders definitely have a better feel when you're bouncing, but all sizes will allow you to perform all exercises.

SoftJoggers have a metallic black and chrome finish, with black Naugahyde spring covers. The SJ4.4H should hold up under very heavy use, even in an institutional environment.

Model: SJ 3.4
Size: 33″ × 45″ × 6″h
Weight: 33 lbs.
Approximate Cost: $149 to $199

Model: SJ 4.4
Size: 45″ × 45″ × 8″ h
Weight: 35 lbs.
Approximate Cost: $249

Model: SJ 4.4H
Size: 45″ × 45″ × 8″h
Weight: 38 lbs.
Approximate Cost: $349

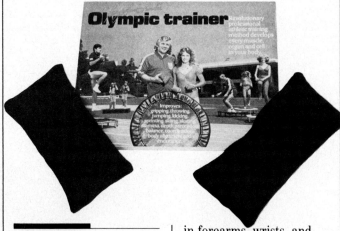

OLYMPIC TRAINER™ WEIGHTS

Olympic Trainer weights are fabric bags filled with sand. They're sold by the pair and come in 1-, 2- and 3-pound sets. Because they're soft and malleable, they can be used by people of any age while doing almost any sort of aerobic exercise (such as rebounding or stationary bike–riding) in which extra resistance is desired. They're excellent for developing grip strength, they increase circulation in forearms, wrists, and hands, and they distribute resistance evenly. They come with a particularly useful training manual, too.

Model: 1 lb.
Size: 6½″ × 3½″
Approximate Cost: $9

Model: 2 lbs.
Size: 6½″ × 3½″
Approximate Cost: $10

Model: 3 lbs.
Size: 7″ × 4″
Approximate Cost: $11

How to Use a
REBOUNDER

Rebounding can be the most delightful of all ways to get and stay in shape—especially if you work out to music. It's like aerobic dancing, but with springs on your feet, and the benefits are just as great. You'll want to do it for 15 to 20 minutes per workout after reaching your target heart rate. Once you're in good condition, you'll probably need sandbags or wrist and ankle weights to attain your target heart rate.

The rebounder is especially effective for people who need a nonstrenuous total body workout: beginners, anyone rehabilitating from an injury or illness, or individuals with a joint/bone/neurological disorder that requires a mild, nonpounding form of exercise. The rebounder is a good choice for older adults who have not been exercising regularly or recently. It's also excellent as a warm-up exercise routine for those on a more strenuous program.

Rebounding in bare feet gives you good traction and even leaves the bottoms of your feet feeling as if they've had a good, brisk massage. The second-best way to rebound is to wear a rubber-soled shoe—tennis shoe, aerobic shoe, "fitness shoe," or something similar. If you're a beginning rebounder, it's probably best to start out wearing such footwear, because they'll help you orient yourself within the limited bouncing area inside the perimeter formed by the springs. Avoid running shoes with flared soles that are significantly wider than the bottoms of the vamps. All that extra rubber can catch the sides of the rebounder on lateral movements, resulting in a twisted or sprained ankle.

Wearing socks or nylons without shoes is a bad idea. They give you no support, and they're much more slippery than your bare feet.

As with all running or bouncing exercises, women should wear support bras. If your balance is a bit shaky, you may want to place your rebounder next to a chair, dresser, or other solid object.

When performing all rebound exercises, stay in a fairly relaxed position with your knees slightly bent. *Never* jump up high and land with your feet together in the middle of the mat. You'll probably "bottom out" and hit the floor, which is not the idea at all.

Again, rebounders should be used for aerobic and warm-up exercises only. You should never use them to propel yourself into the air, or to do acrobatic tricks as you would use a mini-trampoline. We repeat: Rebounders and mini-tramps are *not* the same thing.

The following exercises are designed to be done sequentially: the easier movements are described first, then the more advanced ones.

CALF STRETCHES

STARTING POSITION: Stand on the rebounder mat with heels flat and knees straight. Lean forward, and hold onto a wall, a barre, or a stable chair for support.

MOTION: Lift up on your toes and gently bounce your heels (together) down toward the mat. Keep your back straight while bouncing. Pull in your stomach to keep your back flat.

PRECAUTIONS: If your muscles are tight in the back of your knees and in your calves, you will inadvertently place more weight on your hands and arms. Make sure the object you're leaning on is secure and will not slide.

AREAS STRENGTHENED: Calves, back of thighs.

MUSCLES STRENGTHENED: Gastrocnemius, soleus, hamstrings.

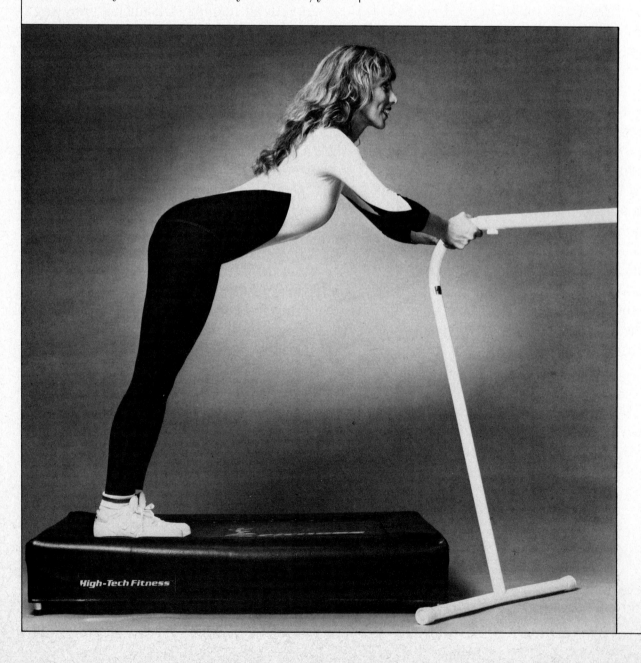

High-Tech Fitness

JOGGING WITH CHEST EXPANSION

STARTING POSITION: Stand on the center of the rebounder mat with your feet shoulder-width apart. Clasp your hands behind your body.

MOTION: Jog in place with your arms straight and raised behind your body.

PRECAUTIONS: Since this movement restricts your regular arm swing and changes your balance from what it would normally be while running, you may at first feel awkward and off-balance. Proceed slowly to get the feel of this different weight distribution.

AREAS STRENGTHENED: All major muscle groups, with emphasis on stretching the front of your chest and toning your upper back and the back of your upper arms.

MUSCLES STRENGTHENED: Stretches pectorals, anterior deltoids. Tones trapezius, rhomboids, triceps.

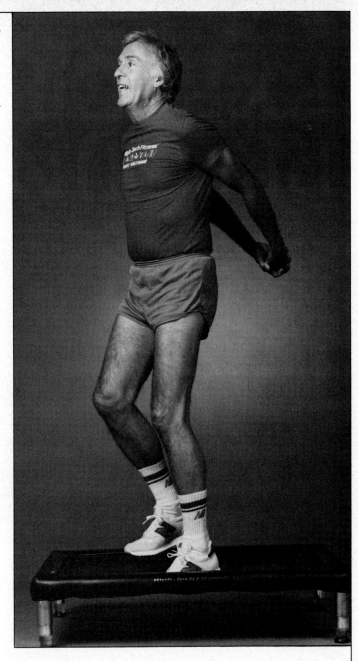

LUNGE SHUFFLE

STARTING POSITION: Stand on the rebounder mat with one leg forward, bent at the knee. Extend the other leg behind, with the knee straight. The arm opposite the bent knee should be slightly bent and reaching forward. The other arm should be bent and pulled backward.

MOTION: Simultaneously bounce and switch leg and arm positions by pulling the straight leg forward and extending the bent leg back behind your body. Reverse the positions of your arms accordingly.

PRECAUTIONS: Avoid propelling your body forward, as you do when running. Remember that your torso remains centered, and that both feet land on the mat and push off from it at the same time.

AREAS STRENGTHENED: Front of thighs, back of thighs, calves.

MUSCLES STRENGTHENED: Quadriceps, hamstrings, gluteus maximus, gastrocnemius, soleus.

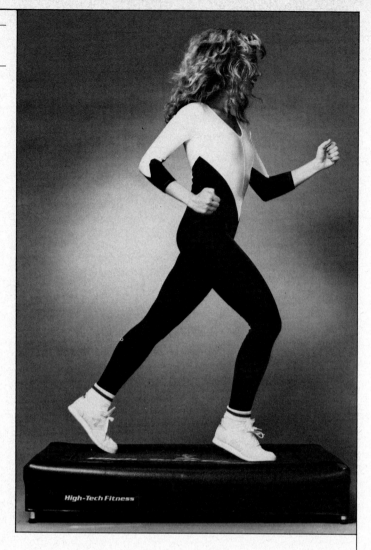

TORSO TWIST

STARTING POSITION: Stand on the rebounder mat with your arms fully extended to the sides at shoulder height. Angle both feet so your toes are pointed either to the right or to the left and your knees are slightly bent.

MOTION: While holding your arms and your upper body (waist to head) still, jump and twist your lower body (waist to feet) to the side opposite your starting position. With each jump/twist, you should land with your lower body twisted toward the alternate side.

PRECAUTIONS: Make sure you jump with enough spring so your feet clear the mat. Wearing thick-soled shoes can make this clearance distance difficult to discern, and the soles may catch on the mat. If balance and coordination don't come easily for you, do this exercise while holding on to a wall or stable chair until you get the feel of it.

AREAS STRENGTHENED: Sides of torso, upper hip, front of thighs, calves.

MUSCLES STRENGTHENED: Internal and external obliques, erector spinae, quadriceps, gastrocnemius, soleus.

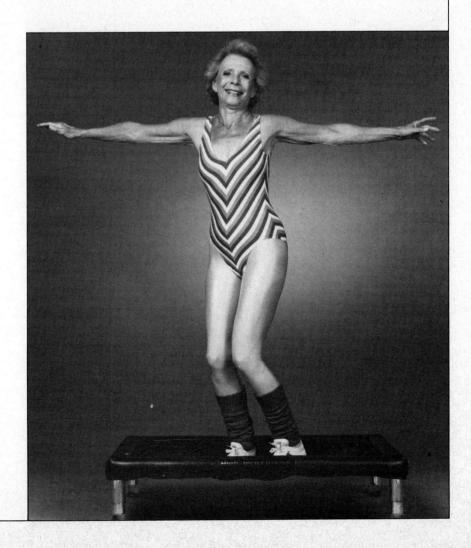

SIDE-BEND BOUNCE

STARTING POSITION: Stand on the center of the rebounder mat with your feet shoulder-width apart. Place one hand on your hip; reach the other over your head toward the opposite elbow.

MOTION: As you bounce (on both feet), bend to the side and at the same time reach with your overhead arm. Try not to lean forward when you bend. Land with your body upright and centered. Bend to alternate sides with each jump.

PRECAUTIONS: Do your side-bend in the air in order not to apply too much force to the back muscles.

AREAS STRENGTHENED: Calves, front of thighs, sides of torso, back.

MUSCLES STRENGTHENED: Gastrocnemius, soleus, quadriceps, internal and external obliques, erector spinae.

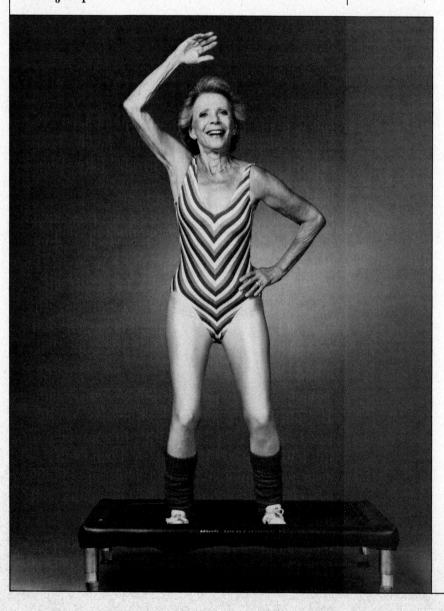

JOGGING WITH WEIGHTS

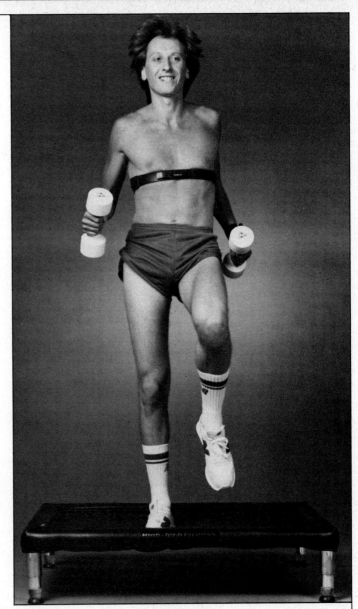

STARTING POSITION: Stand on the center of the rebounder mat with your feet shoulder-width apart. Let your arms hang down at your sides. Grasp the dumbbells firmly.

MOTION: Start jogging in place. As you jog, bring first one dumbbell, then the other, up toward your waist. The dumbbell you're lifting should be the one in the hand opposite the leg you're raising: right dumbbell, left leg; left dumbbell, right leg.

PRECAUTIONS: Adding weight to the upper body while jogging greatly increases the amount of aerobic work you're doing. Don't use too much weight at first. Jogging with weights isn't like weight lifting, because you have to perform the basic movement many, many times. Proceed gradually by first bending the arms only to waist height, then to shoulder height, and finally overhead. Each step/bounce should correlate with one simultaneous arm-bending movement.

AREAS STRENGTHENED: All major muscle groups.

MUSCLES STRENGTHENED: Refer to anatomy chart on pages 22–25.

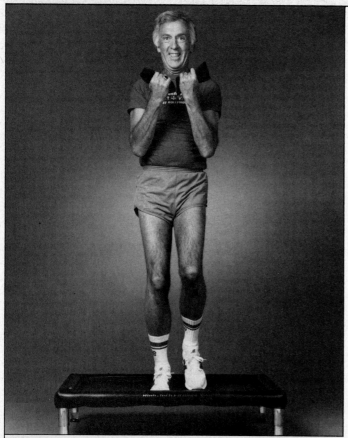

FLYS

STARTING POSITION: Stand on the center of the rebounder mat with your feet shoulder-width apart. Hold the weights in front of your shoulders.

MOTION: While jogging in place, extend both arms out to the sides. Return to the starting position and repeat as you jog.

PRECAUTIONS: Breathe normally, and keep to the center of the mat.

AREAS STRENGTHENED: Calves, thighs, shoulders.

MUSCLES STRENGTHENED: Gastrocnemius, soleus, quadriceps, deltoids.

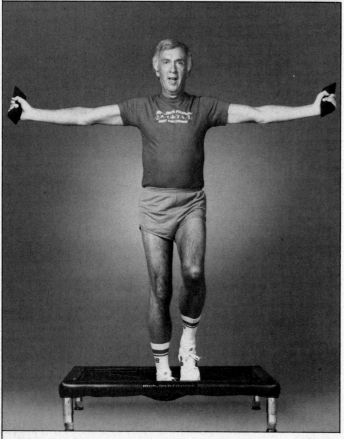

FRONT-KICK

STARTING POSITION: Stand on the rebounder mat with your feet shoulder-width apart and your arms slightly bent.

MOTION: Jump up while kicking one leg up and forward so it crosses in front of your supporting leg. Bring the kicking leg down in time to land with both feet centered under your body. On the next jump, kick with the other leg.

PRECAUTIONS: Be careful when jumping with only one leg for support. Start slowly, and use your arms for balance.

AREAS STRENGTHENED: Calves, hips, thighs.

MUSCLES STRENGTHENED: Gastrocnemius, soleus, iliopsoas, quadriceps.

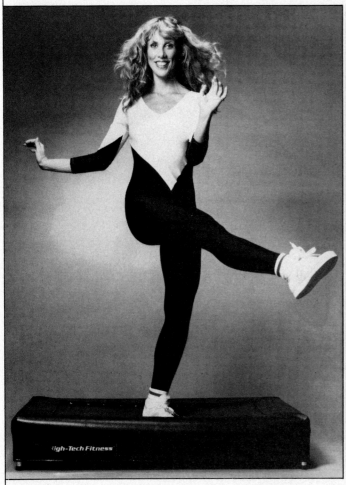
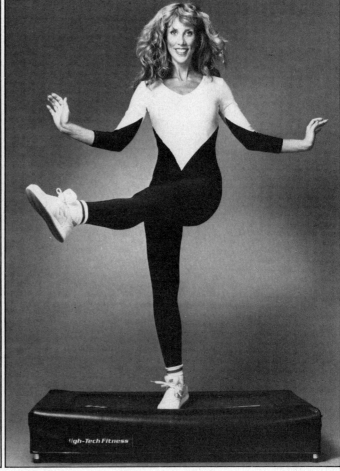

BOUNCING SIDE-KICK

STARTING POSITION: Stand on the rebounder mat with your feet shoulder-width apart, hands on hips.

MOTION: Jump while kicking one leg out to the side. Bring it down in time to land with both feet centered under your body. On the next jump, kick with the other leg. Try to keep your torso straight and hips level during this exercise.

PRECAUTIONS: Bounding on a resilient surface on just one leg can be awkward at first. Start gradually, and take it slowly until you get your "sea legs." Be careful that your support foot lands in or near the center of the mat.

AREAS STRENGTHENED: Calves, front of thighs, outer thighs.

MUSCLES STRENGTHENED: Gastrocnemius, soleus, quadriceps, tensor fasciae latae, gluteus medius.

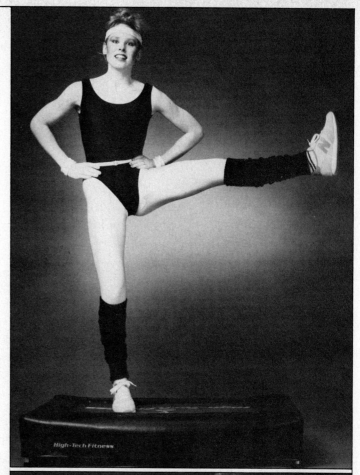

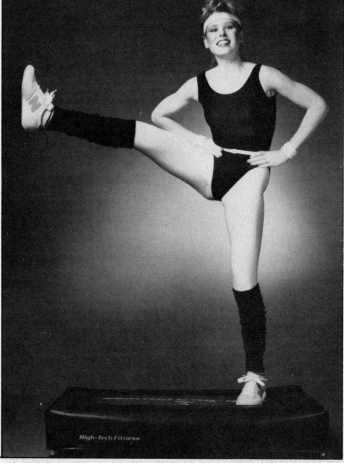

ALTERNATE-SIDE JUMPING JACKS

STARTING POSITION: Stand on the rebounder mat with your feet shoulder-width apart and your arms at your sides.

MOTION: Bounce up on your left leg, kicking your right leg straight out to the side. At the same time, stretch your left arm directly overhead. On the next bounce, alternate legs and arms.

PRECAUTIONS: Be careful when jumping with only one leg for support. Start slowly, and use your arms for balance.

AREAS STRENGTHENED: Calves, hips, shoulders, thighs.

MUSCLES STRENGTHENED: Gastrocnemius, soleus, gluteals, deltoids, quadriceps.

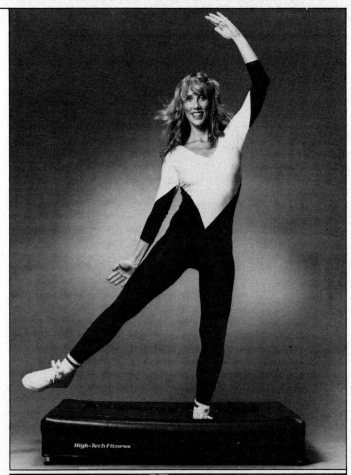

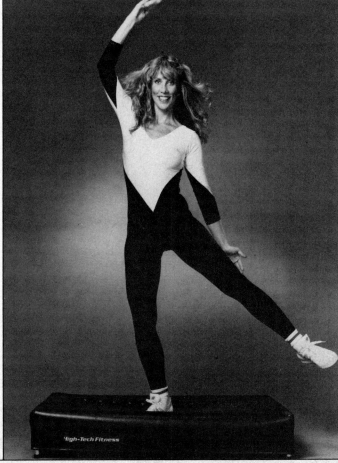

KNEE-CHEST JUMP

STARTING POSITION: Stand on the rebounder mat, feet together, both arms extended in front for balance, your hands made into fists.

MOTION: Pushing off on your toes, jump up in the air while bending both knees and pulling your heels toward your buttocks. Land first on your toes, then on the rest of your feet, remembering to let your knees bend slightly to absorb the shock and prepare for the next jump. Try to keep your torso straight and aligned from hips to head throughout this exercise.

PRECAUTIONS: Don't jump too high or too vigorously at first. Be careful to land in or near the center of the mat. Landing near an edge may propel you out at an angle and cause you to lose your balance. Land with your feet 6 to 12 inches apart.

AREAS STRENGTHENED: Calves, back of thighs, front of thighs, front of torso.

MUSCLES STRENGTHENED: Gastrocnemius, soleus, hamstrings, quadriceps, rectus abdominis.

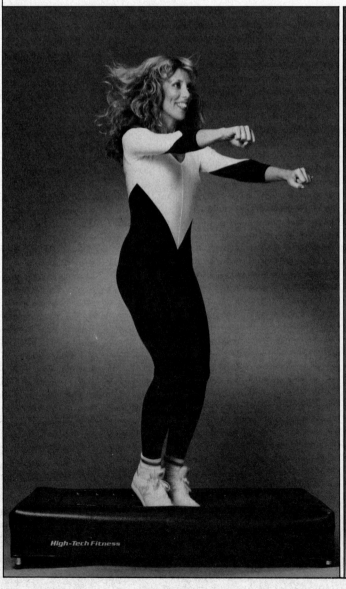
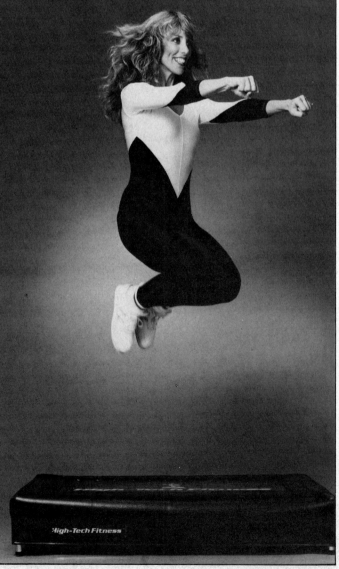

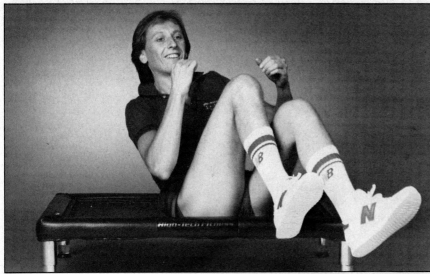

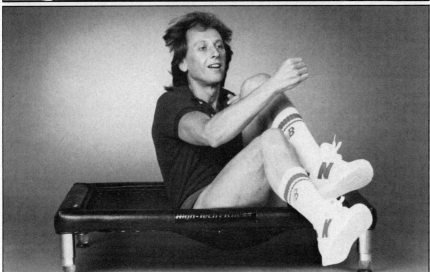

SEATED STOMACH BOUNCE

STARTING POSITION: Sit in the center of the rebounder mat. Place your feet firmly on the floor.

MOTION: Use your feet to start bouncing up and down on your buttocks. Establish a rhythm. Lift your feet off the floor and bring your left knee up toward your right elbow. Alternate knees and elbows as you bounce. Continue to maintain the small bouncing action on the buttocks.

PRECAUTIONS: Because this exercise requires your back muscles to work constantly, people with back problems may have to do the basic knee-and-elbow movements without the bounce for a while. This technique may also help if you're having trouble coordinating your movements.

AREAS STRENGTHENED: Front of thighs, front and sides of torso, entire back.

MUSCLES STRENGTHENED: Quadriceps, rectus abdominis, internal and external obliques, erector spinae.

JUMP-ROPE BOUNCE

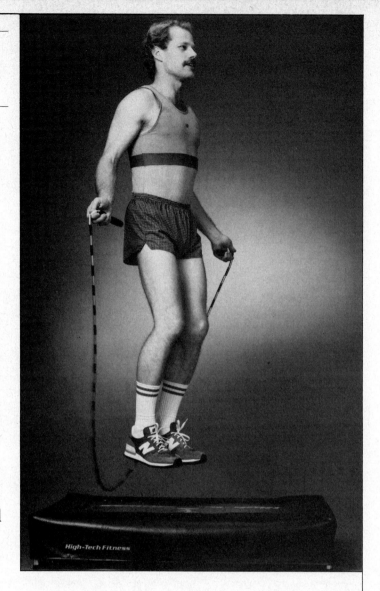

STARTING POSITION: Stand on the center of the rebounder mat with your feet slightly closer together than shoulder-width. Your hands should be at your sides, holding the jump-rope handles.

MOTION: Swing the rope either forward or backward and start jumping rope. Enjoy the additional lift given by the rebounder's resilience.

PRECAUTIONS: Notice that your timing must be somewhat different than when jumping rope on a stationary surface. Since you are bouncing on a resilient surface, you'll go farther up than you're used to. This means that you'll take longer to come down, and that you should turn the rope more slowly than you would when jumping on a stable surface. Keeping your arms fairly stationary and rotating the rope by mainly flicking your wrists will tend to give you a good jumping rhythm and keep the rope from catching the sides of the rebounder.

AREAS STRENGTHENED: Calves, front of thighs, forearms, entire circumference of shoulder joint.

MUSCLES STRENGTHENED: Gastrocnemius, soleus, quadriceps, flexor carpi radialis and ulnaris, deltoids.

SKI-POLE JUMP

The ski-pole jump can help you immeasurably on the slopes. It can improve your technique and add to your endurance for that last run of the day.

STARTING POSITION: Stand off to one side of the rebounder mat, with your feet and knees together. Your knees should be slightly bent. Place your ski poles securely in the inside corners of the rebounder (or if you are using a circular rebounder, place them as wide apart as comfortable.) Be sure to keep the poles stable. Hold the poles' handles in a firm grip.

MOTION: Jump from side to side, keeping your feet and knees together and your knees bent. To reproduce the action and muscular demands of skiing, keep your upper body (waist to head) straight and centered. Only your hips and legs should move from side to side, as you "squeeze" the knees together. Your ski poles should remain firmly in position at all times.

PRECAUTIONS: You should visualize skiing the fall line while you perform this exercise. The closer you can make your movements to actual skiing, the better.

AREAS STRENGTHENED: Calves, front of thighs, inner and outer thighs, sides and back of torso.

MUSCLES STRENGTHENED: Gastrocnemius, soleus, quadriceps, adductors, tensor fasciae latae, internal and external obliques, erector spinae.

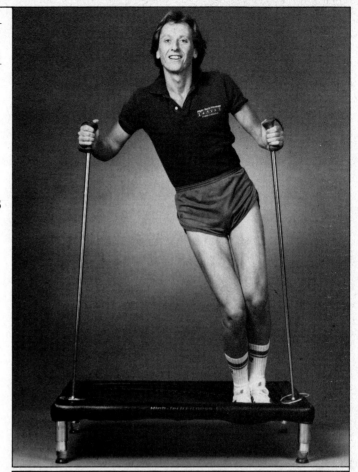

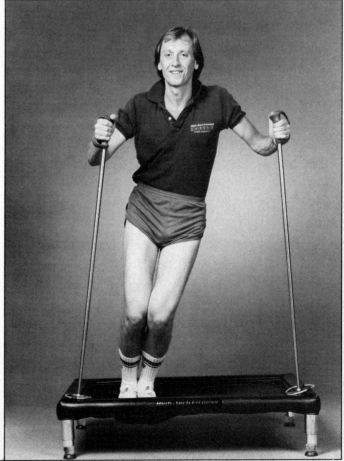

MONITORS AND MEASURING DEVICES

Monitoring is an indispensable part of personal fitness. It's the best way to find out where you're starting from, how hard you're working, and if you're working too hard.

A monitor is *any device that gives you numerical information about the state of your body,* whether the information is about weight, fat content, pulse, or blood pressure. One monitor you probably already have in your home is a bathroom scale. It tells you your weight in pounds or kilograms, and you can use it to chart your daily progress in losing or gaining weight. In this section, you'll find a variety of scales: digital, bathroom-type, and medical balance-beam. The main things to look for in a scale are accuracy and reliability. Once you've found a few that meet these criteria, pick one that fits your decor and budget.

Fat calipers are another measuring device. They measure the percentage of your total body weight that's made up of fat. All other things being equal, it's better to have a lower rather than a higher percentage of body fat. The "ideal" levels are thought to be between 9 and 18 percent for men and between 12 and 23 percent for women. Some physicians recommend hydrostatic weighing, a procedure in which you are lowered into a tub of water and your percentage of body fat is calculated from the amount of water you displace. This procedure can yield a high degree of accuracy, but it's complicated and time-consuming. Besides, who has a tub that large? The fat calipers listed in this section give you virtually the same readings, and at a fraction of the cost and inconvenience.

Approximately 50 percent of our body fat is subcutaneous (under the skin). We can measure our body fat by folding the skin between a pair of calipers, reading out the measurement, and looking up the percentage it corresponds to on a chart. The thicker the skinfold, the greater the amount of fat. The accuracy of such measurement is directly related to the quality of the calipers, and (more importantly) to how carefully you've followed the manufacturer's instructions.

Blood pressure monitors measure your diastolic and systolic blood pressure. Before we talk about them, we're going to digress a little (well, actually a lot) to talk about how your cardiovascular system works and what your blood pressure means.

You probably already know that your heart is a muscle, and that it supplies blood to the rest of your body by contracting, or squeezing. With each squeeze, it squirts blood out through your arteries. During these squeezes (beats), the pressure on your arterial walls rises to a maximum level. Between beats, the pressure falls to a minimum. This maximum pressure point is called the *systole,* and the minimum pressure point is called the *diastole.* When your blood pressure is measured, both pressure points are recorded.

Traditionally, we measure blood pressure with a sphygmomanometer. You've seen these devices in your doctor's office. The doctor wraps a rubber collar around your arm, and the pressure in your arteries forces a column of mercury up into a glass tube. The unit of measure for blood pressure is the millimeter, because what we're actually measuring is how many millimeters up the glass tube the mercury has risen.

We express blood pressure by writing the systolic pressure over the diastolic pressure. Thus, a "normal" blood pressure range would be expressed this way:

$$\frac{110\text{--}135 \text{ mm}}{60\text{--}99 \text{ mm}} \text{(systolic)} \text{(diastolic)}$$

Now that you know what blood pressure is, what does it mean? Your systolic blood pressure tells a medical professional how much energy your heart is expending with each squeeze. This in turn tells him or her something about the level of strain taking place in your arteries. Your diastolic pressure measures how much resistance to blood flow there is in your vascular system (veins and arteries). This can indicate how much tone your blood vessels have.

There are a number of neurological, chemical, and physical situations that can cause your blood pressure to rise or fall. Among them are excessive stress, changes in your blood's pH (level of acidity or alkalinity), adrenal gland activity, changes in certain blood gases, holding your breath, standing on your head, excitement, temperature, and muscular work. Generally, these changes are necessary and temporary adjustments by which the flow of your blood is regulated. For this reason, we recommend that you always monitor your blood pressure at the same time of day and in the same situation (before or after meals, exercise, etc.).

Virtually all the blood pressure monitors on the market also measure your pulse (heart rate), except for the familiar sphygmomanometer, which would be almost as inconvenient to wear while working out as it is to spell and pronounce. Thus we're led to a discussion of one of the most vital and necessary measuring devices around: the pulse monitor (heartbeat monitor).

Pulse monitors can keep you motivated while you exercise. They may just keep your mind off your aching muscles. And we can't overstress the importance of knowing your heart rate during exercise. It's the best single indication of how hard you're working. Aerobically exercising below your target heart rate is like owning a car with a high-compression engine and only driving it below 35 miles an hour. A pulse monitor will also tell you if you're pushing your heart beyond its proper limits, which could cause irreparable damage to the heart muscle. Other muscles can repair themselves, given sufficient rest, but the heart can rest only between beats.

Pulse monitors usually consist of two parts, a sensor (which detects your pulse) and a counter (which records it). They're battery-operated. It's important to remember that, as yet, there's no foolproof way to accurately record your pulse rate every time, except with a stethoscope. This means that any pulse monitor you buy will have certain drawbacks.

There are two types of devices that measure your heart rate: the pulse type and the EKG type. They're distinguished by the way they operate.

The pulse-type monitor has a sensor that's usually placed on your finger or ear lobe, where the capillaries (small blood vessels) are close to the surface of the skin. The sensor operates photo-optically; that is, it shoots a beam of light directly into your capillaries.

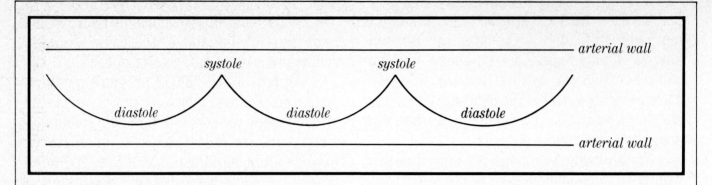

Your blood travels through your vascular system in a wave motion. Each heartbeat causes the wave to crest. With each relaxation of the heart, there's a wave trough. Think of the blood in your arteries as behaving as it does in the diagram above.

When the beam of light from a pulse-type monitor penetrates a capillary, it bounces off the wave crests of blood caused by each beat of your heart. The reflected light then bounces back into the monitor's sensor, where it strikes a photoelectric cell. The monitor's counter records the number of times the light strikes the cell and displays this number—which is, of course, your pulse rate.

The pulse-type monitor is a clever piece of technology, but there are three problems with it. The first is that, since it works by reflected light, it's sensitive to changes in outside light as well. Any change in the ambient light level while you're exercising can affect the accuracy of your pulse reading.

The second problem is that, when your heart is pumping really fast (for example, when you're exercising good and hard), a pulse-type meter can no longer distinguish one wave crest from another. It "sees" the flow of your blood as a steady stream. For this reason, pulse-type monitors are accurate only up to a pulse rate of 160 or 170 beats per minute.

Finally, some sudden movements of the body part (finger or ear lobe) where you're wearing the sensor can give you an erroneous display.

If you're having trouble getting a reading, sometimes it helps to rub the tip of your finger or ear lobe to get your capillary action going.

The other kind of pulse monitor is the EKG type. You wear the EKG's sensor on your chest. It operates by picking up and recording electrical impulses in your body.

Before every heartbeat, your brain sends a strong electrical signal through your nervous system to your heart. This electrical impulse "tells" your heart when to beat (contract). Without such signals, you'd have no heartbeat at all. (Fortunately, this is not a process we have to think about consciously. The brain sends out these electrical pulses automatically.)

Each of these small electric shocks emanating from the brain causes one heartbeat, and it is these impulses that are received, recorded, and displayed by the EKG monitor. Because the EKG doesn't have to "read" your blood's motion, it's usually accurate up to about 200 beats per minute.

The problem is that these heartbeat-causing pulses aren't the only electrical discharges going on in your body. Your brain is sending out other small electric shocks at the same time. After you've eaten lunch, for example, it sends out impulses to your digestive muscles, causing them to contract so that peristaltic (digestive) motion can take place. An EKG-type monitor can also pick up these "artifacts" (conflicting electrical impulses), and they can affect the accuracy of your pulse reading.

An EKG monitor picks up the brain's electrical signals through your skin. The sensor shouldn't move around on your chest. If it does, your pulse reading is more likely to be contaminated by artifacts. The sensor's harness, then, should be tight enough to hold the sensor in place—but not so tight, of course, that it impedes your breathing. People with dry, flaky, or thick skin may also have trouble getting an accurate reading from an EKG-type monitor.

Both types of monitors work by averaging your heartbeat over a 2- to 5-second interval. If your heart flutters, some monitors will automatically reset themselves to zero. People with irregular heartbeats thus won't register at all on these monitors. It's best to test before buying. Having your pulse monitor register zero can be a pretty unnerving experience. Of course, you should consult a physician if a wide range of monitors have trouble picking up your heart rate, or if you're alarmed by the readings you get.

Any monitor will be rendered less accurate by a sudden shock or jar. As a rule, chest-mounted monitors are less susceptible to jarring than ear- or finger-mounted ones. If you're jumping on a rebounder, doing calisthenics, or using a rowing machine, it's wiser to buy a chest-mounted (EKG) unit.

Ear- or finger-mounted monitors, on the other hand, are more comfortable and more convenient to use. If you're riding a stationary bike, you might want to consider a pulse-type monitor.

Monitors come with bicycle mounts, belt mounts, treadmill mounts, and cords from 12 to 72 inches in length. You can determine which one is right for you by taking into account your equipment and the kind of exercises you do, and by testing the monitor before you buy it. In any case, you'll want one that's accurate, reliable, and comfortable. Unfortunately, the ones you order by mail for $39.95 usually fail on the first two counts.

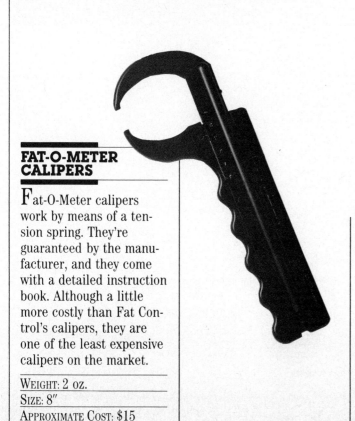

FAT-O-METER CALIPERS

Fat-O-Meter calipers work by means of a tension spring. They're guaranteed by the manufacturer, and they come with a detailed instruction book. Although a little more costly than Fat Control's calipers, they are one of the least expensive calipers on the market.

WEIGHT: 2 OZ.
SIZE: 8″
APPROXIMATE COST: $15

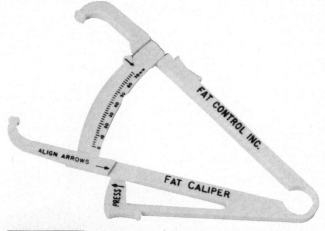

FAT CONTROL, INC., CALIPERS

Dr. Jack Osman, a professor of health sciences at Baltimore's Towson State College, designed these plastic calipers. They come with an instruction manual which is easy to read, and you can look up your fat percentage on a chart, without having to resort to higher mathematics. Fat Control's calipers are the cheapest on the market, and they do roughly the same job as those costing from $100 to $500.

WEIGHT: 2 OZ.
SIZE: 8″
APPROXIMATE COST: $8.95

DATATRIM™ SCALE

The Datatrim gives you a little *more* than everything you wanted from a scale. The vertical scale's LCD shows your weight (up to 300 pounds in ½-pound increments), the date, your weight goal, and the estimated number of days it will take to reach that goal. And that's just the beginning. When you step on the Datatrim, a female voice will greet you with, "Good day, M-1." This may seem a little impersonal, but the Datatrim's memory can keep track of two dieters at a time, and for convenience sake, they're known to the machine as "M-1" and "M-2." A stranger will be asked, "Who are you?" (Datatrim's manufacturer doesn't tell us what the scale does when the stranger answers.) As the LCD flashes the good or bad news, the Datatrim responds with "Fantastic!" or "Congratulations!"—or "Uh-oh!" or "Bad news!" This sort of feedback can be very effective for dieters.

WEIGHT: 10 lbs.
SIZE: 12″ × 11″ × 32″h
BATTERIES: 4 "ERD"
APPROXIMATE COST: $120;
AC adaptor,
$10 extra

POLDER 760 SCALE

This bathroom-type scale is manufactured by Seca, West Germany's leading manufacturer of precision scales. (Polder's the importer.) It has a full-vision dual (pounds/kilograms) dial, steel housing, white baked enamel finish, and textured mat. The 760 measures up to 330 pounds in 1-pound increments.

WEIGHT: 11 lbs.
SIZE: 14″ × 20″ × 5″h
APPROXIMATE COST: $139

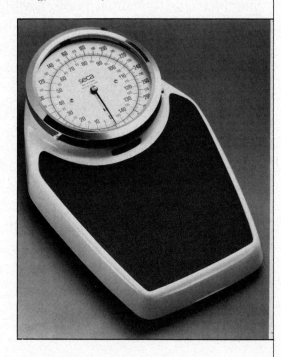

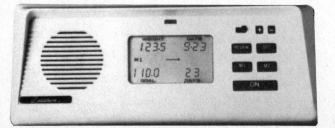

NORELCO® HS10 DELUXE ELECTRONIC DIGITAL SCALE

This one is a rectangular bathroom scale with a rubber footpad, like many others. Its special feature is a detachable LED display with red readout, which you can hang on the wall for easy reading. There's also an instant-on feature (no switches to turn), an automatic lock-in of your reading, a zero weight adjustment, a kilogram conversion switch, and a light that indicates when the batteries are low. Available in white with black platform only.

WEIGHT: 6.5 lbs.
SIZE: 12″ × 14″ × 3″h
BATTERIES: one 9-volt
APPROXIMATE COST: $65

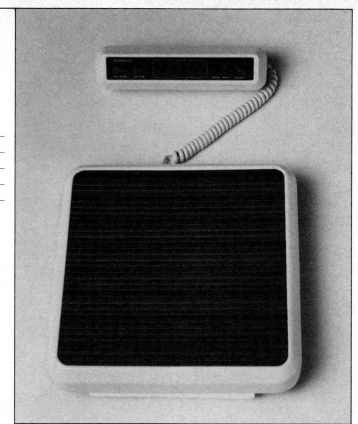

DETECTO MODEL 439 PHYSICIAN SCALE

This mechanical balance-beam device has no electronic gadgetry whatsoever. It is the most accurate type of scale on the market. As the name implies, this is the sort of scale you'll find in your doctor's office.

The 439 measures up to 350 pounds in 4-ounce increments and comes with the familiar height-measuring rod, which extends to 78″. The manufacturer lists the colors as white, cream, walnut spray *(walnut spray?)*, daffodil yellow, jade green, Biscayne blue, gray, and black.

WEIGHT: 40 lbs.
SIZE: 10½″ × 14½″ × 59″h
APPROXIMATE COST: $260

POLDER 755 SCALE

This is essentially an upright professional version of the Polder 760, with the dual dial closer to eye level for easier reading. The platform is cast iron, with a textured mat and white enamel finish. The 755 measures up to 330 pounds in 1-pound increments.

WEIGHT: 34.3 lbs.
SIZE: 11½″ × 18½″ × 36½″h
APPROXIMATE COST: $500

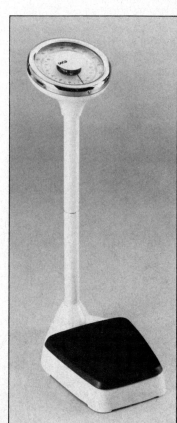

CALTRAC PERSONAL ACTIVITY COMPUTER

It's relatively easy to measure how many calories you're taking in each day. Caltrac measures how many calories you're *burning.* You can enter your weight into the unit, and carry it on your belt or in your pocket. A crystal responds to motion the way a cartridge does to grooves in a record. Your movements are converted into electrical impulses that are displayed on the LCD as numbers of calories burned.

Caltrac works only on movements that include vertical motion, such as walking, jogging, using a rebounder, or playing tennis. "It's not 100 percent accurate," admits the University of Wisconsin's Henry Montoye, one of the device's inventors. "But it's better than anything else on the market." And in fact, we know

of nothing else on the market that gives you an approximate count of the calories you use in daily life.

WEIGHT: 3 oz.
SIZE: 2" × 3" × ½"
BATTERIES: 2 lithium coin-type
APPROXIMATE COST: $80

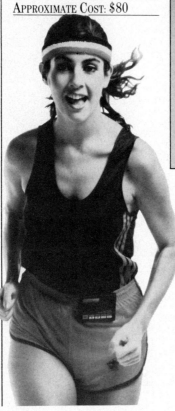

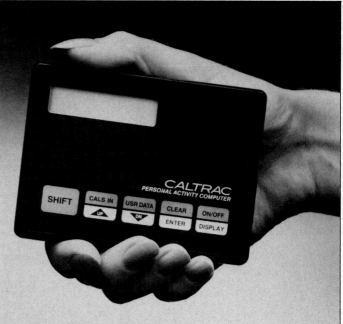

AMEREC 110 PULSEMETER

The 110 is a fairly no-frills pulse monitor. It's similar in design and operation to Amerec's more expensive 130, except that it shows you *either* your pulse or the elapsed time, instead of both simultaneously. If you put the 110 on automatic alternating mode, it will show you approximately five seconds of your pulse, then five

seconds of elapsed time, then your pulse again, etc. You wear the sensor on your ear lobe or finger. This monitor is best suited for stationary bikes.

WEIGHT: 13 oz.
SIZE: 3" × 5½" × 1½"
BATTERIES: 4 AA cells
APPROXIMATE COST: $120

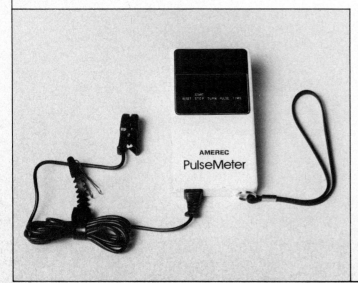

AMEREC 130 PULSEMETER

The Amerec 130 gives you a simultaneous reading of your pulse and the elapsed time (either hour/minute or minute/second). It's accurate to ± one beat per minute. There's a mounting bracket that attaches to most stationary aerobics equipment. The 130's sensor attaches to your ear lobe or finger.

WEIGHT: 5 oz.
SIZE: 2½" × 4½" × 1"
BATTERIES: 4 AAA cells
APPROXIMATE COST: $140

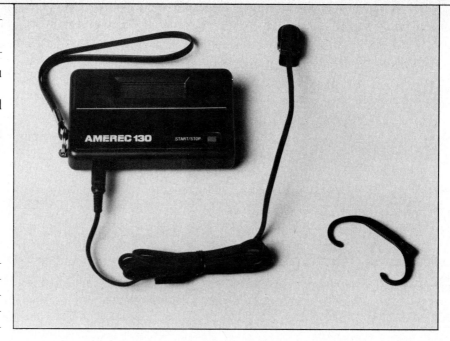

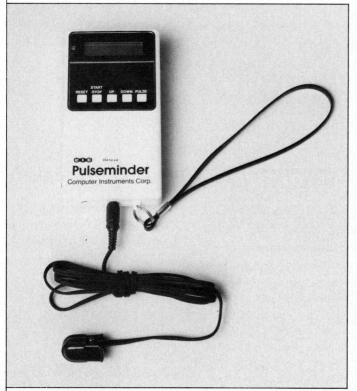

CIC DELUXE PULSEMINDER MODEL 8329

The 8329 features an LED digital pulse display; a programmable high-low heart rate target zone, with an alarm to let you know when you're overworking; colored lights to indicate when you're below, within, or above your target zone; and a digital display that shows elapsed time. You wear the sensor on your ear lobe or finger.

The 8329 is compact, lightweight, and can easily be attached to a stationary bike or other exercise unit with brackets, which are part of the monitor. We don't recommend it for outdoor exercise, but like it for such stationary aerobic devices as bikes.

WEIGHT: 10 oz.
SIZE: 2⅞" × 5³⁄₁₆" × 1⁵⁄₁₆"
BATTERIES: 4 AA cells
APPROXIMATE COST: $160

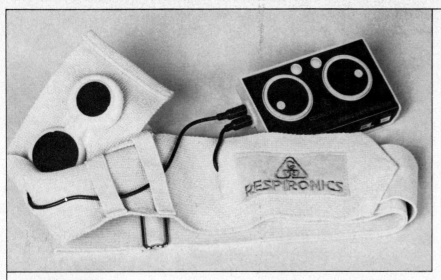

EXERSENTRY™ HEART RATE MONITOR

The Exersentry is a chest-mounted digital unit that will give you continuous feedback on your heart rate. You can set it to your upper and lower target heart rates. It will beep in a low pitch if you're working under your target rate, and in a high pitch if you're over it. If you're working within your target rate, it remains silent.

The Exersentry has an optional wrist attachment (not shown) and bike mount (not shown). There is no time function. No larger than a deck of playing cards, the unit is worn under your clothes and is attached by an elastic chest strap, which some may find slightly uncomfortable. This is a simple, accurate, no-nonsense unit good for virtually all aerobic activity except swimming.

WEIGHT: 3 oz.
SIZE: $4'' \times 2\frac{1}{2}'' \times 1''$
BATTERIES: 1 AAA cell
APPROXIMATE COST: $170

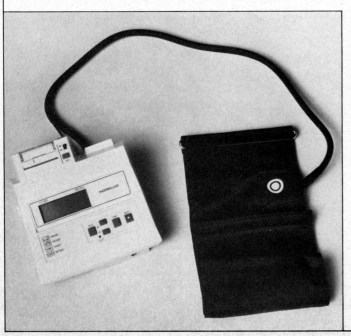

NORELCO® MODEL HC3500 DELUXE DIGITAL BLOOD PRESSURE/PULSE METER

The electric-razor people make this electronic blood pressure monitor which, for simplicity sake, we'll call the HC3500. It gives you a digital readout of your pulse, diastolic and systolic blood pressure, and the time. A printer provides a written record of the readout, including date and time. The cuff inflates at the push of a button, the unit tells you with displays and sounds when it's ready for measuring, and four separate error messages tell you when something's wrong.

WEIGHT: 3 lbs.
SIZE: $6'' \times 6''$; cuff $20'' \times 6''$
BATTERIES: 4 C-cell
APPROXIMATE COST: $195

AMEREC 150 SPORT TESTER™

The Amerec 150 is a heart-rate computer that comes in two parts: a sensor/transmitter, worn over your heart, and a display/receiver, worn strapped to your wrist. The sensor picks up your heart's electrical impulses and transmits them (no wires) to the wrist display unit. This unit displays your heart rate every 5 seconds, memorizes your pulse every 30 seconds, and stores the memory up to 128 times during each workout. Later, you can play back the memory and chart your workout. You can preset the display screen at a maximum and minimum heart rate. If you go beyond your set limits, the computer will flash an alarm.

WEIGHT: sensor, 1.2 oz.; display, 1 oz.

SIZE: chest band, 1″ wide; display unit, size of wrist-watch

BATTERIES: 1 mgh lithium battery

APPROXIMATE COST: $250

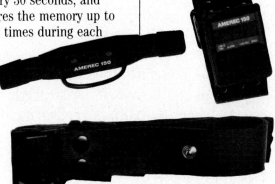

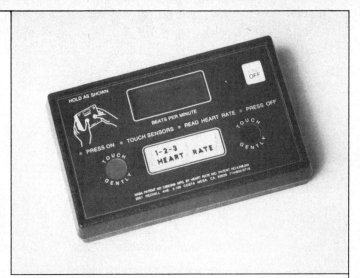

HEART RATE 1-2-3

This small, lightweight pulse meter uses space age technology to give you an accurate (± 2 beats per minute) pulse reading with no wires, straps, or clips. The secret is a pair of electrocardiographic sensors developed for NASA by Texas Tech University. Place your thumbs on the sensor discs, and you get a pulse readout which is cleaner and more interference-free than most. The Heart Rate displays your pulse rate only after it recognizes four consecutive rhythmic beats. It continually monitors and updates the beat per minute average. When your pulse data is erratic, it's rejected, resulting in no display.

WEIGHT: 8 oz.

SIZE: 5⅝″ × 3½″ × 1¼″

BATTERIES: one 9-volt

APPROXIMATE COST: $299

THE COACH

Biotechnology's personal fitness computer performs multiple functions. You enter your sex, age, weight, and target heart rate. As you work out, the Coach tells you your pulse rate, heartbeat, calories burned, fitness quotient, number of strides, miles per hour, and elapsed time. The Coach signals when you've reached your minimum target heart rate, and it beeps for each beat. If your heart rate exceeds your maximum, it warns you with a constant signal to slow down. Although this chest-mounted monitor is a bit tricky to program at first, once you have it set, it will give you more feedback than any of the other pulse monitors available.

WEIGHT: 3 oz.

SIZE: 2½″ × 4½″ × 1″

APPROXIMATE COST: $250

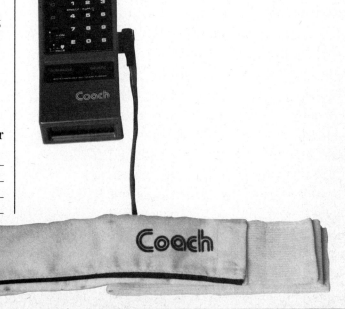

STRENGTH TRAINING EQUIPMENT

Resistance training is still the fastest, most efficient way to develop strength in any single muscle group—or collectively in all muscle groups, depending on how many exercises you want to do. You can isolate muscles that cover areas as large as your entire back, or as small as the fine manipulating muscles of the hand. People have been working out with weights for many years and the result has been a wide and sophisticated array of resistance equipment to assist the exerciser. The sheer number and variety of strength training devices on the market may seem bewildering. Therefore, it is often difficult these days to know what is best, practical, or necessary.

There are machines that supply resistance via gravity by using weights, bars, plates, and pulleys. And there are those that supply resistance by the means of pneumatic or hydraulic cylinders. In recent years, cams have been added to weight equipment that constantly vary the amount of force being applied to the contracting muscle, so that the muscle has to work harder during the entire range of limb movement. Basically, you'll get more resistance at the angle where your muscles are stronger and less resistance at the angle where your muscles are weaker. In the final analysis, though, unless you're training to be a competitive athlete, the results of resistance exercises are the same whether you're pumping iron, water, or compressed air. All can increase your strength, endurance and joint stability, and also improve your overall physical dimensions.

Strength training devices fall into three basic categories:
- *Free weights* is a shorthand term for dumbbells and barbells, which allow you (along with specific types of benches) to work most major muscle groups.
- *Single-station units,* such as those on the Nautilus system, work one major muscle group per machine.
- *Multi-station units* allow you to work more than one muscle group on the same device, like the "Universal-type" and other weight stack machines.

When shopping for single- or multi-station units, the most critical consideration is that the device should be sturdy enough to support the weight it will have to carry. The frame of any kind of resistance unit must be strong enough to bear its load as well as the weight of the person using it. That means that solid construction is all-important. Welded construction is better than bolts, and examine all the welds to make sure they are smooth and clean. Cables, pulleys, and all other parts of the lifting mechanism should be strong and operate smoothly. You'll almost invariably find the cheaper units jerky and wobbly. This can get terribly annoying. Inquire whether the equipment comes with an owner's manual for repair or whether the company has an authorized service agent to help you if there are mechanical problems. Benches should be well padded. Be sure that multi-station units are relatively easy to adjust for doing different exercises for different muscle groups. Some have to be practically knocked down and rebuilt, or you have to redecorate your room each time you wish to change exercises!

Free weights should have knurled grips that rotate freely on the bar. The chrome grips should be of sufficiently high quality so as not to chip. The paint on barbell and dumbbell plates shouldn't come off on the floor. All restraint collars that hold the plates on the bars should be easy to use and effective in securing the weight.

When buying adjustable dumbbell plate sets, make sure you get identical-pound plates in multiples of four. That way both dumbbells can weigh the same. Be careful if you buy sand-filled, plastic-coated plates. If they should fall and crack, you'll probably get sand all over the floor.

Benches for free weights should be sturdily welded (as opposed to using many bolts), and the seats should have enough padding for comfort. The Naugahyde should be of an "expanded" type and quality so it does not stretch or tear easily. The base of the bench should be wide and stable enough so it doesn't wobble on the floor. Also, you'll find on cheaper weight benches that the standards (the two U-shaped holders that support the barbell) are generally a bit narrow. This can make either lifting off or replacing the barbell an awkward experience.

We also recommend such free weight accessories as weight gloves, foam-padded grips, and leather (or similar strength) weight belts. They allow you to reap maximum versatility from your equipment with maximum safety.

Be prepared for the fact that weight "feels" different on different machines, with different proportioned free weights, and with different types of resistance. In general, machines feel easier than free weights, and non-cammed machines feel easier than cammed machines. Dumbbells that are stubby in appearance feel easier to lift than those that are elongated. The reasons for this are a bit complicated, but relate mostly to leverage, the angle at which the resistance force is being applied to the working muscle, and the fact that the muscles are having to control the weight in more space dimensions. Also the types of material used in pulleys, cables, and on weight guides can make an apparent difference in the feel of the weight. The important thing is that you are comfortable with how the equipment feels and that you use the same equipment to judge your progress in strength.

It's important for you to understand some basic concepts about the available machines as well as how your body responds to them. The more serious your training goals, the more you need to know about both. For most recreational exercisers, however, it is enough to grasp that using light weights and high repetitions (anything over 15) tones and shapes the muscles and gives them some degree of muscular endurance. On the other hand, using heavy weights and low repetitions (anything under 8) increases the size (and contours) of your muscles and, in general, creates strength and muscle mass. Women, by the way, don't have to worry about building unattractive amounts of muscle mass since this is determined by the amounts of testosterone (male hormone) in the body. Except in rare cases, women have *little* testosterone and *extra* subcutaneous fat, which makes it pretty difficult to develop biceps like coaxial cables. The commitment for a female to become a bodybuilder requires excessive time (and painful work) to overcome these predispositions.

In spite of much advertising to the contrary, any kind of resistance training will make you stronger and shapelier. All of the various forms and sources of resistance (such as free weight, compressed air or fluids, or cammed weight) do not obviously or significantly affect the strengthening results of strength training exercises. They may, however, make some subtle, sophisticated differences that would show up in a performing, competitive athlete. For example, variable resistance machines (those that use cams and/or cylinders of gas or liquid) have been shown to increase what exercise physiologists call "dynamic strength." This type of strength relates to placing maximum force against an object (bat/ball, club/ball, etc.) throughout every position (degree) of movement (muscle contraction). Although this sounds fancy and all-important it is still only one small aspect in the performance of an athlete. He or she could have all the dynamic strength in the world, but without proper skill, coordination, and summation of forces in movement the dynamic strength would be useless.

It is important to note that using different types of apparatus may be more pleasurable and simpler than using others. Free weights require changing weights, bars, and plates by unscrewing collars and reassembling them. They can be assembled in the form of barbells and dumbbells if you have an assortment of different length and type bars. Free weights also require you to know a little more about what routines work what muscles groups, so that you can position yourself on the bench properly. Free weights also may require a partner as a spotter. Your muscles have to control the free weights in three-dimensional space, which not only requires more from them in terms of work (as in real life movements like lifting a bag of groceries) but also increases instability and the possibility of accidents.

A word about spotters. A spotter is an exercise partner who's responsible for your safety when you lift weights. A spotter helps you lift the weight, helps you balance it, and corrects poor form. You'll see lifters spotting each other in the gym as they work out. When we discuss trampolines, you'll read about spotters again.

Multi- and single-station machines take a lot of the decision-making away from you. A machine designed to work the chest, arms, and shoulders does just that. In addition, the weights tend to be in the form of small, square plates that slide up and down guide rods. Changing the amount of weight you are exercising with is as simple as placing a pin in a hole—no plates to change, move, or assemble. The guide rods decrease the amount of control (and work) your muscles have to do to balance and coordinate the weight you are lifting. From the standpoint of the serious bodybuilder or athlete, this is a drawback because the ability to isolate all the individual muscles (to increase definition) becomes considerably lessened. Keep in mind, though, that the average person, exercising to improve tone, balance the body musculature, minimize injury, and perhaps enhance performance in recreational sports does not have to be concerned with such detail.

There are several principles of exercise training that anyone planning to begin a strength training program should review. In fact, these principles apply to every form of exercise—strength training, aerobic training, speed training, flexibility training, etc. We will introduce you to them here because they are all very obvious to learn and apply within the context of strength training.

• THE OVERLOAD PRINCIPLE. Muscular changes occur only when stress is applied to them beyond a certain threshold—but within the limits of tolerance and safety. In strength training this overload usually takes the form of adding resistance (pounds) to an exercise. In aerobics this would take the form of increasing the pulse rate (workload of the heart). For flexibility the threshold stress is provided by moving a body part just slightly past the point of comfort.

• THE FREQUENCY PRINCIPLE. Workouts should be spaced reasonably so that there is recovery time for tissue growth, nutritional replenishment, biochemical resynthesis, and physiological development. For strength development, clinical evidence has shown that alternate days will bring excellent returns. This means the same muscle group should not be worked out on consecutive days. For aerobic and flexibility training five exercise sessions each week are desirable, and daily workouts can be done if reasonably planned. Do not overdose. Easy/hard workouts must be alternated.

• THE SPECIFICITY PRINCIPLE. Training is highly detailed and specific to a certain kind of activity. No two performances require exactly the same mix of performance factors. Strength can be specific to a given muscle group, performing in a certain range of motion, at a given speed and with a specific type of resistance. This means that the best way to train for a given sport or activity is to mimic the movements of the activity as closely and reasonably as possible, but with added resistance. Thus, you see baseball players swinging two bats, or weighted ones, or you see runners running while wearing or carrying weights on the ankles, wrists, waist, or hands.

• THE VOLUNTARY STIMULATION PRINCIPLE. The best training results come from voluntary neural stimulation, which is a fancy way of saying you should initiate and perform all training movements yourself. Passive exercise, manipulation, and electrical stimulation do not produce results as satisfactory as doing it yourself. In therapy however, these modalities are often used to initially improve the muscles, since the individual may not be able to initiate any movement on his own.

• THE PROGRESSION PRINCIPLE. The threshold mentioned above (under the overload principle) changes as your condition improves. This means if you wish to continue improving you must persistently but gradually increase your workloads.

• THE OVERTRAINING PRINCIPLE. This is a state of overfatigue and body depletion that results from ignoring the previously mentioned principles, as well as not paying attention to your body's feedback. Following the principles only gives us a basic format, which cannot possibly be personalized to fit the dynamic physiology and psychology of every living human being. Overtraining may be more damaging to the body than undertraining.

• THE MOTIVATION PRINCIPLE. The ability to accept fatigue, soreness, discomfort, and monotony of repetitive movements is necessary to be successful in a training program. Although there are ways to add creativity, convenience, rhythm, and diversion to a training schedule, there is no way to make training totally fun. In today's world, this is important to digest. The media seems to be hooked on promoting how much fun exercise is. This approach certainly sells products but frequently produces unrealistic expectations—which causes "dropouts," who then are vulnerable to the next sales pitch, hoping that the new product will be the magical answer to fun in training. Think about it!

• THE RANGE OF MOTION PRINCIPLE—Strength exercises should ideally begin from a position in which a muscle is completely stretched and end at a position where the muscle is fully shortened (contracted). This elicits strength and flexibility through a total range of joint motion and minimizes injury while maximizing performance.

• THE REST PAUSE PRINCIPLE. Heavy exercise can be made more productive if it is broken up with several short rest pauses. A *maximum* of about 3 minutes seems to be best in most situations. During this rest time it has been indicated that moving or massaging a muscle will increase its speed of recovery. Proper body position may also positively enhance overall circulation and expel waste products from the muscles more rapidly.

• THE WARM-UP AND COOL-DOWN PRINCIPLE. Most clinical evidence has shown that a slow warm-up that moves all the body's joints prepares the muscles, tendons, ligaments, joints, and neurological system for the coming movement. This decreases the shock to the body and tends to decrease the chance of injuries. After vigorous exercise, a cool-down period helps to return all those reved-up body processes back toward their normal resting states. This is more critical in aerobic exercise, because blood distribution in the body is usually skewed to the lower body. (This is termed "blood pooling.") Without a walking-type of cool-down, blood may pool in the lower half of the body and dangerously deprive the heart and brain of oxygen-rich blood.

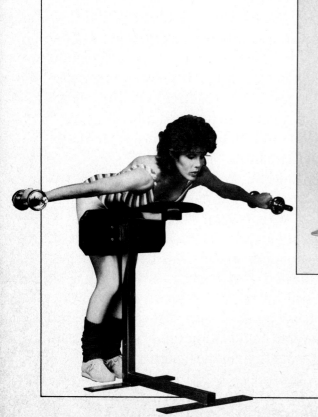

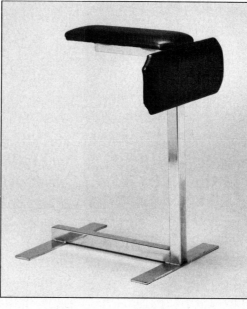

QUALITY SPIDER BENCH

The Quality Spider Bench is a device to support your back, abdominals, and arms during weight lifting, allowing you to use heavier weights. You use it by bending over it and either facing the end pad, or bending sideways and using the end pad for elbow support. The Quality Spider helps you do full extension barbell and dumbbell curls, barbell and dumbbell rowing, flys, and other upper back exercises. This bench comes in chrome or black gloss finish, with black Naugahyde upholstery.

WEIGHT: 20 lbs.
SIZE: 32″ × 20″ × 32″ h
APPROXIMATE COST: $100

QUALITY ADJUSTABLE INCLINE BENCH

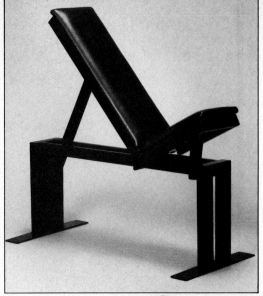

This heavy-duty (all welds, no bolts) bench has heavier padding than most. The serious lifter will be able to work out in any of four incline positions, plus supine. Comes in chrome or black, with black upholstery.

WEIGHT: 30 lbs.
SIZE: 1½′ × 3′ × 1½′ h
APPROXIMATE COST: $160

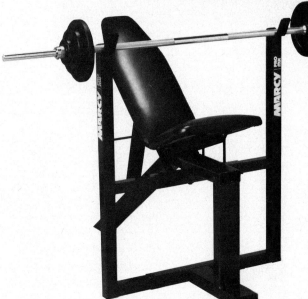

575 MARCY® PRO-MX BENCH

On most weight benches, the weight is behind the user. The Marcy 575 puts it in front. Some people will find this a convenient feature. This unit has adjustable supports for incline and decline presses and sit-ups. Its welded crutch supports adjust to three widths to accommodate standard or Olympic barbells. There's a leg flexion/extension, and an abdominal board position for straight-leg or bent-knee sit-ups. The Pro-MX Bench is made of 2″ × 4″ rectangular and 2″ × 2″ heavy-gauge steel tubing, with powder coat finish, welded support, and heavy padding covered with vinyl. An arm curl accessory is available as an option (shown with optional barbell).

WEIGHT: 76 lbs.
SIZE: 65″ × 34″ × 46″ h
APPROXIMATE COST: $198

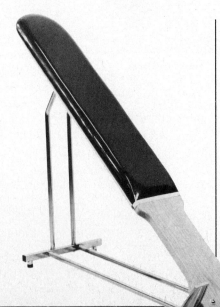

CAL GYM B-11 2 INSTITUTIONAL INCLINE BENCH

This traditionally styled standing incline bench is tough enough to stand up to virtually any weight training program. As the name suggests, it was designed for use in gyms and health clubs, but is suitable for home use. The bench itself is made from kiln-dried douglas fir, the padded Naugahyde is tan. The footplate assembly is solid cast; brace tubes are chrome-plated steel.

WEIGHT: 90 lbs.
SPACE: 64″ × 14″ × 48″ h
APPROXIMATE COST: $239

EXCEL BRUTUS® BENCH

This unit has a three-position incline with self-locking pins. Attachments include a squat rack, an optional leg extension unit, and an adjustable arm curl device. The Brutus Bench is made from 2″ heavy steel tubing and finished in black-textured powder paint that's impervious to ordinary use and weather. Its versatility and lifetime guarantee on everything but the vinyl and foam padding make it a good buy.

WEIGHT: unit, 61 lbs.; leg extension, 25 lbs.
SIZE: 48″ × 24¾″ × 5′ h
APPROXIMATE COST: unit, $280; leg extension, $59.95

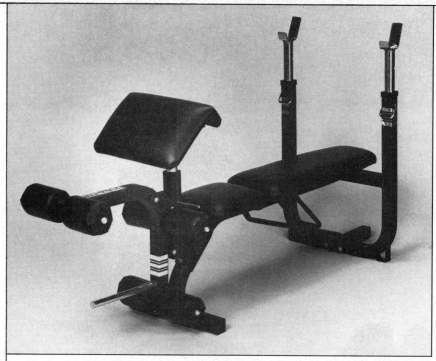

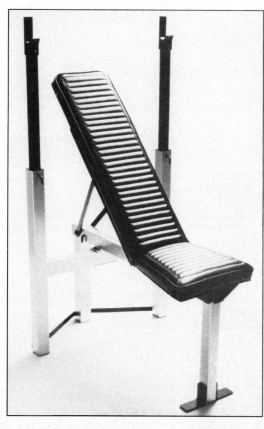

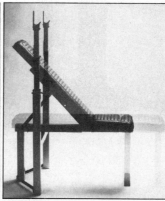

AMF® LIFE STYLER 700 MODULAR BENCH

AMF's heavy-duty weight bench is the only one whose frame telescopes when raised to an incline (up to 45°). Thus, the uprights are always correctly positioned in relation to your shoulders. It features custom-fit nylon guides between the bench and the vertical supports to prevent wobbling. The seat is flared for extra support during inclined lifting, and there's a molded bar-catch to make removing and replacing the weights safer and easier.

The Life Styler 700's uprights adjust in two-inch increments from 39″ to 61″. The unit's stress points are welded for strength, and its two-inch polyethylene padding won't lose shape.

WEIGHT: 68 lbs.
SIZE: 28″ × 36½″ × 49″ h
APPROXIMATE COST: bench, $290; leg extension, $90 (option not shown)

DUMBBELL PULL-OVER

STARTING POSITION: Lie supine on a bench, with knees bent and feet dangling. Hold dumbbells in each hand, at full arm extension above the chest.

MOTION: Keeping arms extended, slowly lower the weights behind your head until your arms are parallel to the ground. Return the weights to the starting position by bringing your arms forward. Keep your elbows locked during the entire motion.

PRECAUTIONS: Due to the leverage involved, use relatively light weights, and raise and lower them slowly. Inhale as you lower the weights, exhale as you raise them. If you have problems with your back arching, place your feet, with knees bent, on the end of the bench.

AREAS STRENGTHENED: Back, shoulders, back of upper arms.

MUSCLES STRENGTHENED: Latissimus dorsi, anterior deltoids, triceps.

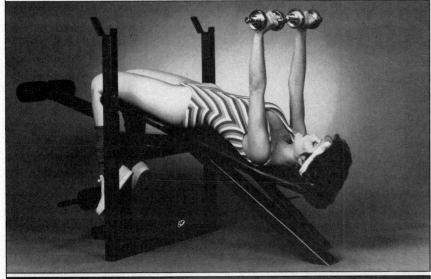

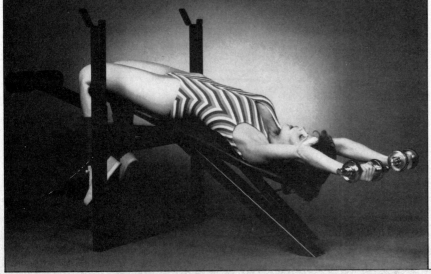

DUMBBELL BENCH PRESS

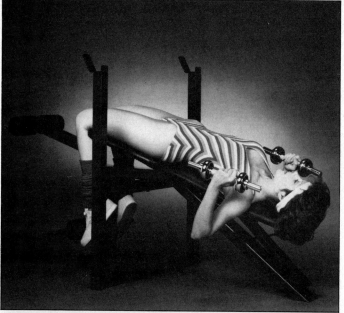

STARTING POSITION: Lie supine on a bench, with knees bent and feet dangling. Hold dumbbells in each hand, a little wider than shoulder-width apart. Hold elbows perpendicular to the body and low enough to comfortably stretch chest muscles.

MOTION: Press both dumbbells upward simultaneously to full arm extension. At that point, the two dumbbells should make slight contact. Then slowly lower the weights to starting position.

PRECAUTIONS: Keep head, shoulders and buttocks in contact with the bench at all times. *Don't arch your back.* If you have problems with your back arching, place your feet, with knees bent, on the end of the bench. Lower the weights slowly. Don't bounce them at the bottom position, in order to prevent overstretching your chest muscles. Inhale as you lower the weights, exhale as you raise them.

AREAS STRENGTHENED: Front of shoulders, chest, back of upper arms.

MUSCLES STRENGTHENED: Anterior deltoids, pectoralis majors, triceps.

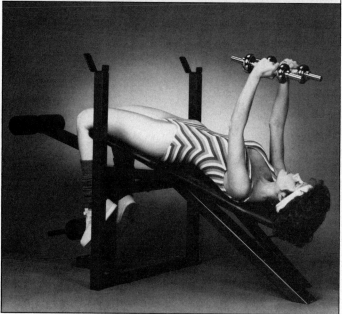

BARBELL BENCH PRESS

STARTING POSITION: Lie on a flat bench with your head, shoulders, and buttocks in contact with the bench, knees bent and feet flat on floor. With a grip slightly wider than shoulder width, remove the barbell from the standards and hold it with arms fully extended.

MOTION: Slowly lower the weight until it touches your chest at a point in line with the nipples. Hold the weight motionless for a moment, then press it upward to full arm extension.

PRECAUTIONS: *Always use a spotter for this exercise.* Keep feet flat on floor. Don't raise the buttocks off the bench by arching your back. If you have problems with your back arching, place your feet, with knees bent, on the end of the bench. Don't bounce the weight off your chest—this could cause bruising and injury. Inhale as you lower the weight, exhale as you raise it.

AREAS STRENGTHENED: Front of shoulders, chest, back of upper arms.

MUSCLES STRENGTHENED: Anterior deltoids, pectoralis majors, triceps.

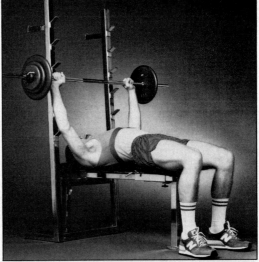

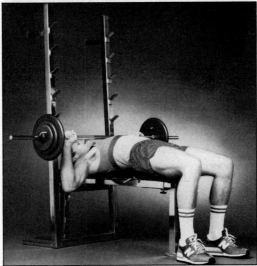

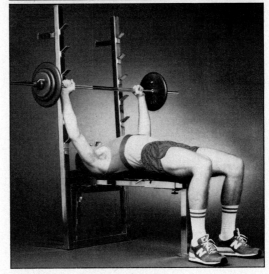

INCLINED DUMBBELL PRESSES

STARTING POSITION: Recline on the inclined bench with head, shoulders, and buttocks touching the bench. Grasp the dumbbells and hold them close to your shoulders. Your elbows should be held about 45° away from your trunk.

MOTION: Press the dumbbells straight upward to full arm extension. Slowly lower the weights to the starting position.

PRECAUTIONS: Don't arch your back in such a way that the buttocks lose contact with the bench. After you lower the weights, pause a moment before raising them again. Inhale as you lower the weights, exhale as you raise them.

AREAS STRENGTHENED: Upper chest, front of shoulders, back of upper arms.

MUSCLES STRENGTHENED: Pectoralis majors, anterior and middle deltoids, triceps.

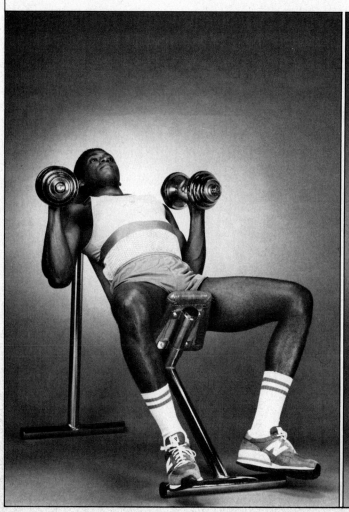 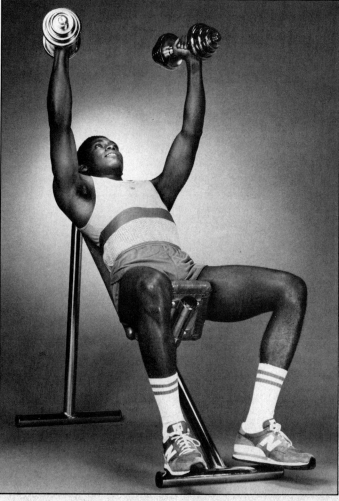

ISOLATED DUMBBELL CURLS

STARTING POSITION: Sit on any bench. With arms fully extended at your sides, grasp a dumbbell in each hand.

MOTION: Slowly bend your elbows and bring the dumbbells as close to your shoulders as possible. Slowly extend your elbows to the starting position.

PRECAUTIONS: Stabilize your upper body as much as you can during this exercise. Lower the weights slowly. Don't swing the dumbbells with your upper arms, as this will reduce the effectiveness of the exercise. Exhale as you raise the weights, inhale as you lower them.

AREAS STRENGTHENED: Front of upper arms, forearms.

MUSCLES STRENGTHENED: Biceps, brachialis, brachioradialis, flexor carpi ulnaris, flexor carpi radialis.

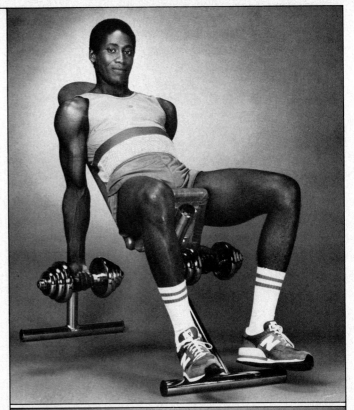

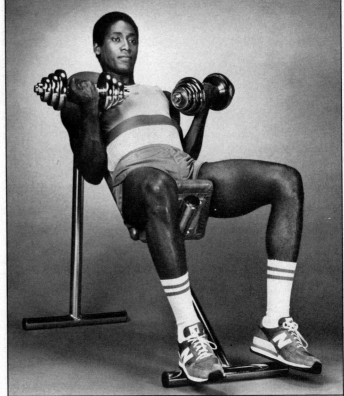

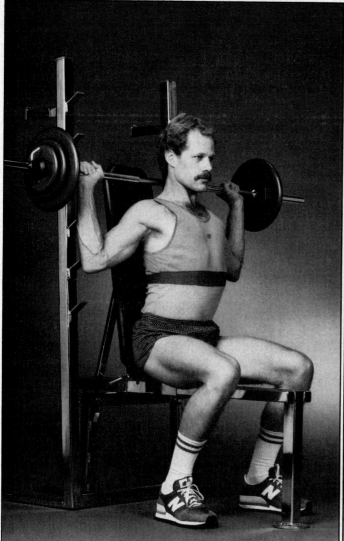 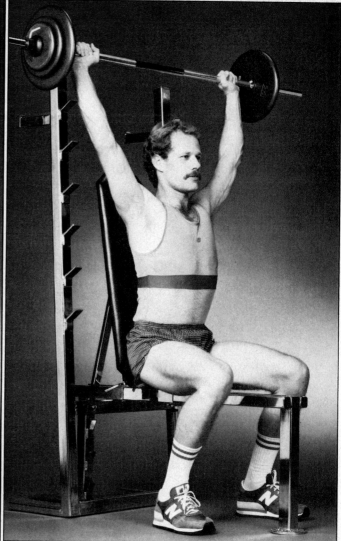

SEATED BEHIND-THE-NECK PRESS

STARTING POSITION: Sit upright on the bench, using the back support. With a relatively wide grip (to enhance the utilization of your shoulder muscles), remove the barbell from the standards and rest it on your shoulders behind your neck.

MOTION: Press the weight directly upward until your arms are fully extended. Then slowly lower the weight back to the starting position.

PRECAUTIONS: *Always use a spotter.* Stabilize your upper body to prevent hyperextension and possible lower back strain. You may want to use a weight belt for lower back support. Inhale as you lower the weight, exhale as you raise it.

AREAS STRENGTHENED: Shoulders, upper back, upper chest, back of upper arms.

MUSCLES STRENGTHENED: Anterior, middle, and posterior deltoids, trapezius, pectoralis majors, triceps.

INCLINE PRESS

STARTING POSITION: Adjust the inclined bench to about a 45° angle. Lie on it, with your head, shoulders, and buttocks in contact with the bench. Your knees should be bent and your feet flat on the floor. With a grip slightly wider than shoulder width, remove the barbell from the standards and hold it overhead, arms extended.

MOTION: Slowly lower the weight until it touches your chest between nipples and collarbones. Hold the weight motionless for a moment, then press it upward to full arm extension.

PRECAUTIONS: *Always use a spotter for this exercise.* Don't raise your buttocks off the bench by arching your back. Don't bounce the weight off your chest. Inhale as you lower the weight, exhale as you raise it.

AREAS STRENGTHENED: Front and middle of shoulders, upper chest, back of upper arms.

MUSCLES STRENGTHENED: Anterior and middle deltoids, pectoralis majors, triceps.

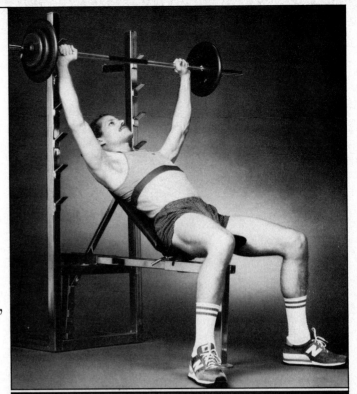

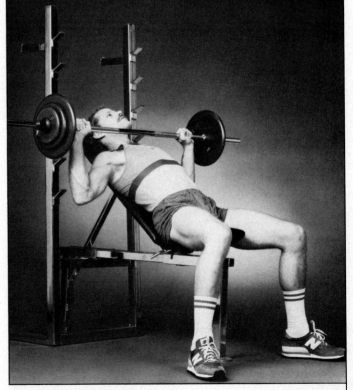

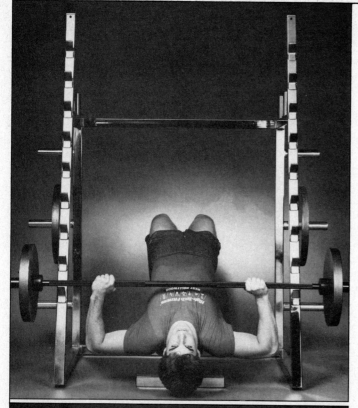

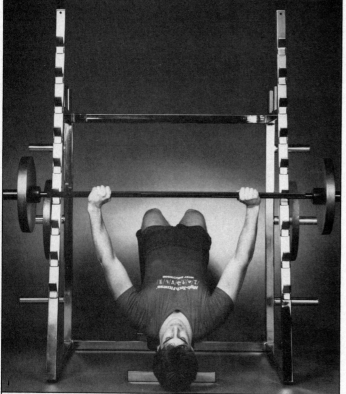

DECLINE PRESS

STARTING POSITION: Lie on the decline bench with your head lower than your knees. With a grip slightly wider than shoulder width, remove the barbell from the standards and rest it on your lower chest between your nipples and navel.

MOTION: Press the weight directly upward to full arm extension, then lower it back to the starting position.

PRECAUTIONS: *Always use a spotter.* Lower the weight slowly. Don't bounce it off your chest. Inhale as you lower the weight, exhale as you raise it.

AREAS STRENGTHENED: Lower chest, back, back of upper arms.

MUSCLES STRENGTHENED: Pectoralis majors, latissimus dorsi, triceps.

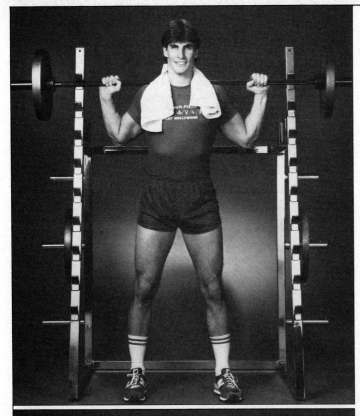

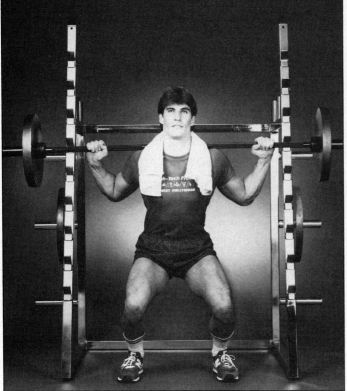

PARALLEL SQUAT

STARTING POSITION: Stand straight, with feet about shoulder-width apart and toes pointed slightly outward. With a relatively wide grip to help your balance, lift the barbell from the standards and rest it on your shoulders behind your head.

MOTION: Bend your hips and knees to lower your body until the tops of your thighs are nearly parallel to the ground. Return to the starting position by extending your hips and knees.

PRECAUTIONS: *Always use a spotter.* Keep your head up and your back flat to avoid lower back strain. We strongly recommend a weight belt for this exercise. Don't incline your torso forward more than 30°. Lower the weight slowly, keeping it fully under control, and do not bounce back after you've reached the squat position. Don't go down to a *full* squat, where your hips are lower than your knees. Inhale while lowering your body, exhale while raising the barbell to the return position.

AREAS STRENGTHENED: Legs, hips, lower back.

MUSCLES STRENGTHENED: Quadriceps, hamstrings, gluteals, erector spinae.

We like Ivanko weights and bars for several reasons. The first is that they're precision-made, so the weight you ask for is the weight you get. Some manufacturers cast their plates 5 to 8 percent underweight. Ivanko's average weight tolerances are zero on the down side, and 2 percent on the up side.

Ivanko's bars are 1¹⁄₁₆″ in diameter, which gives them 13 percent more strength than 1-inch bars. Some manufacturers make their bars from 1010 steel, which has very little carbon. Ivanko uses 1018- to 1045-grade steel, which is higher quality for greater strength. This is important when you're lifting heavier weights.

Ivanko uses polyester paint on their products. They bake it on, then chill it for better adhesion. The result is a finish that's less likely to chip or crack. The coating on Ivanko's rubber-coated weight plates is molded on, and it contains no recycled rubber. Some manufacturers use as much as 40 percent recycled, which doesn't adhere as well. Ivanko's chrome barbells and dumbbells are made of steel, not cast iron.

Another U.S. manufacturer we find to have the same quality-oriented goal and philosophy is the York Barbell Company. Their products are also precise and well made.

You can generally buy weights from various manufacturers in any size

or quantity, from a 1½-lb. dumbbell plate for under a dollar, to a complete 310-lb. Olympic weight set for about $350. We've used Ivanko prices and equipment merely as typical models for the quality types of free weights and bars you're likely to find.

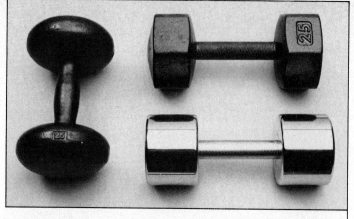

IVANKO® SOLID DUMBBELLS

Solid dumbbells by Ivanko and most other companies generally come in three configurations: solid round, black-painted; solid hexagonal, black-painted, knurled-handled; and solid round, chrome, knurled-handled.

The following are typical weight ranges and prices for each type:

BLACK ROUND

WEIGHT	APPROXIMATE COST
3 lb.	$5 pair
5 lb.	$25 pair

BLACK HEXAGONAL

WEIGHT	APPROXIMATE COST
5 lb.	$9 pair
100 lb.	$169 pair

CHROME ROUND

WEIGHT	APPROXIMATE COST
3 lb.	$15 pair
50 lb.	$150 pair

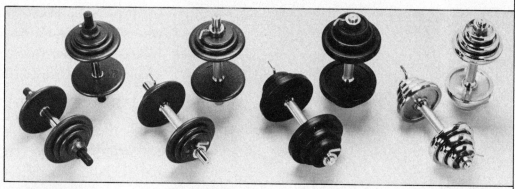

IVANKO® ADJUSTABLE DUMBBELL PLATE SETS

The following dumbbell sets all come with two 14″ dumbbell handles, collars, and 12 individual plates—four at 5 lbs., four at 2½ lbs., and four at 1¼ lbs. The differences lie in the type of collar, quality of handle, and kind of coating over the plates—paint, rubber, or chrome. All sets weigh a total of 45 lbs., including handles and collars.*

MAXIMO—black-painted, standard collars and handles
APPROXIMATE COST $30

ULTIMO—black-painted, deluxe collars and handles
APPROXIMATE COST $45

RUBIMO—black, rubber coated, deluxe collars and handles
APPROXIMATE COST $65

DELUXE—chrome, deluxe collars and handles
APPROXIMATE COST $120

Left to right: Maximo, Ultimo, Rubimo, Deluxe.

*Also available are 110-lb. barbell-dumbbell sets (not shown). These are the same as the 45-lb. dumbbell sets with the addition of one 5½-ft. barbell and collars and four 10-lb. plates. Prices range from $50 to $190, depending on the quality of the handles, collars, and plate finish.

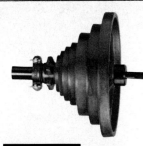
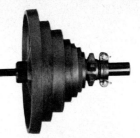

OLYMPIC PLATES AND BARS

Bars and barbell plates come in two configurations: the more ordinary "regular" and the Olympic size.

Olympic plates are calibrated in kilograms (and sometimes in kilograms and pounds). They're designated as "Olympic" because, as you might suspect, international weight lifting competitions, including the Olympics, use kilogram plates.

Olympic plates have larger holes than the kind most often found in American home gyms. As a result, Olympic bars have two-inch hubs to fit the plates. Olympic bars are also longer than standard bars—about 86″ instead of the usual 60″ to 66″—and they weigh 45 pounds.

Are Olympic bars and plates better? No. Weight is weight, however you lift it. If you're training for the '88 Olympics in Seoul, however, you'll probably want to use Olympic equipment.

OLYMPIC BARBELL

SIZE: 86″

WEIGHT: 55 lbs. with collars; 45 lbs. without

APPROXIMATE COST: $195 (including collars)

OLYMPIC PLATES (available in various weights from 1¼ lbs. to 100 lbs.)

APPROXIMATE COST: 1¼ lbs., 75¢; 100 lbs., $70

COMPLETE 310-LB. OLYMPIC SET

APPROXIMATE COST: $350 (including bar, collars, and plates)

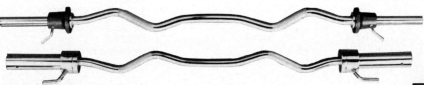

CURLING BARS

The curling bar takes the place of an ordinary barbell during biceps curls and triceps extensions. The bar is bent so the wrists are in a properly supinated position, allowing for better alignment of the biceps with the radius and ulna, the two long bones of the lower arm. The result is that you are able to do the biceps curl and triceps extension more efficiently. It's quite possible to do both these exercises with an ordinary barbell, but some people complain of pain and forearm splints when using a straight bar.

The curling bar comes in regular and Olympic sizes and includes collars.

REGULAR

SIZE: 48″ long

WEIGHT: 10 lbs.

APPROXIMATE COST: $20

OLYMPIC

SIZE: 48″ long

WEIGHT: 20 lbs.

APPROXIMATE COST: $65

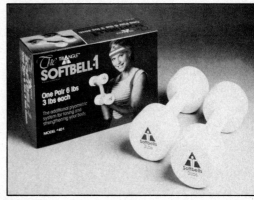

TRIANGLE MFG. CORP. SOFTBELLS

These innovative lightweight dumbbells are made of pressure-packed lead particles encased in padded white vinyl. They look nice, and they won't chip your floors if you drop them. They will, however, still land hard on your toes. Softbells are sold by the pair, and come in three different sizes.

WEIGHT:	APPROXIMATE COST
3 lb.	$19.99
6 lb.	$23.99
10 lb.	$32.99

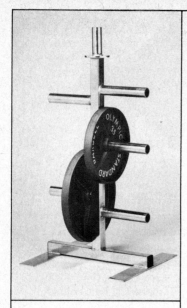

QUALITY OLYMPIC PLATE RACK

This compact rack allows you to store over 1,000 lbs. of Olympic barbell plates neatly in a confined space (as opposed to laying them on the floor). It's durable, made of polished chrome, and it has six weight pegs. We like it for its good looks and its all-important space-saving design.

WEIGHT: 40 lbs.

SIZE: 2′ × 2′ × 3′4″h

APPROXIMATE COST: $110

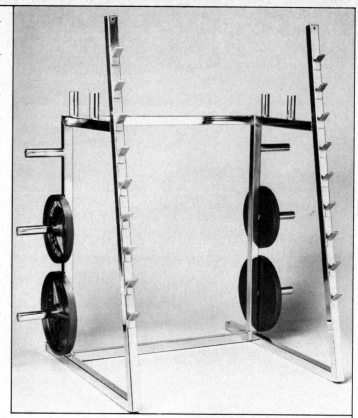

CAL GYM APOLLO SERIES DUMBBELL RACKS

We have to confess that what first attracted us to these all-chrome racks was that they look so sharp. But they're also durable and functional products. Their wire tops (a new design) hold each pair of dumbbells individually. They're designed for institutional use, but they're compact enough to fit in your home.

R-23 Single Tier Rack (holds 6 pairs of weights)

WEIGHT: 45 lbs.

SIZE: 50″ × 18″ × 30″h

APPROXIMATE COST: $225

R-22 Double Tier Rack (holds 12 pairs of weights)

WEIGHT: 60 lbs.

SPACE: 54″ × 18″ × 32″h

APPROXIMATE COST: $325

QUALITY PROFESSIONAL MULTI-PURPOSE RACK

This heavy-duty, all-welded, multipurpose weight rack will suit even the most serious body-builder. Depending on which bench you use, it allows you to perform virtually all the Olympic-style free weight exercises in the standing, seated, incline, decline and supine positions. This rack comes in chrome or black.

WEIGHT: 140 lbs.

SIZE: 6′ × 4′ × 5′h

APPROXIMATE COST: $450

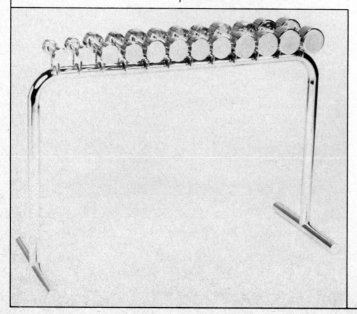

590 MARCY® PRO ABDOMINAL BOARD

This slant board adjusts to five positions and features handles to provide balance when doing leg raises. It's heavily padded with black Naugahyde and made of 2″ steel tubing with a blue powder-coat finish. It folds away for carrying and storage.

WEIGHT: 25 lbs.
SIZE: 80″ × 19″ × 38″h
APPROXIMATE COST: $79

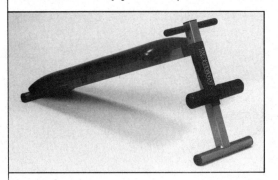

EXCEL BRUTUS SLANT BOARD

You can use this slant board for sit-ups or abdominal exercises. It's made of 2″ steel tubing finished in camel or black. The 5½′ pad is 12-gauge vinyl over foam padding. The board adjusts to any of 15 positions and locks in place with self-locking steel pins.

WEIGHT: 50 lbs.
SIZE: 6′ × 13″ × 49″h
APPROXIMATE COST: $110

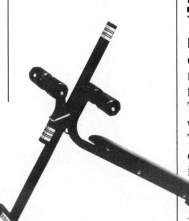

DECLINED SIT-UPS

STARTING POSITION: Lie supine on the abdominal board, with your knees bent and your lower legs hanging straight down. The fronts of your ankles should touch the padded rollers. Clasp your hands behind your head with the fingers interlocked.

MOTION: Keeping your torso straight, raise your upper body to a sitting position by bending at the hips. Slowly lower your torso to the starting position.

PRECAUTIONS: Avoid jerky, bouncy movements. Concentrate on contracting your abdominal muscles during the exercise. Return to the full supine position before repeating the movement. Don't bounce back up. Exhale as you raise your torso, inhale as you lower it.

AREAS STRENGTHENED: Abdomen, front of hips.

MUSCLES STRENGTHENED: Rectus abdominis, internal and external obliques, rectus femoris, iliopsoas.

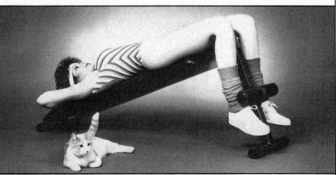

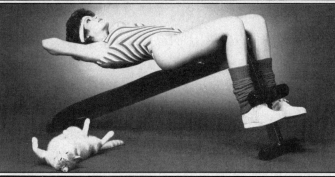

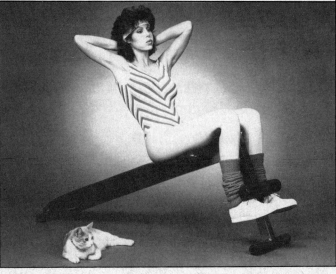

M + R DIP STAND

This stand is made of heavy chrome-plated steel. It lets you do the standard dip and five other exercises (such as push-ups and knee-ups) for your arms, shoulders, and upper-body muscle groups. Using gloves or rubber pads makes it easier to grip.

WEIGHT: 15 lbs.
SIZE: 18″ × 48″ × 40″h
APPROXIMATE COST: $99

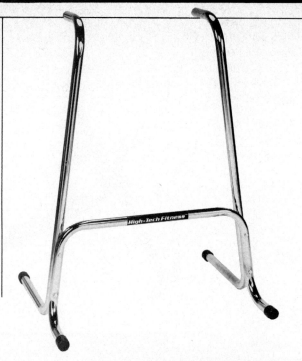

DIP BAR PUSH-UPS

STARTING POSITION: Grasp bars with arms extended. Your body should be at an approximately 45° angle to the floor, with your toes on the ground.

MOTION: Lower your body as far as possible by bending your elbows. Return to the starting position by extending your elbows to push your body upwards.

PRECAUTIONS: Keep your body straight while performing this exercise. Don't lower only your upper body by bending at the waist. Don't arch your lower back by lowering your hips. Exhale as your body is pushed upward, inhale as you lower yourself.

AREAS STRENGTHENED: Chest, front of shoulders, back of upper arms.

MUSCLES STRENGTHENED: Pectoralis majors, anterior deltoids, triceps.

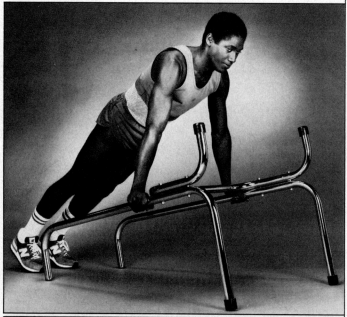

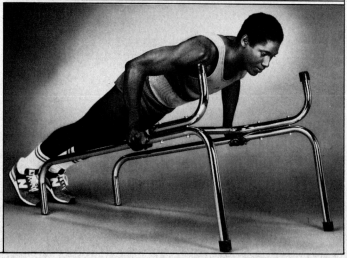

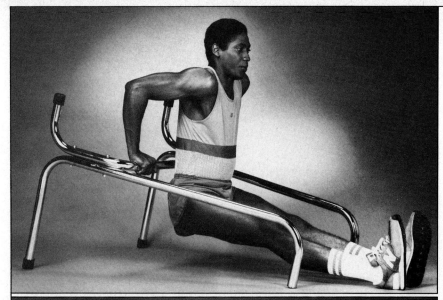

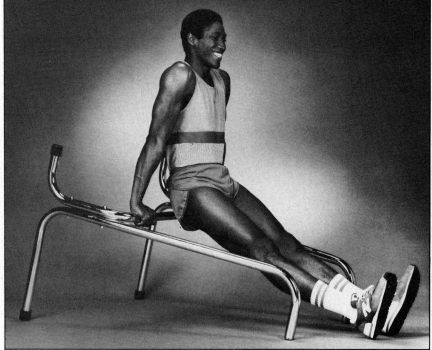

DIPS

STARTING POSITION: Sit upright with your buttocks off the floor, your hands grasping the dip bar behind your back, and your legs fully extended in front of you.

MOTION: Push your torso straight upward by extending your arms. After reaching full arm extension, lower your body slowly to the sitting position. When you return to the sitting position, your elbows should reach at least a 90° angle.

PRECAUTIONS: This exercise is similar to bar dips, but offers less resistance for the novice. Inhale as you lower your body, exhale as you raise it.

AREAS STRENGTHENED: Chest, back, front of shoulders, back of upper arms.

MUSCLES STRENGTHENED: Triceps, pectoralis majors, anterior deltoids, latissimus dorsi.

BAR DIPS

STARTING POSITION: Support your body in a suspended position, with your hands on the hand grips, arms fully extended.

MOTION: Lower your body by bending your arms. The goal is to have the fronts of your shoulders below the level of your elbows, with your arms bent at a little more than a 90° angle (not shown). Return to the starting position by pushing your body upward to full arm extension.

PRECAUTIONS: Try to keep your torso as upright as possible during this exercise. If neces- sary, bend your knees to prevent your feet from touching the ground at the lowered position. Do not arch your lower back. Inhale as you lower your body, exhale as you push upward. For a better grip, you may want to wear weight gloves or use a rubber grip.

AREAS STRENGTHENED: Chest, back, front of shoulders, back of upper arms.

MUSCLES STRENGTHENED: Pectoralis majors, triceps, anterior deltoids, latissimus dorsi.

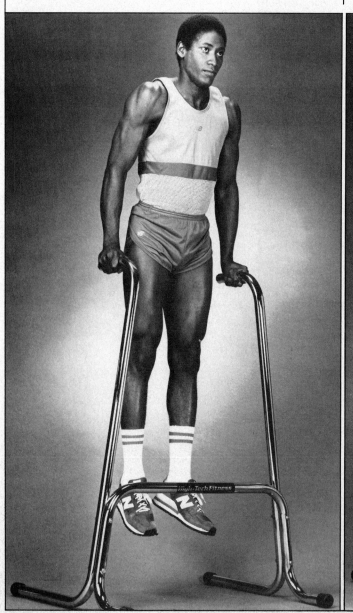
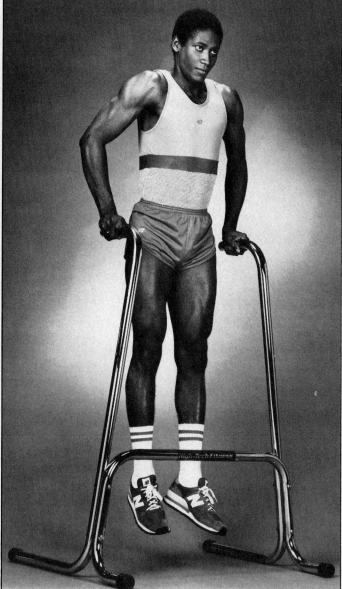

1930 MARCY® HIP FLEXOR

This abdominal-conditioning unit has contoured pads for elbows and arms, and an angled back rest for greater contraction of your abdominals. It's made of 2½″ structural steel tubing, chrome plated with a satin finish. The upholstery is black vinyl.

WEIGHT: 95 lbs.
SIZE: 36″ × 25″ × 62″ h
APPROXIMATE COST: $360

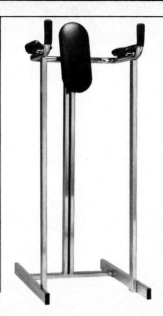

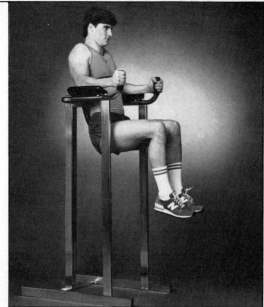

KNEE-UPS

STARTING POSITION: Support your body by resting your forearms on the padded supports and gripping the hand grips. Your body should be fully extended, with the legs hanging straight downward (not shown).

MOTION: Bring your knees up as close to your chest as possible by flexing the hips and knees. Hold this position momentarily, then return to the starting position with your legs fully extended. For a variation, the same movement can be performed with the knees straight.

PRECAUTIONS: Keep your upper body as motionless as possible during this exercise, in order to isolate the working muscles. Don't let your legs drop suddenly. Exhale as you raise your legs, inhale as you lower them. People with back problems should avoid the straight-knee version of this exercise. Beginning exercisers may feel fatigue and tension in their necks and shoulders due to weak muscles in the upper back and shoulder regions.

AREAS STRENGTHENED: Abdomen, front of hips.

MUSCLES STRENGTHENED: Rectus abdominis, internal and external obliques, quadriceps, iliopsoas.

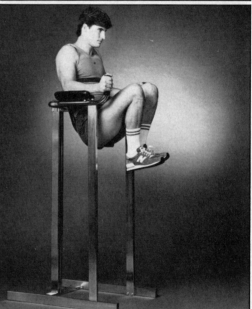

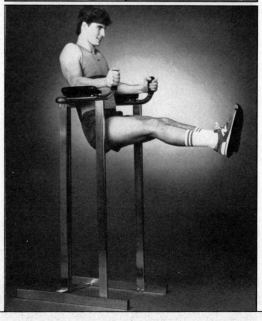

QUALITY ADJUSTABLE ROMAN CHAIR

This type bench is welded for strength and adjustable to almost any body size. Its unique design allows such additional functions as gravity traction, abdominal crunch, and external oblique exercises, as well as the traditional abdominal and lower back exercises. This Roman chair comes in chrome or high-gloss black.

WEIGHT: 90 lbs.
SIZE: 2½' × 4½' × 34"h
APPROXIMATE COST: $280

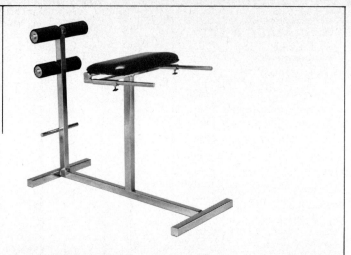

ROMAN CHAIR SIT-UP

STARTING POSITION: Sit upright on the hip pad with your legs extended and the fronts of your ankles under the padded rollers. Hold your hands behind your neck, with your fingers interlocked.

MOTION: Slowly lower your torso so that your body is parallel to the ground. Return to the upright starting position by flexing your hips and torso.

PRECAUTIONS: Don't place excessive strain on your lower back by hyperextending your torso—that is, by lowering your body beyond the point where it's parallel to the ground. When you return to the starting position, you *may* bend farther forward than a 90° angle. If you have any lower back problems, do not attempt this exercise. Exhale while lowering your body, inhale while returning.

AREAS STRENGTHENED: Abdomen and front of hips.

MUSCLES STRENGTHENED: Rectus abdominis, internal and external obliques, rectus femoris, iliopsoas.

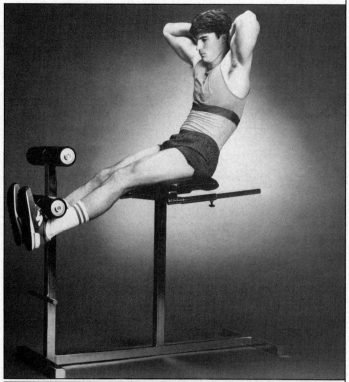

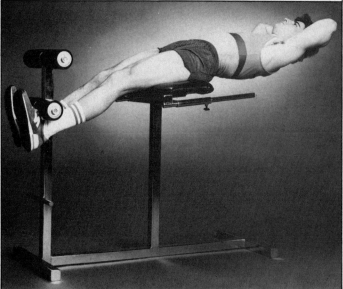

ROMAN CHAIR BACK EXTENSIONS

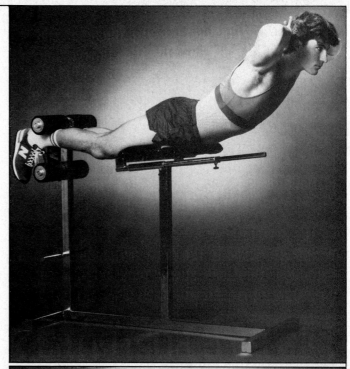

STARTING POSITION: Lie prone on the Roman chair, with your body parallel to the floor. Put your upper thighs and abdomen on the hip pad and the backs of your ankles under the rollers. Hold your hands behind your neck, fingers interlocked.

MOTION: Slowly lower your upper body until the torso is almost perpendicular to the ground. Return to the starting position by extending your hips and back. Keep your head in a neutral position and your elbows out.

PRECAUTIONS: Lower the upper body slowly to avoid excessive lower back strain. If you have any lower back problems, do not attempt this exercise. Inhale while lowering your body, exhale while raising it.

AREAS STRENGTHENED: Lower back and buttocks.

MUSCLES STRENGTHENED: Erector spinae, gluteals.

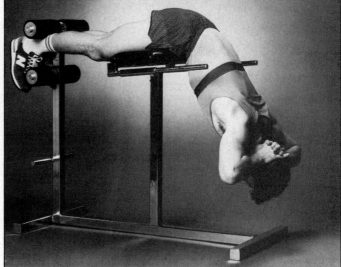

ROMAN CHAIR SIDE BENDS

STARTING POSITION: Lie on your side on the Roman chair with your body extended. One hip should rest on the padded seat, with your feet crossed and your ankles under the padded rollers. Clasp your hands behind your head, with fingers interlocked.

MOTION: Bend your torso upward as far as possible. Hold this position for a moment, then lower yourself to the starting position.

PRECAUTIONS: Don't excessively lower your trunk, which can cause lower back and sacral strain. Exhale as you raise your trunk, inhale as you lower it.

AREAS STRENGTHENED: Sides of torso, hips.

MUSCLES STRENGTHENED: Internal and external obliques, gluteals.

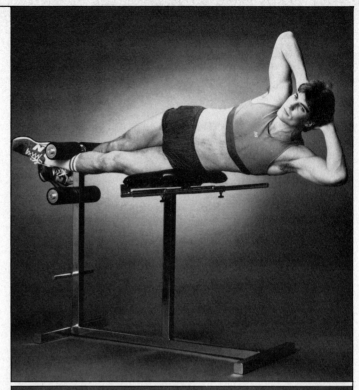

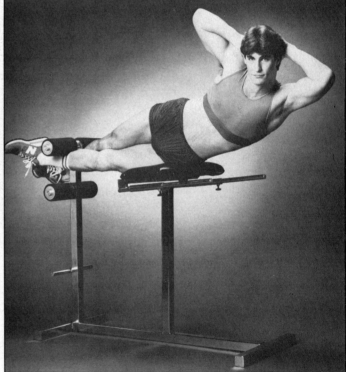

NAUTILUS® LOWER BACK MACHINE

This Nautilus has nine graduated resistance settings. Its outstanding feature is that it lets you work your lower back with no spinal compression, because it exerts its resistance perpendicular to your spinal column. It's the only machine on the market that strengthens your back without vertical loading. The Nautilus is made of painted beige tubular steel, padded with black Naugahyde, and assembles in 15 minutes (its manufacturer promises) with screwdriver and wrench.

WEIGHT: 150 lbs.
SIZE: 51″ × 34½″ × 54″h
APPROXIMATE COST: $475

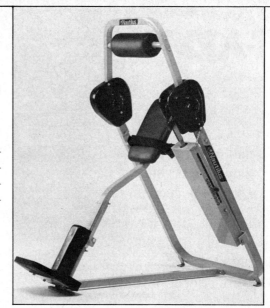

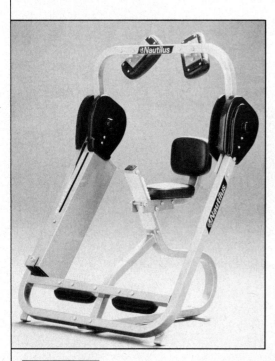

NAUTILUS® ABDOMINAL MACHINE

This Nautilus isolates the abdominal muscles without working the hip flexors—the muscles that do much of the work in situps and leg lifts. There are nine graduated resistance settings, and as with other Nautilus equipment, the "vector of resistance" is maintained at a 90° angle to the body parts being worked in order to reduce the risk of strain. This unit is made of painted beige tubular steel with thick black Naugahyde padding.

WEIGHT: 150 lbs.
SIZE: 38″ × 35½″ × 48″h
APPROXIMATE COST: $485

7050 MARCY® VERTICAL BUTTERFLY

This weight stack machine isolates the pectorals and deltoids. You can increase weight resistance through its selectorized weight stack system up to 190 lbs. The seat adjusts to various heights and angles, and seat and handles are padded for comfort. The unit is made of 4″ × 2″ structural steel tubing, finished in satin chrome, with black Naugahyde.

WEIGHT: 480 lbs.
SIZE: 50″ × 32″ × 76″h
APPROXIMATE COST: $1,250

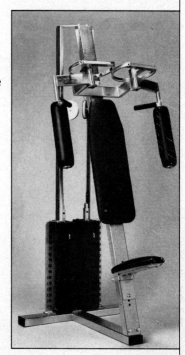

BENT-ARM FLYS

STARTING POSITION: Sit upright with head, shoulders, and buttocks in contact with the back support. Flex your elbows to a 90° angle and place them behind the padded rollers. Your elbows should be far enough back to comfortably stretch the chest muscles.

MOTION: Bring your arms forward, pushing with the elbows, until the padded rollers come together in front of your face. Slowly return to the starting position by bringing your arms backward.

PRECAUTIONS: Don't arch your back or raise your buttocks off the bench. Avoid pushing the rollers together with your hands. Release the weight slowly and under full control, so you don't overstretch your chest muscles. Exhale as you bring your arms forward, inhale as you return to the starting position.

AREAS STRENGTHENED: Front of shoulders and chest.

MUSCLES STRENGTHENED: Anterior deltoids, pectoralis majors.

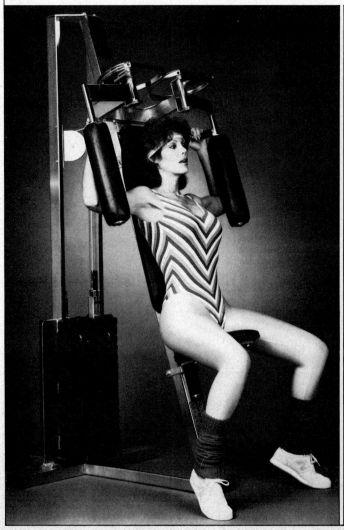
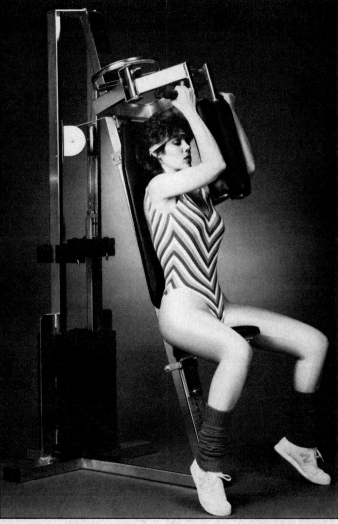

LEG EXTENSIONS

STARTING POSITION: Sit upright on the leg machine, with your legs hanging straight down over the machine's edge. Place the fronts of your ankles under the padded rollers. Position your body so that your back is straight and your knees are right at the edge of the bench. Grasp the sides of the bench to stabilize your body.

MOTION: Fully extend your knees until your lower legs are straight and parallel to the floor. Return to the starting position by slowly lowering the weight.

PRECAUTIONS: Prevent any upper body motion in order to isolate the working muscles. Move only your lower leg. Lower the weight slowly; don't bounce it at the bottom in order to prevent unnecessary strain on your knee joints. Exhale when extending your knees, inhale when bending them.

AREAS STRENGTHENED: Front of thighs.

MUSCLES STRENGTHENED: Quadriceps (rectus femoris, vastus lateralis, vastus medialis, vastus intermedius).

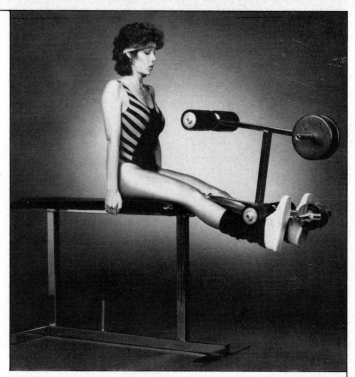

QUALITY LEG EXTENSION/LEG CURL BENCH

This all-welded unit's variable resistance is determined by the placement of the dual weight stacks, allowing for a more intense isolation of quadriceps and hamstrings. It comes in chrome and black, with black upholstery. Its thick padding gives you more comfort when using heavier weights.

WEIGHT: 150 lbs.
SIZE: 2' × 5' × 3'h
APPROXIMATE COST: $350

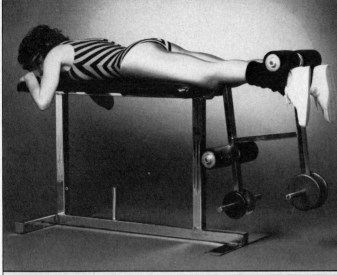

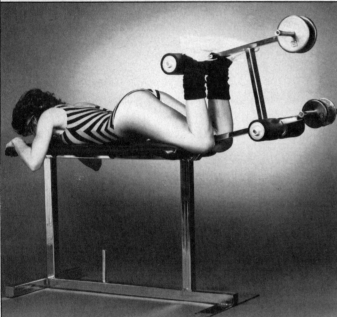

LEG CURLS

STARTING POSITION: Lie prone on the leg machine, with your legs extended and the backs of your ankles under the padded rollers.

MOTION: Bend your knees to bring the rollers up and forward until the rollers touch your buttocks. Return to the starting position by slowly lowering the rollers until your legs are fully extended.

PRECAUTIONS: Try not to raise your buttocks in the air, and keep your front thighs in contact with the bench in order to effectively isolate the working muscles. Lower the weight slowly; don't bounce it at full leg extension. Exhale when bending your knees, inhale when lowering the weight.

AREAS STRENGTHENED: Calves, back of upper legs.

MUSCLES STRENGTHENED: Gastrocnemius, hamstrings.

QUALITY SEATED CALF BENCH

The Quality Seated Calf bench allows you to exercise calf muscles in a way they can't be worked standing up. Calf exercises require high weights. The calf block allows you to stretch your hamstrings and extends your range of motion. This unit is built for durability. It comes in chrome or high-gloss black.

WEIGHT: 80 lbs.
SIZE: 2½′ × 3′ × 1½′h
APPROXIMATE COST: $300

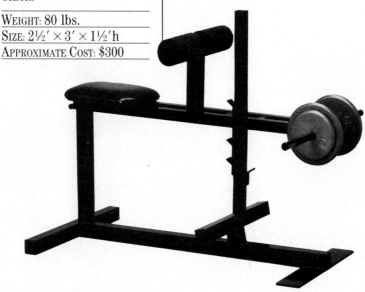

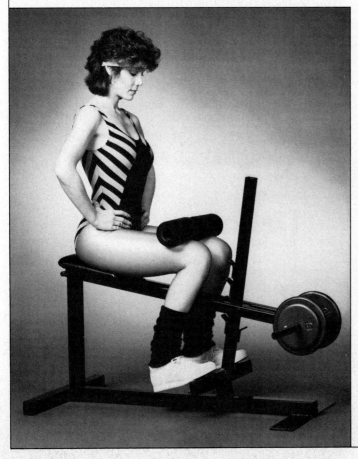

CALF RAISES

STARTING POSITION: Sit upright on the calf machine, with the balls of your feet on the footrest and the padded rollers on the lower part of your upper legs, just above the knees.

MOTION: Push the rollers upward by pointing your toes downward as far as possible. Keep your feet parallel to each other; don't toe in or out. Return to starting position by slowly lowering the weights.

PRECAUTIONS: Lower the weight slowly and under full control, in order to avoid overstretching your calf muscles. Exhale as you lift your feet, inhale as you lower them.

AREAS STRENGTHENED: Calf.

MUSCLES STRENGTHENED: Gastrocnemius, plantaris, soleus.

QUALITY LEG PRESS

This sturdy steel weight machine allows you to do various leg-pressing exercises. Its inclined bench is set at a measured angle to relieve back stress. We like the Quality Leg Press because it has easily reachable handles to let you operate its safety-stop feature. If you feel the weight on your legs becoming too much for you to support, just grab the handles and give them a turn. The weight will automatically be locked in place, and you can save yourself a possible painful back injury. This machine comes in chrome or black-gloss finish, with black Naugahyde upholstery.

WEIGHT: 80 lbs.
SIZE: 2′ × 3½′ × 4½′h
APPROXIMATE COST: $376

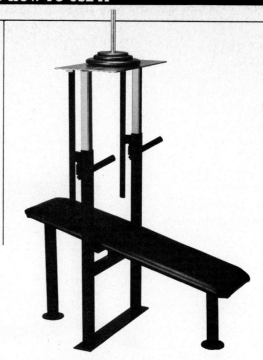

VERTICAL LEG PRESS

STARTING POSITION: Lie supine on a bench, with knees fully bent. Place your feet directly against the weight stack, four to six inches apart. Your hips should be directly below your feet.

MOTION: Extend your hips and knees to press the weight stack upward until your legs are fully extended. Then point your toes to fully shape the calf muscle. Keep your knees about four inches apart. Then slowly lower the weights back to the starting position.

PRECAUTIONS: This exercise allows the use of relatively heavy weights without causing undue strain on your lower back or upper body. Spotters aren't normally required. Exhale as you press the weights upward, inhale as you lower them.

AREAS STRENGTHENED: Legs, hips.

MUSCLES STRENGTHENED: Quadriceps, hamstrings, gluteals, gastrocnemius, soleus.

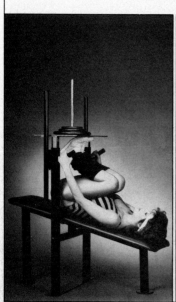
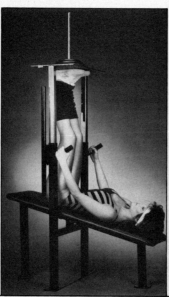
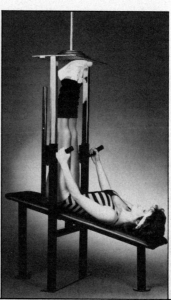

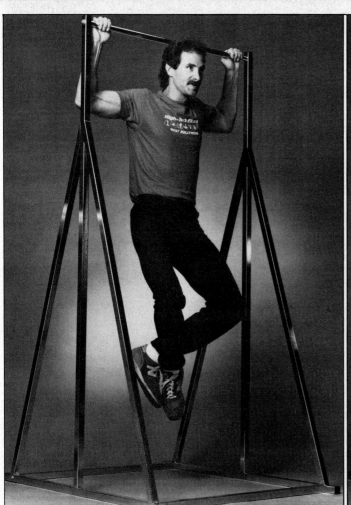
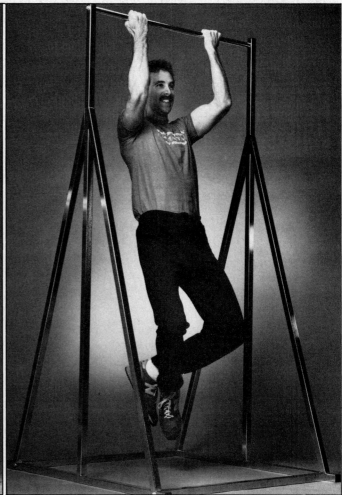

PULL-UPS

STARTING POSITION: Grasp any chinning bar (a free-standing chinning bar is shown) with your hands placed 10 to 12 inches wider than shoulder width, palms facing outward. Allow your body to hang. For a variation of this exercise, grasp bar with palms facing inward, about shoulder-width apart (this is called a chin-up).

MOTION: Pull your body upward so that the bar passes either in front of or behind your head. You should raise your body until the bar touches either the top of your shoulders or your upper chest. Then lower your body slowly to the starting position.

PRECAUTIONS: Don't swing your body—this reduces the effectiveness of the exercise.

When returning to the starting position, extend your arms completely before pulling up again. Don't bounce when you get to the bottom. Inhale when lowering your body, exhale when raising it.

AREAS STRENGTHENED: Front of upper arms, back.

MUSCLES STRENGTHENED: Biceps, brachialis, brachioradialis, trapezius, latissimus dorsi.

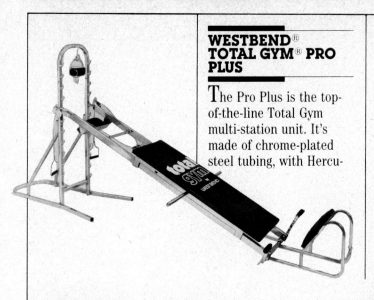

WESTBEND® TOTAL GYM® PRO PLUS

The Pro Plus is the top-of-the-line Total Gym multi-station unit. It's made of chrome-plated steel tubing, with Herculite vinyl covering on the glideboard. The cables are 2000-lb. test, the arm pulley has bronze self-lubricating bushings, and the board moves on nylon rollers. You can choose one of eleven different resistance levels. The Pro Plus comes with a two-handle pulley system, swivel foot holder, deluxe weight cuff, squat stand, and weight lifting frame. It even folds up for easy storage.

The Total Gym operates by making you work against your own body weight. You lie down on the glideboard and pull yourself up an incline with smooth, rolling motions. Because the glideboard supports your weight, the strain on your joints is greatly reduced.

WEIGHT: (shipping) 110 lbs.
SIZE: 24″ × 108″ × 53″h
APPROXIMATE COST: $595, including deluxe attachments

INNER THIGH PULL

STARTING POSITION: Lie on your side on the glideboard. Attach the cable strap to the ankle of your upper leg. Bend your elbow to support your head, and bend your lower leg to steady your body.

MOTION: Raise your working leg straight up. Slowly bring it down until it rests on your supporting leg.

PRECAUTIONS: Keep your working leg fully extended from the knee. In order to isolate the working muscles, don't use your body or your support leg to perform this motion. Inhale as you raise your leg, exhale as you bring it down.

AREAS STRENGTHENED: Hips, thighs.

MUSCLES STRENGTHENED: Adductors.

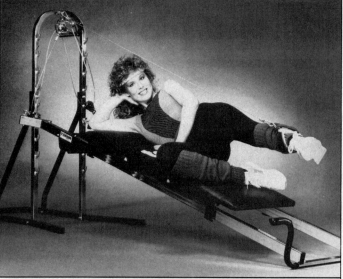

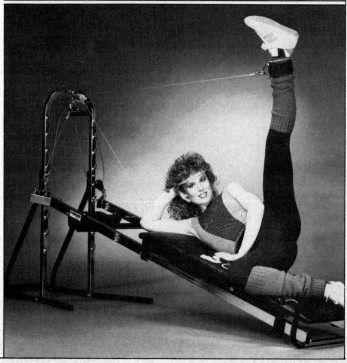

BUTTERFLY

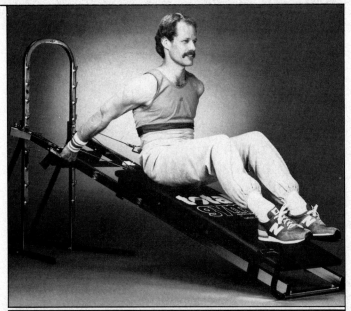

STARTING POSITION: Sit upright on the glideboard, facing away from the ladder, with your knees slightly bent. With arms stretched out behind you, grasp the cable handles with your palms facing backward.

MOTION: Pull yourself up the rails by bringing both arms in a half-circle from behind you until your handles touch in front of your body. Return to the starting position.

PRECAUTIONS: Keep your torso stable and straight while performing these movements. Exhale as you bring your arms forward, inhale as you return them to the starting position.

AREAS STRENGTHENED: Chest, shoulders, upper arms.

MUSCLES STRENGTHENED: Pectoralis majors, anterior deltoids, biceps.

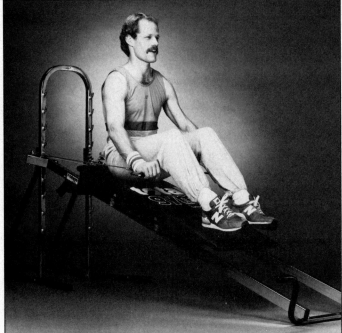

HAMSTRING PULL

STARTING POSITION: Lie on the glideboard on your back. Attach the cable strap to the ankle of your working leg and raise it until it is perpendicular to the floor and fully extended. Let your arms rest at your sides. Bend your free leg at the knee, and place the foot at the bottom of the glideboard. Slightly raise your head off the glideboard.

MOTION: Keeping your working leg fully extended, slowly bring it down until it touches the glideboard.

PRECAUTIONS: Keep your working leg fully extended throughout the entire movement. Exhale as you bring your leg down and forward, inhale as you raise it.

AREAS STRENGTHENED: Thighs, buttocks.

MUSCLES STRENGTHENED: Hamstrings, gluteals.

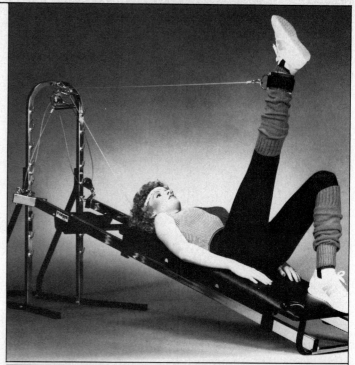

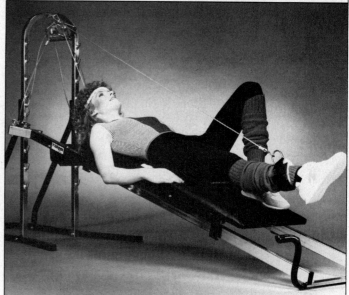

LEG EXTENSION

STARTING POSITION: Lie prone on the glide-board, with your head raised and your arms folded. Hook the ankle strap around the ankle of your working leg. Bend your free leg at the knee and keep it in a bent position throughout the exercise.

MOTION: Bend your working leg from the knee until you bring it up as close to your thigh as possible. Slowly straighten it, extending it from the knee as far as you can.

PRECAUTIONS: While performing this exercise, the motion should occur only at the knee joint. Keep your free knee bent during the entire movement. Exhale as you straighten your leg, inhale as you bend it.

AREAS STRENGTHENED: Front of thighs.

MUSCLES STRENGTHENED: Quadriceps.

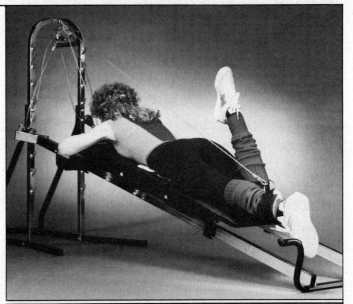

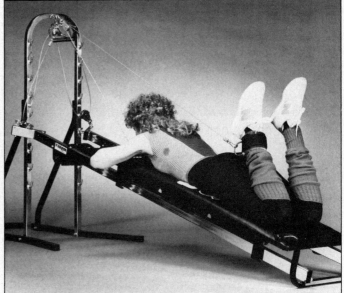

TENNIS BACKHAND

STARTING POSITION: Sit sideways on the glideboard, supporting yourself by grasping the edge of the board with your free hand. With your working arm extended, grasp the cable handle.

MOTION: Keeping your arm straight, pull the cable across your chest until your arm is directly lateral to your body. Slowly return it to your starting position.

PRECAUTIONS: Keep your working arm as fully extended as possible during the motion. Exhale as you pull your arm across your body, inhale as you return it to the starting position.

AREAS STRENGTHENED: Shoulders, forearms, upper arms, upper back.

MUSCLES STRENGTHENED: Posterior deltoids, triceps, rhomboids.

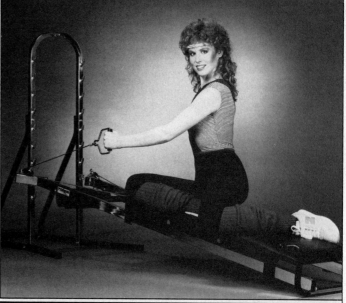

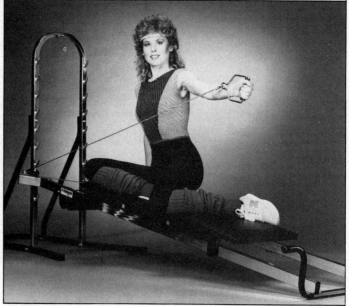

KONG PRO FORM 2000

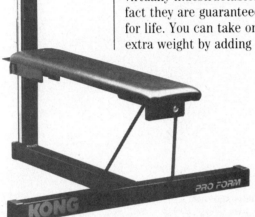

This is a highly compact multi-station unit that offers up to 24 standard weight lifting exercises. Instead of a selectorized weight stack system, its solid steel springs provide you with up to 200 lbs. resistance. The springs are virtually indestructable. In fact they are guaranteed for life. You can take on extra weight by adding conventional disc barbell plates to the resistance arm extensions. The full-length bench is heavily padded for comfort. The Kong Pro Form 2000 comes in black and has an optional leg extension

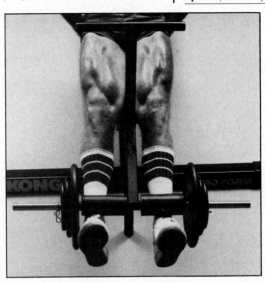

unit. It is a relatively solid unit and a good buy for the price.

WEIGHT: 150 lbs.
SIZE: $48'' \times 42'' \times 73''$h
APPROXIMATE COST: $599
($675 with leg extension option, shown)

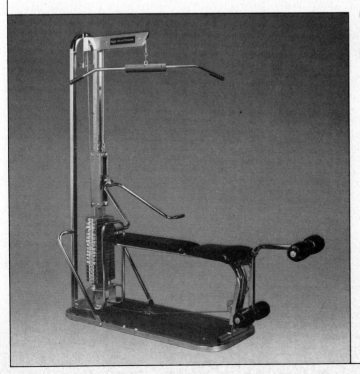

CAL GYM MASTERLINE 500

This space-efficient weight machine allows the user to do all the popular strength training exercises, including bench presses, standing presses, lat pull-downs, leg curls, and rowing.

The Masterline 500 is built of reasonably heavy steel tubing, with a wood-grained base and a tan bench cover. Each weight on the stack weighs 10 pounds and locks into place with a selector key. The unit comes with a color exercise chart, and you can choose from three weight stacks weighing 130, 170, or 200 pounds.

The Masterline 500's action does not have the fluidity of the more expensive institutional machines you'll see in gyms or health clubs. But as a conventional multi-purpose home weight stack machine, this unit is a good value for the money.

WEIGHT: 300 lbs.
SIZE: $60'' \times 25\frac{1}{2}'' \times 87''$h
APPROXIMATE COST: $995
($1,200 with chrome weight stack)

CAL GYM WP-250FS QUAD PULLEY SYSTEM

Cal Gym has been making quad pulleys for 14 years. This two-pulley unit is their best model. It's entirely chrome-plated, with two 100-lb. weight stacks. The weights lock down in a selectorized system, and the cable action is very smooth. The WP-250FS is so durable that it's used in a lot of gyms. The parts are guaranteed for a year, and the frame carries a lifetime warranty.

WEIGHT: 175 lbs.
SIZE: 32″ × 35″ × 70″ h
APPROXIMATE COST: $930

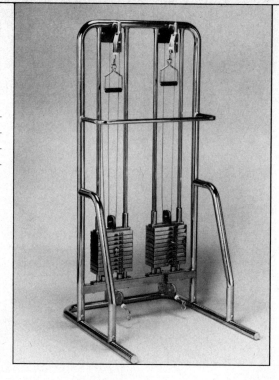

FORWARD THIGH PULL

STARTING POSITION: Stand facing away from the machine, with arms fully extended backward and hands grasping the handrail at shoulder width. The cuff of a lower cable should be fastened to one ankle.

MOTION: Move the working leg forward and upward as far as possible, while keeping it fully extended from the knee. Slowly lower the weight to return to starting position.

PRECAUTIONS: Stabilize the entire body during this exercise, in order to effectively isolate the working muscles. Exhale as you raise your leg, inhale as you return to the starting position. Don't "crunch" your torso in at the waist when you lift your leg forward.

AREAS STRENGTHENED: Hips, thighs.

MUSCLES STRENGTHENED: Iliopsoas, quadriceps.

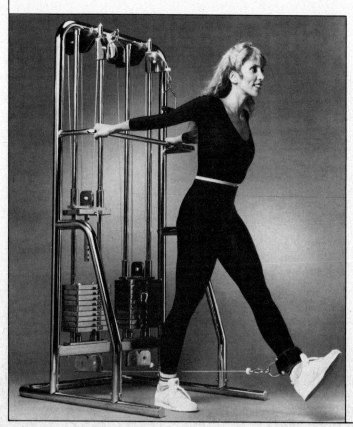

BUTTOCKS PULL

STARTING POSITION: Stand facing the machine, with arms fully extended and hands on the handrail, shoulder width apart. The cuff of a lower cable should be fastened to one ankle.

MOTION: Bring the working leg back and up as far as possible, keeping it fully extended from the knee. Your torso should remain straight. Slowly lower the weight by bringing your leg forward to the starting position.

PRECAUTIONS: Don't arch your lower back during this movement. Exhale as you raise the weight, inhale as you lower it.

AREAS STRENGTHENED: Back of thighs and buttocks.

MUSCLES STRENGTHENED: Hamstrings, gluteals.

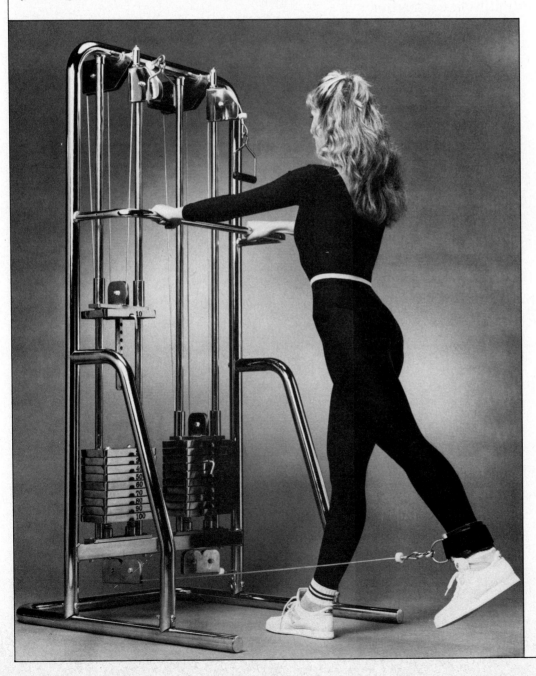

PULLEY ROW

STARTING POSITION: Sit upright on the floor, facing the machine, with legs fully extended. Place your feet in contact with the machine to stabilize your body. Grasp the handles of the lower cables, with your arms fully extended forward.

MOTION: Keeping your torso straight, bend your elbows and pull the handles as close to your torso as possible. Slowly lower the weight by extending your arms to the starting position.

PRECAUTIONS: Don't bend at the waist or knees while performing this exercise. Exhale as you raise the weight, inhale as you lower it.

AREAS STRENGTHENED: Upper back, front of arm, and shoulders.

MUSCLES STRENGTHENED: Trapezius, biceps, posterior deltoids, rhomboids.

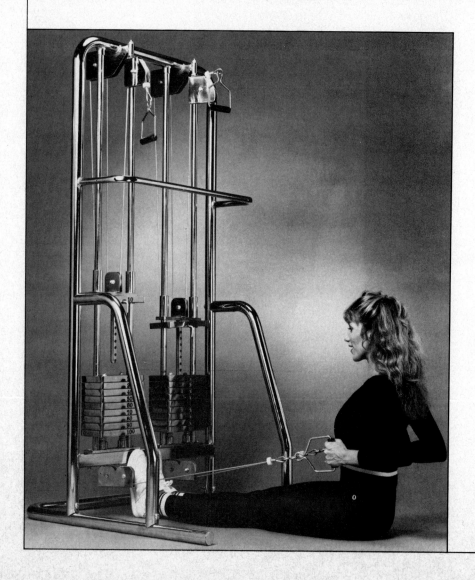

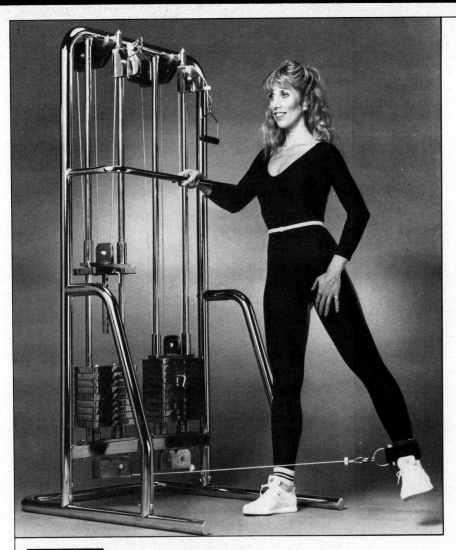

OUTER THIGH PULL

STARTING POSITION: Stand sideways in front of the machine, with the hand nearest the machine grasping the handrail. The cuff of one of the lower cables should be attached to the ankle of the leg that's farther from the machine.

MOTION: Move the exercising leg outward and upward as far as possible, keeping it fully extended from the knee. Slowly lower the weight to return to the starting position.

PRECAUTIONS: Stabilize the entire body when performing this exercise, in order to isolate the working muscles. Keep the knee of the working leg facing directly forward throughout the exercise. Exhale as you raise the weight, inhale as you lower it.

AREAS STRENGTHENED: Hips, thighs.

MUSCLES STRENGTHENED: Gluteus medius, tensor fasciae latae.

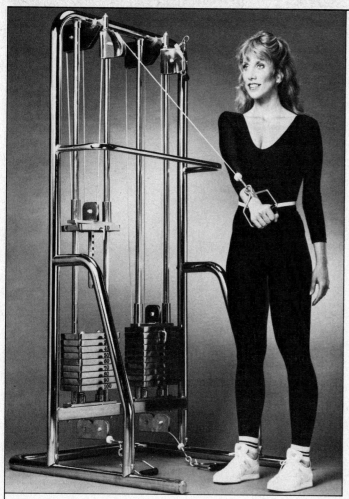

CHEST PULL

STARTING POSITION: Stand sideways in front of the machine, with the arm nearest the machine raised and the hand grasping the handle of an upper cable. The opposite arm remains at your side.

MOTION: Pull the cable diagonally across your body, keeping your working arm fully extended from the elbow. Lower the weight slowly to return to the starting position.

PRECAUTIONS: Stabilize your torso as much as possible during this exercise, using only the arm and shoulder to perform the motion. Exhale as you raise the weight, inhale as you lower it.

AREAS STRENGTHENED: Shoulders, chest.

MUSCLES STRENGTHENED: Pectoralis majors, anterior deltoids.

PARAMOUNT FITNESS EQUIPMENT CORP. FITNESS MATE ™

This machine features a chest press/shoulder press bar; rollers for leg extensions and leg curls (not shown); a high pulley for lat pull-downs and triceps extensions; and a low pulley for biceps curls, rowing, and leg kicks. It's one of the best built and best priced multi-station units of its kind, from a company that specializes in both home and commercial gym equipment. This is an unusually smooth working unit.

WEIGHT: 430 to 490 lbs. (depending upon weights)

SIZE: $3\frac{1}{2}' \times 8\frac{1}{2}' \times 6'11''$h

APPROXIMATE COST: $1,500 with black weights (chrome weights extra)

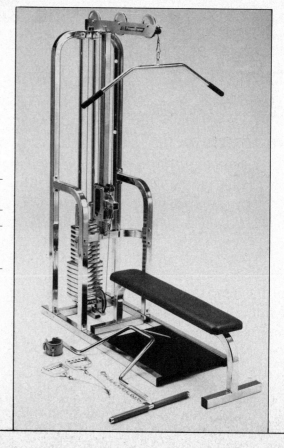

1350 MARCY® MASTER GYM

Four people can work out on this unit at the same time. It features a barbell press station, with 220 lbs. of weight and an eight-position lifting arm; a quad pulley, with two 50-lb. adjustable weight stacks, four handles, padded ankle straps, and nonslip support grips; a lat station, with a 180-lb. weight stack; and a four-position abdominal board and exercise bench. It's chrome with black Naugahyde upholstery.

WEIGHT: 1,010 lbs.	
SIZE: 8' × 12' × 7'2"h	
APPROXIMATE COST: $2,650 (chrome weight stacks $800 extra)	

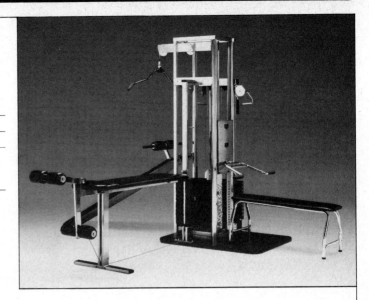

LAT PULL-DOWNS

STARTING POSITION: Face the machine and kneel directly under the lat bar. Your back should be straight, your hips forward, and you should grasp the bar with a wide grip.

MOTION: Pull the bar down until it touches the back of your neck, then let the weights pull the bar upward until your arms are fully extended above your head.

PRECAUTIONS: The motion of this exercise should be smooth. Exhale as you pull the weight down toward your neck; inhale as the bar returns to its starting position.

AREAS WORKED: Back, upper arms.

MUSCLES WORKED: Latissimus dorsi, biceps.

SHOULDER PRESS

STARTING POSITION: Sit facing the machine, with your back straight and your feet on the floor. Grasp the shoulder press bar handles, which should be resting on your shoulders at the beginning of the exercise.

MOTION: Extend your arms full-length from the elbows in a smooth movement, then pull the bar back down to shoulder height.

PRECAUTIONS: Exhale as you press the weight upward, inhale as you pull it down. You can also do this exercise facing *away* from the machine.

AREAS WORKED: Front of shoulders, back of upper arms.

MUSCLES WORKED: Deltoids, triceps.

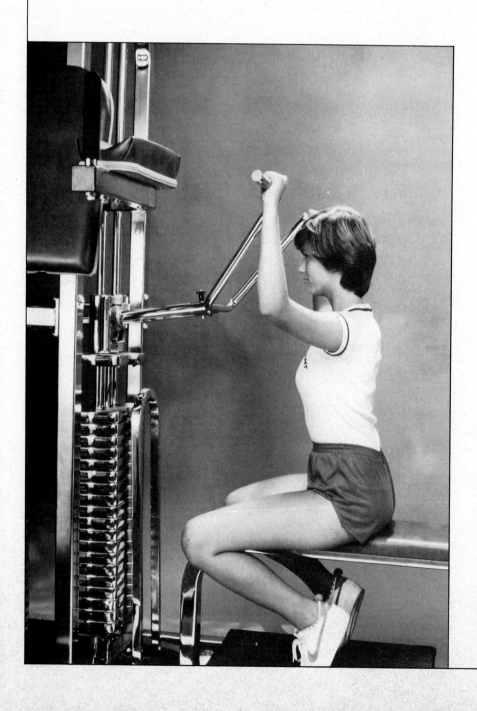

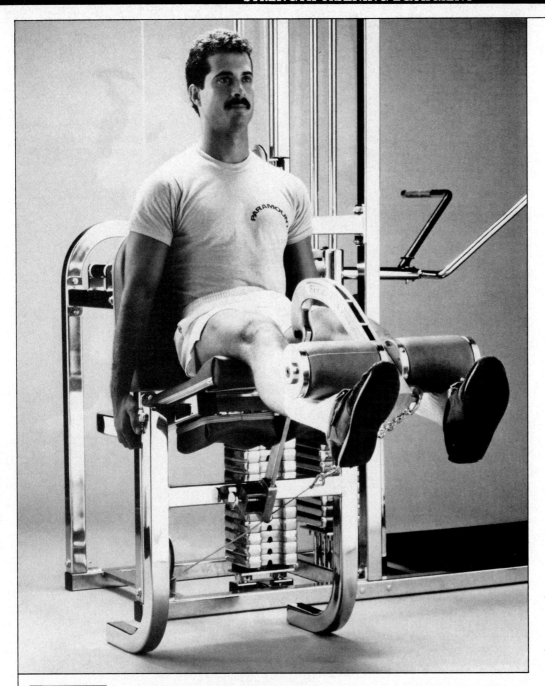

LEG EXTENSIONS

STARTING POSITION: Sit straight, with the backs of your knees at the edge of the bench, and your ankles directly under the padded rollers. Grip the edge of the bench for support.

MOTION: Extend both legs evenly until they're completely horizontal. Then lower them back to the starting position.

PRECAUTIONS: The motion of this exercise should be smooth and even. Exhale as you extend your legs, inhale as you lower them.

AREAS STRENGTHENED: Front of thighs.

MUSCLES WORKED: Quadriceps.

SQUATS

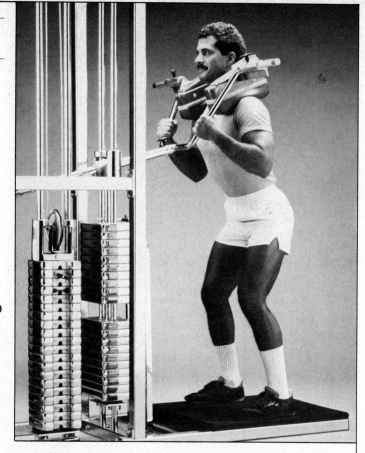

STARTING POSITION: Stand facing the weight stack, with your feet shoulder-width apart underneath the shoulder pads.

MOTION: Slowly lower your body downward by bending the hips, knees, and ankles toward the floor as far as you can while keeping your heels on the floor and your knees aligned over the center of your feet. Return to the starting position by straightening your legs and standing up.

PRECAUTIONS: This exercise is very similar to the leg press except that the body is maintaining its upright stance. Consequently there is a tendency to contort or arch the lower back to assist the movement. This should be avoided. The spine should remain straight as possible. We recommend a weight belt for this exercise.

AREAS STRENGTHENED: Front and back of hips and thighs, back of calves, overall back musculature.

MUSCLES WORKED: Quadriceps, gluteus maximus, hamstrings, gastrocnemius, soleus, erector spinae.

GYM-IN-ONE™ DELUXE QUAD KICK

Gym Equipment International's multi-station unit gives you 320 lbs. pressing resistance and 220 lbs. pulley resistance from the front weight stack. The quad kick pulley station offers two weight stacks of 50 lbs. each. This good quality unit includes the standard attachments, plus two stirrups, two ankle straps, quad kick pulley station, thigh/knee bench, sit-up board, leg press and leg squat. The weights come in black or (optional) chrome.

WEIGHT: 906 lbs.

SIZE: 10′ × 10′ × 8′4″h

APPROXIMATE COST: $4,000 (depending on black or chrome weights and options)

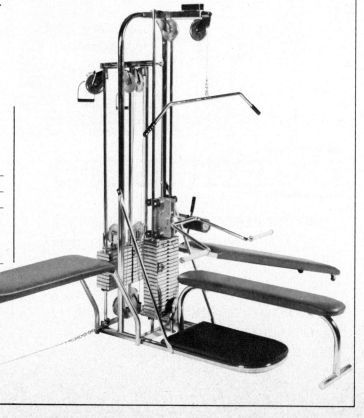

UNIVERSAL® POWER PAK 400

Years ago Universal gym equipment helped set the standard for quality in the institutional gym equipment industry. Both their commercial and home products are no-nonsense and solidly built.

This machine has six separate stations. Three people can work out on it simultaneously. It offers more than 100 different exercises, yet takes up only a few feet of floor space. This versatility makes the Power Pak 400 one of the top-of-the-line home exercise systems.

The stations include a combination chest/shoulder press, a high pulley, a low pulley, a thigh/knee extension, an abdominal conditioner, a leg squat attachment and a leg press attachment.

WEIGHT: 700 lbs.
SIZE: 96″ × 112″ × 84″h
APPROXIMATE COST: $2,700 (chrome weight stacks $800 extra)

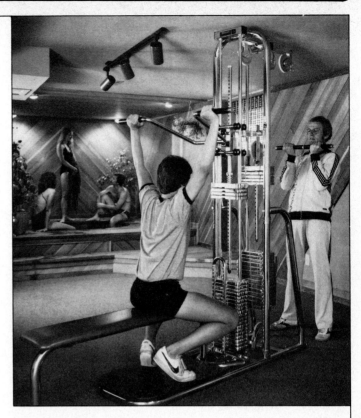

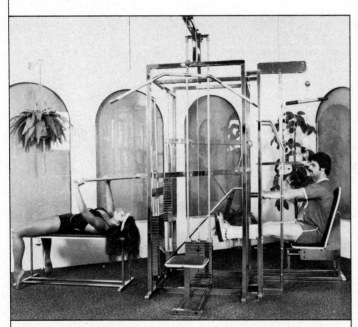

HOGGAN HEALTH EQUIPMENT, INC. COMPACT FITNESS CENTER

Hoggan has developed a reputation in the commercial gym equipment field for extremely polished-looking chrome weights, clean welds, and heavy solid steel construction. Their upholstery is well crafted and you can choose from dozens of colors. This multi-station, selectorized weight stack machine is actually a cut-down version of their larger commercial unit. This unit features four basic stations: a bench/shoulder press station, a seated-leg press, a lat and triceps pull-down, and a versatile single high-low pulley station good for biceps curls and inner/outer leg exercises. Various attachments like a low-row pulley, pivotal curl bar, and leg extension/leg curl bench are also available.

WEIGHT: 1,700 lbs.
SIZE: 6½′ × 11′ × 8′h
APPROXIMATE COST: $4,500 with black weights; $4,900 with chrome weights (optional leg extension/leg curl attachment, $500)

HEART RATE, INC. VERSA-CLIMBER

This unique machine lets you work most of your major muscle groups by duplicating the motion of vertical climbing. The device itself consists of a pole, set at a 75° angle, with hand grips and foot pedals. To exercise, you place your feet in the stirrup-style foot pedals and take hold of the hand grips. Then you step down on one pedal, while pulling down on the grip on the same side. On the opposite side, you push up on the grip and pull up on the pedal. The pedals and grips on opposite sides move synchronously, and the effect is much like that of climbing a ladder by lifting your body weight hand over foot at a selected time, rate, and distance.

Using the Versa-Climber gives you the same benefits you'd get by doing chin-ups, shoulder presses, leg presses, and weighted leg lifts simultaneously. You can set the machine for fast step rates and low resistance to give yourself an aerobic workout, or low rates and high resistance for isokinetic conditioning, similar to pumping iron. You can also stand on the base plate and work only your arms, or grasp the stationary hand grips and work just your legs.

The Versa-Climber's electronic metronome paces you from 25 to 95 beats per minute in five-beat increments. Its 10-digit LCD displays your exercise time, rate of climb (feet/minute), total feet climbed, strokes/minute, total strokes, and stroke length. Unorthodox as it looks, the Versa-Climber will give you a thorough, basic workout.

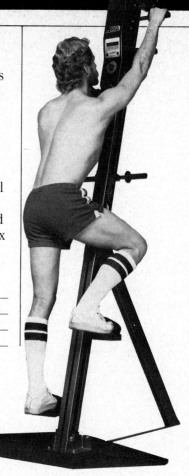

WEIGHT: 140 lbs.
SPACE: 4′ × 4′ × 7′10″h
APPROXIMATE COST: $2,795

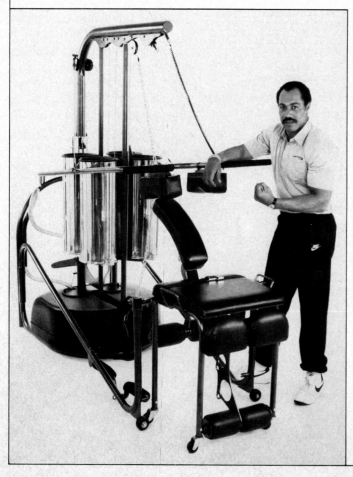

QUESTSTAR™ SELECTRONIC 2100

The Queststar looks like a Lunar Excursion Module and is nearly as impressive a piece of technology. This machine's weight medium is water. It's transferred by a valve-and-pump system from the reservoir in Queststar's base to the four weight cylinders. You initiate the transfer by touching a hand-held switch. What makes Queststar unique among weight machines is that the switch enables you to adjust your resistance *during any single repetition* of an exercise movement.

The Selectronic 2100 is Queststar's home fitness machine. You can do over 100 different exercises on it, varying resistance from zero to 360 pounds. This unit operates on ordinary household current. Its colors are chrome and dark pewter, with upholstery available in black and oxblood. (Other colors are extra-cost options.) Pulleys and cables are aircraft quality.

Queststar also offers a computerized version of the Selectronic 2100. If you already have a computer, they'll sell you their customized compatible software for it.

WEIGHT: (shipping) about 636 lbs.
SIZE: 4′ × 10′ × 7′3″h
House Current
APPROXIMATE COST: $4,995; software and computer components run from $500 to $4000 extra

FITNESS™ F602 POSITIVE RESISTANCE GYM

The Fitness Gym uses no weights or pulleys. Instead, there's an adjustable resistance cylinder (shock absorbent-type system) which supplies maximum resistance at each leverage point during each exercise. The roller glide system and pull-pin design lets you switch from leg to arm exercises easily. The padded foot-ankle bar adjusts within a full 360° range to accommodate any alternative force requirement. An optional electronic monitor called a potentiometer attaches to the resistance cylinder and reads out time in seconds and work in watt-seconds.

WEIGHT:	160 lbs.
SIZE:	62″ × 40″ × 59″h
APPROXIMATE COST:	$2,500

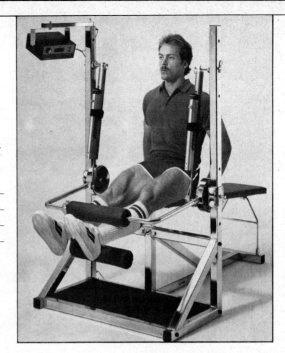

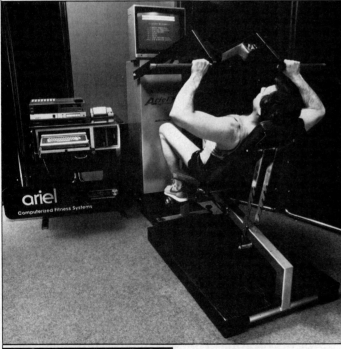

Left: Ariel 4000 #110A.
Below: Ariel 4000 #110B.

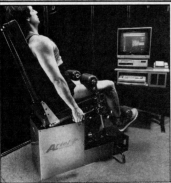

ARIEL 4000

Dr. Gideon Ariel developed the Ariel Computerized Exercise Machine for the Olympic athletes he trains at his own research center. You operate it by putting a fitness program disc into the unit's computer. The computer then adapts the equipment to the best speed, range of motion and weight resistance for your needs. As you work out, the computer's display screen gives you information on your progress as measured against your past performance and shows you how many calories you're burning. There's even a little Pac-Man–like character who eats a cheesecake— the harder you work, the quicker he eats. And while you're resting between sets, you can use the display screen to check out the latest stock quotations or catch the news.

There are two separate versions of the Ariel 4000. The #110A is a multi-function unit that allows you to do a wide range of exercises. The #110B is designed to concentrate on working your arms and legs. Each unit is hooked up to its own computer console—that is, one computer per unit.

Perhaps the Ariel 4000's price makes it more suited for rehabilitation and sports testing facilities than for individuals. But if it's high-tech you're looking for, this machine is just about the ultimate.

#110A (multi-function)	
WEIGHT:	400 lbs.
SIZE:	93″ × 30″ × 53½″h
House Current	

#110B (arm and leg)	
WEIGHT:	250 lbs.
SIZE:	42″ × 28″ × 54″
House Current	

APPROXIMATE COST:	about $16,500 for each unit. Options can run an additional $4,000.

Computer console for either unit:	
WEIGHT:	60 lbs.
SIZE:	23″ × 29″ × 45″h

FLEXIBILITY, STRETCHING AND GRAVITY INVERSION

You are probably aware of the need for regularly stretching your body in order to stay limber. It's not only important to feeling youthful, but it can help keep you from getting injured during sports and everyday activities.

Although we show you flexibility and stretching routines that use no equipment later in this book, in this section you'll find a number of devices to facilitate your quest for a supple body.

Two pieces of equipment, the SportStick and the Rack, are designed to stretch various major muscle groups. They are particularly useful for pre-sports training and warm-ups. When evaluating these kinds of devices, look for solid construction and safe design. Stretching should always be a slow, deliberate activity and you do not want any sudden or unexpected body movements.

All the other devices have to do with a somewhat new concept of *inversion* as it relates to a very old concept of *gravity*.

Gravity presses us all inexorably toward the center of the earth. This is generally a good thing—if you put something down, it's almost always in the same place when you come back for it.

But some of gravity's effects on our bodies are not so good. It compresses our spinal discs, slows our circulation, causes all our soft tissues (including our stomachs) to sag downward, and creates stressful twisting on our joints as they try to maintain a stable, upright posture against its unceasing force.

It's just good, old-fashioned common sense to try to use the force of gravity to our advantage. After all, that's what calisthenic exercise does: It forces us to work our bodies (or parts thereof) relative to gravity in ways in which they aren't normally exerted. (We're assuming that your job requires you to remain vertical most of the time. The rest of you know who you are.)

Now modern fitness technology has given us the inversion device, which enables us to use gravity in a new and helpful way.

An inversion device is a frame (either freestanding, ceiling/floor attached, or doormounted) from which you can hang yourself upside down. As you hang, you stretch your entire body in the opposite direction from the way it's compressed by gravity. This pulling is called traction.

Various inversion devices are designed to let you hang from either the thighs, the knees, or the ankles. You can hang completely upside down (that is, at a 180° angle from the upright vertical), or choose some lesser angle of decline. These devices may permit you to hang free (straight down from the ankles), or they may incorporate a bed or table that rotates around an axial bar. This swinging back and forth is called oscillation.

You may have seen these devices used, and you've probably seen them advertised. Unfortunately, there's been a lot of misinformation in the air about their "magical" effects. Here's what inversion devices really do for you—and what they don't:

• They remove pressure from and decompress the discs and, in some cases, the knee and ankle joints.

• They increase the flow of blood to the brain and head region.

• They seem to reduce stress considerably.

• They do not, by themselves, strengthen your muscles. Many inversion devices allow you to exercise while you hang, but in some cases, the exercises you're doing can be performed more efficiently when you're right-side-up.

Are there any problems that go with inversion? Yes, there can be. Hanging upside down temporarily increases your blood pressure. The increase is generally small, and blood pressure usually returns to normal immediately on return to the upright, seated position. But if you have hypertension or if you're a stroke or coronary risk, you should consult a physician—*not* just a coach or trainer—before you start an inversion program.

Other conditions that could preclude you from engaging in an inversion (or other fitness) program would include serious heart, vascular, or pulmonary disease; hypertension; detached retina; glaucoma; recent surgery; certain types of hernia; extreme obesity; diabetes; pregnancy; and the use of certain drugs (such as anticoagulating medications).

The major danger inversion poses to an otherwise healthy person is, as you've probably suspected, falling on your head. So when you look for inversion equipment, look for frame stability, specific accessories you feel are important to your overall program, safety and comfort of the ankle collars or thigh pads, quality of the welds on stress-bearing joints, general comfort while in an inverted position, and a reliable manufacturer who'll provide a reasonable warranty and instruction manual.

Table-style devices (oscillating bed-types) that rotate on a central axis are easier to mount and dismount than the free-hanging units from which you hang by your ankles (inversion boots and doorway bar). They also leave you with less chance of getting stuck upside down, and they allow you to choose your angle of decline. Most units are also collapsible for fairly easy storage.

Look out for any doorway-mounted inversion device whose mounting brackets don't *bolt into* the door frame. Avoid units with only pressure-mounted door bars. These are usually designed only for chin-ups and pull-ups. Also, look out for free-hanging (ankle-suspension) units whose boots or straps are uncomfortable or too large for your feet. The idea is to be able to hang totally relaxed without slipping out of the ankle collars.

It should be noted that most oscillating inversion devices are not intended for use by children or people under 4'5" and weighing less than 85 pounds. If you are unusually tall or obese you may also have difficulty finding a unit that works for you.

When using free-standing or oscillating-type units, here are some tips to keep in mind before inverting:

• Units should be on a hard surface for stability during operation. Thick pile carpeting is generally not recommended.

• Rotate the oscillation bed to make sure

there is sufficient ceiling clearance, and make sure it is able to operate away from windows, sliding glass doors, and other obstacles.

• Units can generate dynamic force when operated too rapidly. Move slowly, always keeping elbows close to the body. Rapid rotation coupled with body weight may cause the device to tip over.

• Check the exercise unit over carefully, making sure it is properly installed, with the pin securely in the lowest hole.

• Use a spotter your first time. Inversion can be a bit confusing until you become familiar with the sensation of being upside down. Another person can assist you in case of difficulty during your initiation.

How much inversion is good for us? You can hang yourself (upside down, that is) every day, both before and after exercise. Spending from 10 seconds to 10 minutes each day in an inverted position can bring you noticeable results. As with all exercise, you should start at the lower limit and work up to the maximum. Too much stretching too soon can be as traumatic to your body as too much of anything else. In addition, inversion can increase the blood pressure and other fluids in your head, so some people will find it uncomfortable to hang for very long at first. But again, as with any other exercise, you can build up a tolerance to this new, positive physical stress by proceeding gradually.

According to Drs. Mark D. Grabiner and Leroy Perry, Jr., members of the High-Tech Fitness Team, inversion is primarily a mechanism by which we can apply traction to stretch our lower backs. Its greatest effects are on our "passive" tissue, such as cartilage (specifically discs) and ligaments. (These tissues are passive because, unlike muscle tissue, they don't actively cause motion).

Our discs are pieces of cartilage which act as shock absorbers between our vertebrae. They undergo constant compression by gravity. As we grow older, they degenerate and become less elastic. One result of this process of degeneration is that people grow shorter as they grow older. Their discs are compressed thinner and thinner and become less efficient at distributing stresses on the spinal column. Thus, they (and we) become less resistant to injury. That's one of the reasons why most Americans suffer from backache at some time in their lives.

Inversion relieves gravity's compression effect on our discs by making gravity pull on the spine in the opposite direction. It gives our hard-working spines a rest from their daily toil.

Can inversion relieve back pain? Research indicates that it sometimes can. One Ohio State University study, for example, showed that over 80 percent of patients with back pain felt an improvement after inversion.

Indeed, it has been suggested that most backaches result from weak muscles that cannot counter the effects of gravity on the body. Fortunately, muscle weakness can be rectified through appropriate strengthening exercises, which often leads to the relief of back pain.

Some research has suggested that bent-knee (forward) inversion *may* stretch your lower back better than straight-leg (from the ankles) inversion. Hanging from the ankles *may* have a negative effect on people with ankle, knee, or hip joint problems. On the other hand, straight-leg inversion allows you to do different kinds of exercises while you're hanging around and may be easier for you. More clinical research is being conducted to further study the effects of inversion on the body.

ANATOMY OF A GRAVITY INVERSION DEVICE

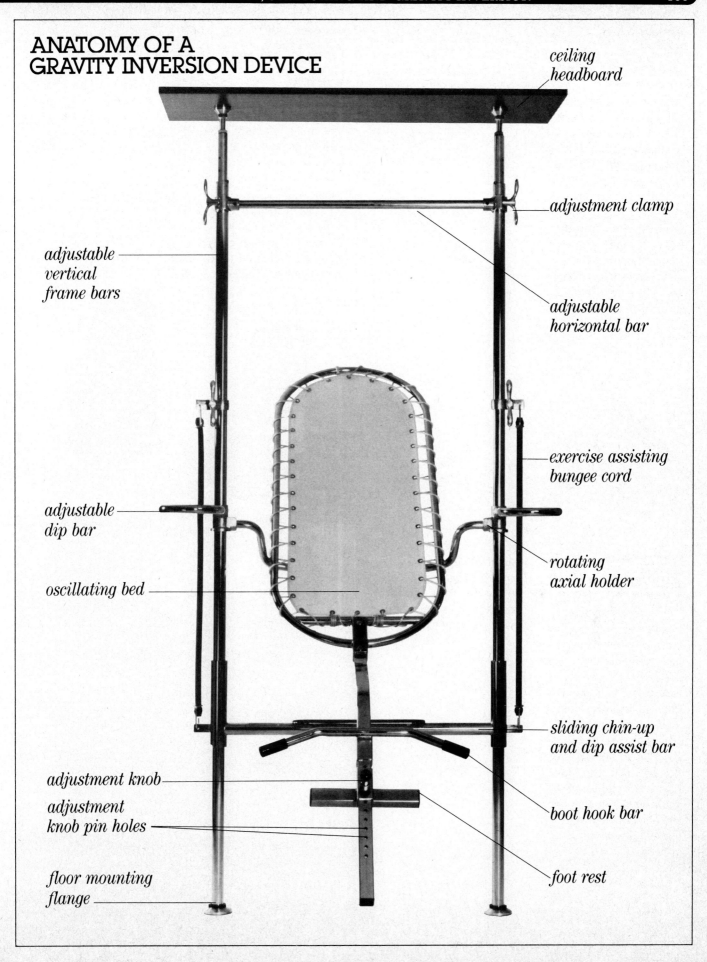

ceiling headboard

adjustment clamp

adjustable vertical frame bars

adjustable horizontal bar

exercise assisting bungee cord

adjustable dip bar

rotating axial holder

oscillating bed

sliding chin-up and dip assist bar

adjustment knob

adjustment knob pin holes

boot hook bar

floor mounting flange

foot rest

GRAVITY GUIDANCE INC. INVERSION BAR®

You can pair this chrome bar with your inversion boots for the most economical inversion exercise system possible. The bar is also ideal for such standard upright exercises as chin-ups and pull-ups. Designed to fit doorways from 30″ to 36″ wide, it supports up to 300 lbs. and is safer than ordinary pressure bars using no screwed-in brackets.

Mounting hardware is included in the package. You can easily remove the Gravity Guidance bar for storage.

WEIGHT: 2½ lbs.
SIZE: 1⅛″ × 30″ to 36″
APPROXIMATE COST: $24.95

GRAVITY GUIDANCE INC. INVERSION BOOTS®

Gravity Guidance was the first to manufacture inversion boots, and their products are still the "Rolls Royce" of the upside-down business.

Their boots are durable and chip-resistant. They're black, with copolymer foam lining for maximum comfort. One size fits all, but you can vary the comfort level by adding one or more of the provided spongy foam inserts. These are the top-of-the-line inversion boots on the market. They can be used with any bar or machine that requires boots, although the manufacturer prefers you use them with Gravity Guidance equipment.

WEIGHT: 5½ lbs. per pair
SIZE: 9″ × 6″ × 10″ h
APPROXIMATE COST: $59.95 black; $79.95 chrome

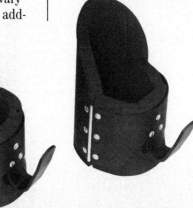

H.W.E. GRAVITATOR®

This well-constructed, functional, oscillating inversion system comes with padded lumbar back support, automatic safety lock, safety belt, hand grips for leg raises and dips, a chinning and stretching bar, and a shiatsu foot massager/reflexology pad. The Gravitator features adjustable ankle collars of high-density foam; no boots are required. This easy-to-assemble unit comes in brown Naugahyde. H.W.E. also has a lighter-weight, portable unit, complete with carrying case.

WEIGHT: 60 lbs.
SIZE: 30″ × 51″ × 79″ to 92″ h
APPROXIMATE COST: $499; portable unit with carrying case (not shown), $299

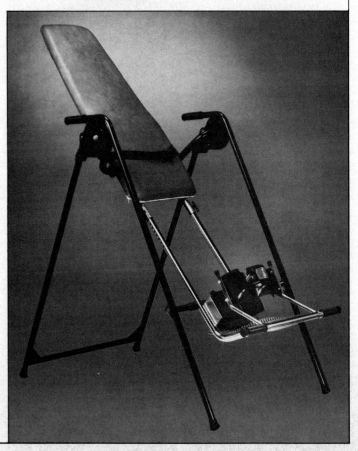

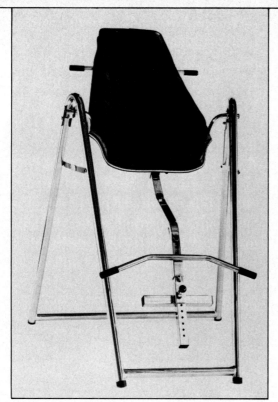

GRAVITY GUIDANCE INC. 1121 GRAVITY GUIDING SYSTEM®

This well-designed, full-length oscillating unit is one of the best units on the market. It sports a heavy-gauge steel A-frame, and a custom-upholstered oscillating bed for optimum comfort. The color scheme is chrome and black.

The 1121 is adjustable for the user's weight (from 100 to 300 lbs.) and height (from 5′ to 6′7″).

It's portable and folds easily for storage. You need inversion boots with this unit and must buy them separately.

WEIGHT: 40 lbs.
SIZE: 43″ × 26″ × 6′h
APPROXIMATE COST: $589.95

GRAVITY GUIDANCE INC. 1130 GRAVITY GUIDING SYSTEM®

This is the most comprehensive full body traction device you can buy for home or professional use. The fully integrated traction/inversion system provides both intermittent traction through oscillation (swinging), and sustained traction through free-hanging inversion by its top horizontal bar.

The unit features a comfortable, removable oscillation bed, an adjustable horizontal bar, a toggle bar (pivotal fitness bar) that attaches to the horizontal bar to give you an upper body workout, an assist mechanism, and parallel grip bars for knee-ups and dips.

The 1130 comes in chrome and white canvas. It requires some (actually, quite a bit of) assembly, but it's well worth the effort.

WEIGHT: 106 lbs.
SIZE: 88″ × 35″ × 10½′ (adjustable to ceiling height)
APPROXIMATE COST: $1,195

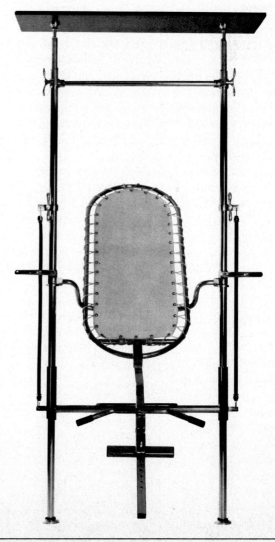

MARCY ORTHOPOD® GRAVITY TRACTION SYSTEM

The Orthopod is a bent-knee (forward) inversion device—you hang from your thighs instead of your ankles. It's an effective way to relieve gravitational compression of the upper and lower back. This free-standing unit requires no bolts, no accessories, and comes in basic black. It will handle up to 300 lbs., and has two height adjustments and thick, comfortable thigh pads. The Orthopod is lightweight, portable, relatively easy to use, and folds for storage.

WEIGHT: 35 lbs.
SIZE: 24″ × 30″ × 4′h
APPROXIMATE COST: $329

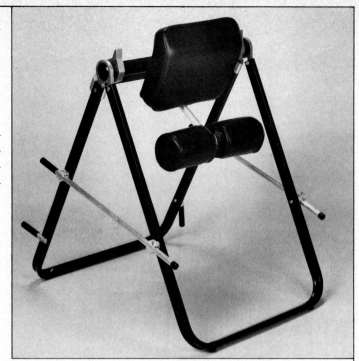

GYM-MOBILE™ EXERCISE AND INVERSION SYSTEM

You'll note from the photograph that this device looks quite different from most inversion systems. The Gym-Mobile consists of a square steel bracket that hangs from your doorway header or any sturdy wood beam. When not in use, the bracket stores away upright on door hooks. There are no inversion boots. Instead, a flexible, cushioned thigh support (like a sling swing in a schoolyard) hangs from the bracket by a chain.

The Gym-Mobile's design allows you to hang from your upper thighs with your legs bent, a position some people find more comfortable than hanging from a boot-system gravity device. Because it is not stationary, it may take you a few times of inverting to get "the hang of it." You can do more than 25 exercises, some of which you can't do with other systems. You can thus stretch and strengthen every muscle group, even the hard-to-reach ones—just be careful not to over-stretch.

The Gym-Mobile is adjustable for people of almost any height. It's lightweight, sturdy, and requires less than a square yard of floor space. If you don't have doors, or if they're too narrow, there's a free-standing Gym-Mobile with a vertical frame. Both models come with illustrated exercise charts.

DOORWAY MODEL
WEIGHT: 13 lbs. (shipping)
SIZE: 3″ × 25″ × 26″h
APPROXIMATE COST: $199

FREE-STANDING MODEL
WEIGHT: 40 lbs. (shipping)
SIZE: 30″ × 29″ × 60″h
APPROXIMATE COST: $275

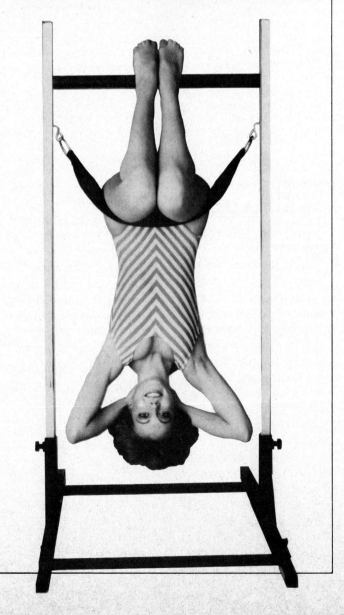

BED-STYLE INVERSION

STARTING POSITION: With the inversion bed in the upright position, stand with your back against the bed. Secure your ankles and feet in the provided brackets, boots, or collars. Lie on the bed and lean backward against it at the same time. Adjust the foot mechanism by raising or lowering it until you are at an approximate 30° angle to the floor, with your head higher than your feet. Your arms should be at your side, your head back (not shown).

MOTION: Extend arms slowly overhead until you achieve your desired angle of inversion. Hold the position. Return by slowly swinging your arms back to your sides.

Most machines have hand assists to help in the backward rotation, so you can easily control speed and extent of the movement. You have the option to hang completely inverted, at a lesser angle of decline, or to oscillate back and forth. Some apparatuses require you to balance in less-than-vertical angles, while others offer a locking device to hold you firmly at different angles of decline. Some people start with as little as 10 to 30 seconds of inversion. Only invert as long as it feels comfortable.

PRECAUTIONS: Make sure the feet and ankle supports fit and you feel secure without pressure or pinching. You may want to use the additional foam lining pads provided with the better boots. Let the foam hang down a bit below the bottom of the boot to give your feet better cushioning. Invert slowly to allow blood flow and pressures to adjust gradually. You may want to return to the neutral position for a moment before dismounting. Although bed-style inversion has the advantage of lesser angles of inversion and oscillation, it does place some pressure on the ankles, knees, and hips that may be contraindicated for some conditions. Check with your doctor as to the best form of inversion for you.

AREAS STRETCHED: Back, hips, knees, ankles.

MUSCLES STRETCHED: Erector spinae, deep posterior group, rectus abdominis, all leg muscles.

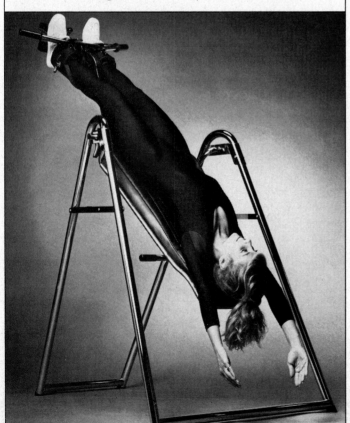

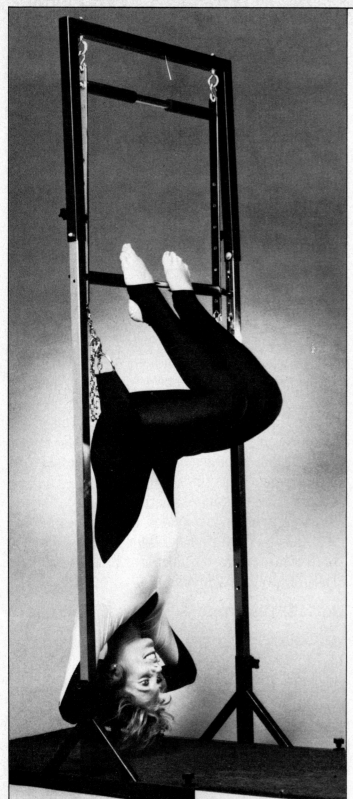

BENT-KNEE (FORWARD) INVERSION

STARTING POSITION: Face the padded bar or sling that will be supporting the pressure of your hips and thighs.

MOTION: Using whatever hand assists are provided by your machine, lean forward to drape your body over the bar or sling. As your torso approaches the vertical position, intercept the restraining foot or calf bar. It is the mechanism which "holds" you securely in the machine so you can relax without feeling you are going to slip out. Hang for a time, then use hand assists to push your torso back to the upright position.

PRECAUTIONS: Take your time to fully invert, as your body needs a little time to adjust to the temporary changes in blood flow and pressure. Although you'll feel like a pro at mounting and dismounting in no time, try to have someone assist and watch you in the beginning.

AREAS STRETCHED: The lumbar (lower) spine as well as the upper back.

MUSCLES STRETCHED: Erector spinae, deep posterior group, quadratus lumborum, iliopsoas.

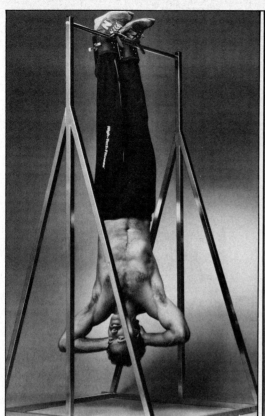
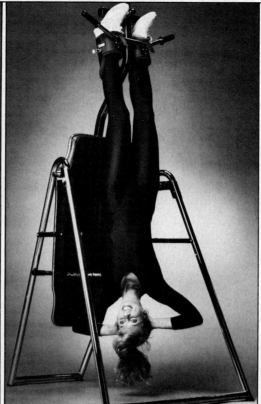
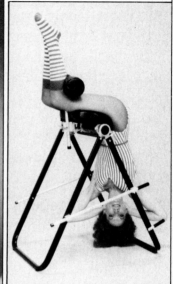

INVERTED TORSO TWISTS

STARTING POSITION: Once comfortably inverted, clasp your hands behind your neck.

MOTION: Twist your upper torso (from waist to head) toward one side, and then to the other. Perform this motion smoothly, without jerking your shoulders or rib cage. Breathe normally and rhythmically.

PRECAUTIONS: Twisting the spine gives mobility to all the vertebral joints, but should be done smoothly, slowly, and with caution. Since the spine is already experiencing a substantial stretch due to the inverted position, it is in a somewhat vulnerable state and could easily be overstretched. Therefore, *do not force* the twisting movement. More twisting range of motion can be achieved when hanging from the ankles than from the pelvis. However, it is important to realize that this increase is mainly due to the greater freedom of the overall body to move. Most of the increased twist is occurring in the hips, thighs, and knees—not in the spine. If you have a back problem, check with your doctor or therapist about twisting movements in general.

AREAS STRETCHED: Sides of torso and back.

MUSCLES STRETCHED: Erector spinae, internal and external obliques.

INVERTED SIT-UPS

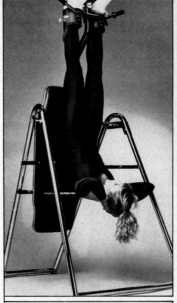
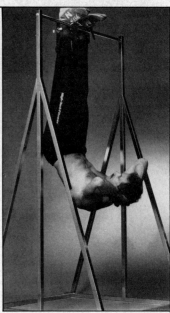
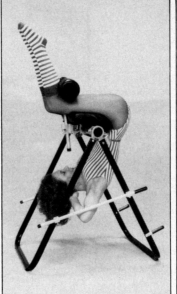
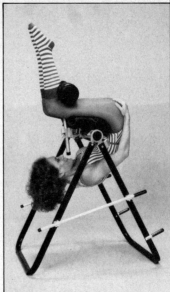

STARTING POSITION: Once comfortably inverted, clasp your hands behind your head.

MOTION: Slowly curl your torso upward so that your head is being pulled closer toward your slightly bent knees. Do this segmentally by first lifting your head, then your neck, shoulders, and rib cage. To return to the original position, lower your body segmentally in reverse order. Exhale as you curl your torso upward, and inhale as you lower it to the vertical hanging position.

PRECAUTIONS: Do the movement slowly with a lifting motion rather than a yanking one. By all means, do not pull your neck to assist the exercise. If you have upper back or neck problems, you may want to cross your arms over your chest rather than place your hands behind your head. Concentrate on using only the muscles of your torso and keeping the muscles on the front of your thigh as relaxed as possible.

Exercises for increasing abdominal strength can be done on all inversion machines. The straight-legged form, which is done on the machines that hang you from the ankles, demands greater work from the hip flexors, quadriceps, iliacus, psoas majors and less from the abdominal muscles (rectus abdominis, internal and external obliques). When hanging from the pelvis, hips, or thighs with the hips flexed, the contribution of the hip flexors is reduced considerably and the exercise works the abdominal muscles almost solely.

If you have lower back pain, these exercises could aggravate the condition.

AREAS STRENGTHENED: Front of thighs, front and sides of torso, front and sides of neck.

MUSCLES STRENGTHENED: Quadriceps, rectus abdominis, internal and external obliques, sternocleidomastoids.

CHIN-UPS

STARTING POSITION: Face the bed of the inversion machine and grasp the overhead handles in an underhand grip.

MOTION: Keeping your body fairly motionless, pull your chin up toward the handles by bending your elbows and pulling your upper arms down toward the sides of your rib cage. Return to the starting position by straightening your elbows and fully extending your arms. Exhale as you pull your body up, and inhale as you lower it downward.

PRECAUTIONS: Make sure the bed is securely locked into the upright position. The bed position diminishes the swinging motion of regular chin-ups and makes the movement a bit more difficult and isolated. If you are too weak to do a chin-up, you can gain strength by doing the "lowering" portion of the movement only. Get up on a step or crate to get to the top position (chin at bar), and then lower the body as slowly as possible until you build strength and control.

AREAS STRENGTHENED: Front of forearms and upper arms, upper chest, back of upper arms, sides of upper back.

MUSCLES STRENGTHENED: Brachioradialis, biceps, pectorals, triceps, latissimus dorsi, teres majors.

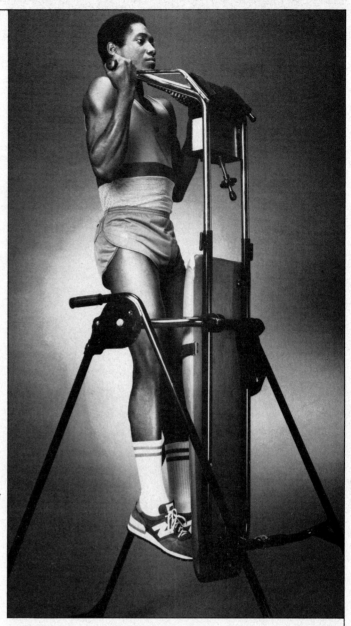

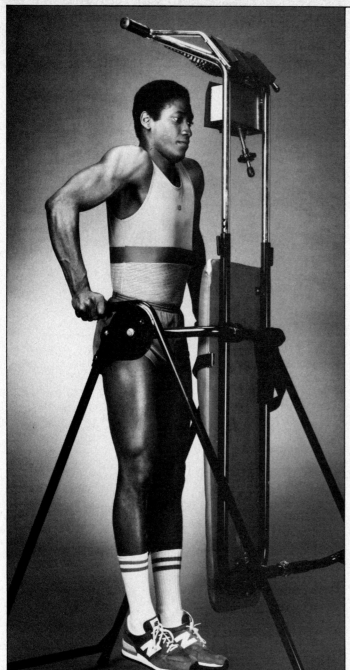

DIPS

STARTING POSITION: Face the bed of the inversion machine and place your hands on the lower set of horizontal handles.

MOTION: With a small jump, elevate your body off the floor, arms completely straight at the sides and torso hanging between the handles. Holding your entire body vertical, lower yourself toward the floor by bending your elbows and letting your upper arms move backward behind your body. Return to the upright hanging position by straightening your elbows and pressing your upper arm down and forward toward the sides of your rib cage. Inhale as your body is lowered toward the floor, and exhale as you push upward.

PRECAUTIONS: This is typically a very difficult exercise for most people. If you need an easier version, do the lowering phase only, and use a step or crate to get back up to the starting position. Try to keep your head and neck as relaxed as possible so that the chest, arms, and shoulders can recruit maximum energy.

AREAS STRENGTHENED: Front of shoulder and chest, back of upper arms, middle and sides of mid-back.

MUSCLES STRENGTHENED: Anterior deltoids, pectoralis majors, triceps, subclavius, pectoralis minors, trapezius.

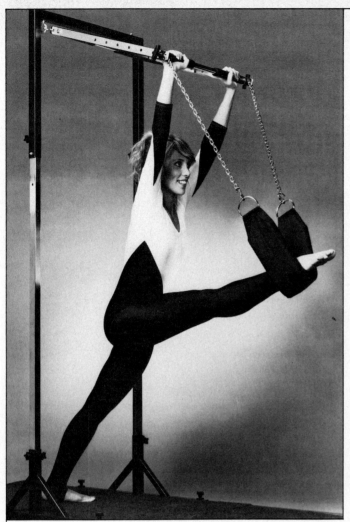

SPLIT STRETCH

STARTING POSITION: Stand with your back to the machine. Grasp the bar in an overhand fashion. Place one foot in the sling and the other directly underneath the machine's frame.

MOTION: Allow your body to lean forward until your arms are straight overhead and your front leg in the sling is straightened in front of your body. Keep the foot of your support leg flat on the floor to give your calf the maximum stretch possible. Hold the stretch, and then return to the starting position by bending your support leg and leaning backward.

PRECAUTIONS: The exercise is to be done with the simultaneous control of the arms and the legs, so you don't stretch further than you are capable. Make sure your front leg and arms are straight and the foot of your support leg is flat. Any *one* of these areas may be tighter than the others and may limit the extent to which you can perform the entire movement. Let the tightest area govern the movement until you eventually stretch it out and can move further into your stretch. Exhale into the stretch; otherwise breathe normally.

AREAS STRETCHED: Back of calves, front of thighs and hips (support leg), back of thighs and hips (suspended leg), inner thighs, front of torso, back of upper arms, front of shoulders, and sides of upper back.

MUSCLES STRETCHED: Soleus, gastrocnemius, quadriceps, iliopsoas, hamstrings, gluteus maximus, adductors, rectus abdominis, triceps, deltoids, latissimus dorsi, teres majors.

SHOULDER AND CHEST STRETCH

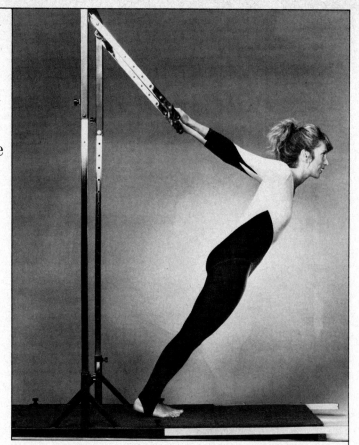

STARTING POSITION: Stand with your back to the machine and situated so that the trapeze will swing toward your back. Heels should be placed about one foot in front of the machine frame. Reach behind your body and grasp the trapeze bar in an overhang grip.

MOTION: Keeping your body straight from your shoulders to your heels, lean forward as far as you can. Hold the stretch, then return to the starting position by leaning backward to a normal standing position.

PRECAUTIONS: Lean forward slowly at first, so you do not jerk on your shoulder joints. The shoulders and chest may be very tight, especially on individuals who are round-shouldered or who spend a great deal of time doing desk work. Also, your calves may be so tight that your heels tend to lift up from the floor. Whichever area is the tightest, let it govern the degree to which you perform the entire exercise. As you become more limber, you can move further into the stretch. Exhale into the stretch; otherwise breathe normally.

AREAS STRETCHED: Front of chest and shoulder, front of torso, front of thighs, and rear of calves.

MUSCLES STRETCHED: Pectorals, anterior deltoids, rectus abdominis, quadriceps, gastrocnemius, and soleus.

THE RACK

This unique and innovative Y-shaped device lets you increase the flexibility of your lower body by allowing you to stretch both legs, either independently or together, against controlled resistance. You set the angle against which your legs are to stretch (from 0° to 195°) by manipulating the handcrank, then push the handcrank assembly forward or pull it back to provide resistance. You can work one leg at a time by moving a shift lever that renders either leg immobile. The idea is to increase the elasticity of your leg muscles to give yourself a longer stride, a wider stance, a higher kick or

a more complete follow-through. A side benefit is that the more flexible you are, the less prone to sports injuries you'll be.

The Rack is made from tubular steel, welded at the joints, with a baked-on, metallic-colored epoxie finish. Upholstery is one-inch polyurethane foam, covered by black elastic-backed vinyl. The device folds for convenient storage. There's a somewhat larger institutional model, Biostretch, made of stainless steel and designed for injury rehabilitation.

WEIGHT: 52 lbs.
SIZE: 17″ × 42″ × 9½″ h
APPROXIMATE COST: $295;
Biostretch, $300 to $600

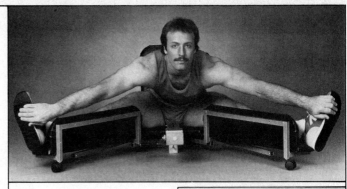

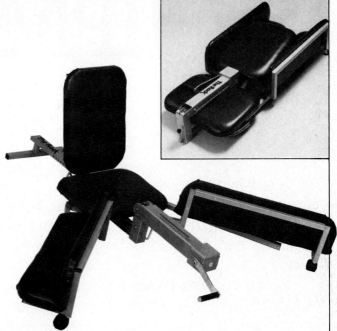

BODY SLANT

This is the most conservative of all inversion units. It's a favorite with the older generation, many of whom are uncomfortable hanging upside down. The Body Slant unfolds into four different positions, so it can double as a single bed, ottoman, or lounger. In one posi-

tion, you can lie down with your feet elevated above your head. The Body Slant comes in nine colors.

WEIGHT: 14 lbs.
SIZE: 6′ × 22″ × 7″ to 14″h
APPROXIMATE COST: $139.95

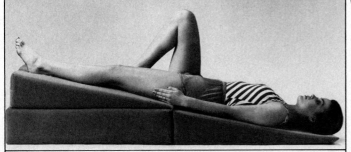

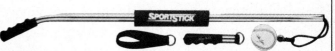

SPYMARK SPORTSTICK™

This baton-size exercise device consists of a lever with a stretching cord. It comes with a baseball grip, a handgrip, and a foot sling. It's designed to help you stretch major muscle groups to avoid

soreness and sports injuries by using the isometric/isotonic principle. To get maximum benefit from the SportStick, however, you must *already* be relatively flexible.

WEIGHT: 2½ lbs.
SIZES: 33″ × 3¼″
APPROXIMATE COST: $29.95

BALANCE AND COORDINATION EQUIPMENT

Skiing and gymnastics require a good sense of balance. Football, baseball, and the racquet sports demand a high degree of hand-eye coordination. In fact, good balance and coordination are prerequisites to success in any sport.

What's less well known is the importance of balance and coordination in everyday life. There is a direct relationship between the high incidence of household accidents among the elderly and the general decline in balance and coordination that often comes (but need not) with age. Educators have found that the acquisition of balance and coordination skills at an early age correlates with scholastic achievement, especially in math and languages. In fact, some educators and therapists use trampolines to improve the motor skills of students whom they're treating for learning disabilities. Clearly, even if you don't want to be an Olympic pole-vaulter or an NFL running back, balance and coordination are useful traits to have.

We've chosen five kinds of home gym equipment that will help you in these areas: the ballet barre, the balance beam, rings, the JetStar, and the backyard trampoline.

The first three items have no moving parts. You just need to pay attention to the quality of the materials and the way the units are con-structed. The fourth item, the JetStar, is one of a kind.

But there are many different makes and models of trampolines, and before you shop for one, there are a few things you should know. The first is that backyard trampolines are probably the most underrated fitness devices ever made. Their use will improve your balance, co-ordination, timing, rhythm, and poise more effectively than any other piece of fitness equipment.

We've all heard the horror stories about people incurring serious injuries on trampolines. Such injuries have happened, but the trampoline isn't an inherently dangerous device. If you're careful, it can be safe enough for everyone, even the very young.

If you've never used a trampoline, the sensation of walking or standing on the mat may surprise and even disorient you at first. It's not at all like standing on solid ground. You may even be a little afraid of the power of the springs as you bounce. That's why it's very important to take time to get used to the trampoline before you begin an exercise program. You should become completely familiar with and proficient at the simpler trampoline moves before attempting the harder ones. You should *always* jump with one or more spotters around, and only one jumper should use the tramp at any given time.

Once you get used to the feel of a trampoline, you'll realize that no other form of exercise is more fun. As you become more acclimated, your confidence and capabilities will develop. You'll find that simply jumping up and down for 15 or 20 minutes gives you a fantastic aerobic workout.

If you're looking for a trampoline, be sure to get one with sturdy safety pads that cover the entire frame and butt right up to the mat. Most trampoline injuries occur when someone comes down between the frame and the mat.

In terms of construction, look for heavy-duty springs (although you can easily replace low-quality springs with better ones), a welded frame, and an ultraviolet-resistant polypropylene bed (jumping surface). White nylon web beds give you more rebounding resilience, but they won't last as long in the sun and the weather.

The general rule about trampolines is: the larger the jumping surface, the better. Why? On a physical level, a larger bed gives you more room to make a mistake. On a psychological level, you'll feel more secure with a larger bed.

A 14- or 16-foot octagon is probably the best shape and size for general use or for beginning jumpers. Octagons are better than round units for two reasons. First, the bounce is more even all over the mat, not just in the center. Second, the eight sides can be used as reference or spotting points. The drawback to the octagon is that these larger units will have a somewhat slower, mushier bounce than similar-size circular models. You won't be able to bounce quite as high. Large square units have a slightly livelier bounce. These are fine, too.

For more serious or experienced jumpers, the standard 6 × 12- or 7 × 14-foot rectangular trampolines are probably a better choice. (Incidentally, the dimensions refer to bed sizes. To get the overall size, add 1 or 2 feet per side.) The big rectangles are "hotter," that is, livelier and more resilient when you bounce. But they don't have as much working area as the larger octagons.

If you have enough room in your backyard (or if you have 14-foot ceilings), a trampoline is the most fun way we can think of to keep fit.

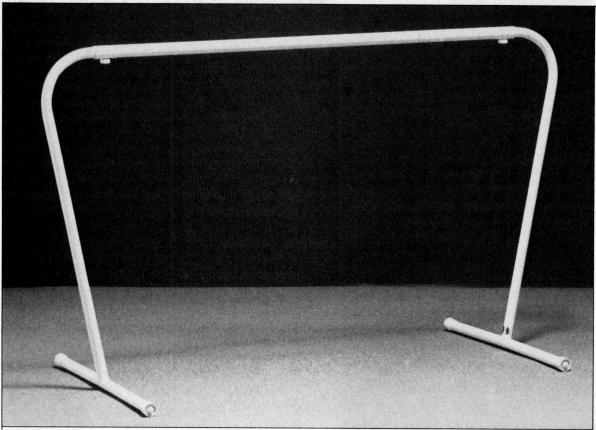

NU-BARRE ®

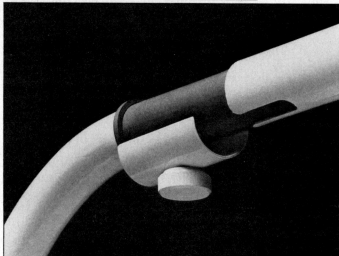

Millions of Americans dance for fun, for fitness, and for artistic expression. Yet very few of us can afford a mirrored rehearsal room with an attached ballet barre. That's why Nu-Barres are an idea whose time has come.

The Nu-Barre is a portable stretching barre which supports your entire weight. The barre's feet are rubber, to protect your floor and remain stationary on the floor. Nu-Barre's force-lock principle keeps the barre totally stable and enables you to use the device for both upper and lower body toning.

The barre is coated with electrostatically applied epoxy powder, baked on in your choice of white, black, strawberry red, peacock blue, gray, chocolate, or midnight blue. The epoxy gives you a reliable grip and a durable finish that's easy to clean.

The Nu-Barre's feet connect with a single bolt. The upper section requires no tools, and the unit can be quickly set up or taken down.

Nu-Barres come in a standard height of 42 inches unless otherwise specified, and in 5-, 8- and 10-foot lengths. Double barres are also available.

SIZES	WEIGHTS
5′	32 lbs.
8′	34 lbs.
10′	38 lbs.

APPROXIMATE COST:

SIZES	SINGLE BARRE	DOUBLE BARRE
5′	$149	$199
8′	$169	$229
10′	$189	$249

COLORS (other than white): $15 extra

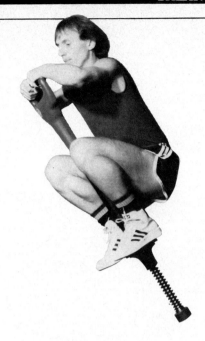

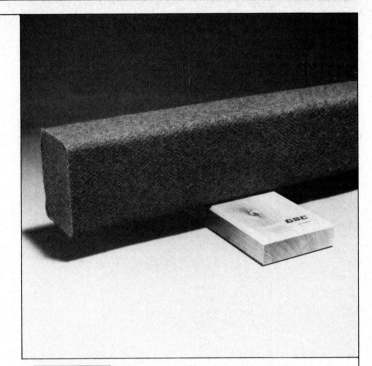

JETSTAR™ SUPERTRAINER

A high-tech pogo stick, the West German–made JetStar features a heavy-duty steel spring, rubber foot and handgrips, non-skid rubber footrests, and a six-month warranty. You can jump as high as 35 inches on the JetStar (the current world's record), and it will support a 300-pounder.

You may be surprised to learn that jumping on a JetStar will actually give you an aerobic workout as well. This activity requires you to constantly adjust your balance, thus strengthening all muscle groups, tendons, ligaments, and joints. When you pogo on one of these devices, you improve your take-off power, your mobility, your posture, your reaction ability, and your balance. It helps you lessen the risk of injury in any sport you play.

To decrease the risk of injury in *this* activity, you should be careful to take it slowly the first few times you use the JetStar. Jumping on a pogo stick is like riding a bike—you have to learn how to do it before you attain any degree of competence.

WEIGHT: 8 lbs.
SIZE: 12″ × 3½″ × 51″ h
APPROXIMATE COST: $119

GSC CARPETED PRACTICE BEAM SYSTEM

The balance beam is a long, narrow piece of wood that helps you develop your balancing skills and your kinesthetic sense and awareness.

What kind of exercises can you do on a balance beam? Just one: you can walk on it—barefoot, in socks, or in shoes for extra support. When you get tired of walking forward you can walk backward, and when you tire of *that,* you can hop or skip. That's what a balance beam was designed to be used for. It's one of the oldest and simplest pieces of fitness equipment.

We've chosen to illustrate the GSC Carpeted Practice Beam System. AMF makes a good model as well. The GSC has a 4-inch working surface (that is, the top of the beam is 4 inches wide), with a quarter-inch of rubber padding on top of it. It's covered with a layer of red carpeting. The beam sits on wooden blocks at either end, putting the top of the beam 8 inches off the floor.

WEIGHT: 70 lbs.
LENGTH: 12′
APPROXIMATE COST: $164

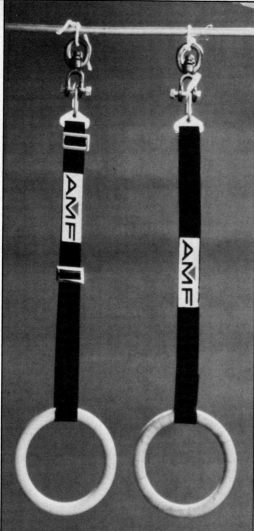

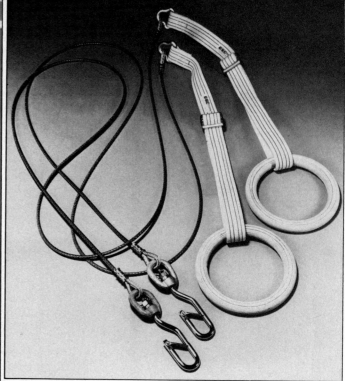

RING SETS

You've probably watched gymnasts work out on the rings. They're good for swinging and support, and there are many coordination-enhancing gymnastic routines you can do on them. If you're looking for simpler exercise, you can do chin-ups, pull-ups, and bar dips on the rings.

The rings themselves are made of laminated hardwood. They're attached to cotton webbing or nylon straps, usually 2 inches wide, and the straps are attached to stainless steel aircraft cable.

If you're using the rings inside, be sure to attach them to a ceiling beam—a heavy one. Outdoors, you can put up your own frame made from pipe. Be sure to sink the ends of the pipe in concrete. Either way, it's important to provide some sort of padding underneath the rings as a safety measure.

Adjustable ring sets (not shown) include a cable-and-pulley arrangement that lets you vary the height of the rings. The international regulation length for rings and cables is 18 feet 4 inches.

GSC and AMF both make good ring sets. Our figures are for GSC equipment. Prices for AMF are similar.

OFFICIAL RING SET (clamps, snap swivels, cable, webbing, rings)

WEIGHT: 25 lbs.

APPROXIMATE COST: $240; rings alone, $58

ADJUSTABLE RING SET (pulleys, chain, snap swivels, webbing, rings, mounting cleat)

WEIGHT: 115 lbs.

APPROXIMATE COST: $630; webbing straps alone, $18.80

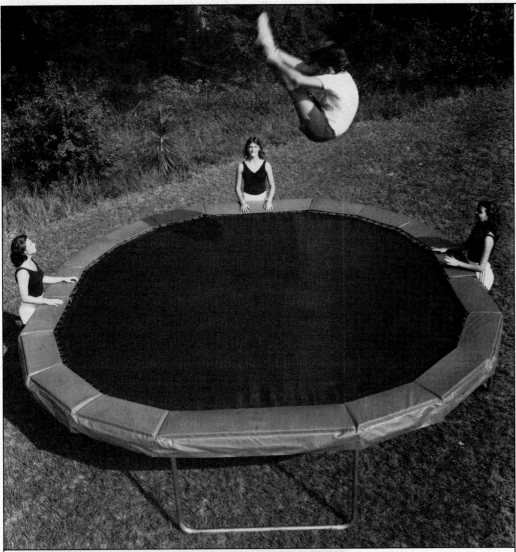

TRAMPOLKING TRAMPOLINES

TrampolKing is like the General Motors of the trampoline industry. Their products are well built, reliable, and carry a five-year limited warranty. These tramps are made with zinc-coated steel tubing (the kind used for chain-link fenceposts), 8-inch zinc-plated, heat-tempered steel springs, zinc-plated V-rings with 1,800-pound-test webbing, and 1,400-pound-test polypropylene beds.

Other reputable manufacturers include Sidlinger, American Playworld, AMF, and Round Trampolines.

We repeat our recommendation that you always buy heavy-duty frame and spring bumper pads with your trampoline. And again, never work out on your tramp without a spotter. The following are TrampolKing sizes and prices:

MODEL:	APPROXIMATE COST:
5′ octagon	$344.95
14′ octagon	$639.95
16′ octagon	$739.95
5′ × 10′ rectangle	$519.95
6′ × 12′ rectangle	$559.95
7′ × 14′ rectangle	$789.95

HEAVY-DUTY BUMPER PADS
APPROXIMATE COST: $149.95 to $209.95, depending on the size and shape of your trampoline

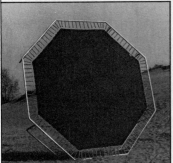

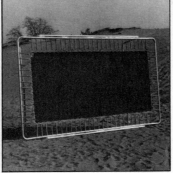

RELAXATION AND STRESS REDUCTION EQUIPMENT

The most dangerous aspect of our modern environment isn't dioxin or smog or even *Gilligan's Island* reruns. It's stress. Stress has been linked to virtually every illness that plagues mankind, from the common cold to cancer and heart disease.

There's nothing new about stress. Our Neolithic ancestors experienced plenty of it when chasing after their dinner, or running like crazy to avoid becoming something else's dinner. That kind of stress requires us to pump out a lot of adrenalin over a very short period of time. It's the kind of stress the human body was designed to cope with.

Modern stress is an entirely different proposition. The stresses caused by high-pressure jobs, bad marriages, financial difficulties, and such inescapable environmental factors as traffic and noise persist for weeks, months, even years. Our bodies have no effective mechanism for dealing with the incessant stress levels of the modern world, so stress takes its toll on us in the form of ulcers, migraines, and heart attacks.

Many stress-inducing factors are simply beyond our control. There's nothing we can do about freeway traffic, and it's not practical to expect the president of a large corporation to quit and find work as a potter or batik designer. But we can all improve our physical condition to help our bodies deal with the stress in our lives.

A vigorous fitness program is an excellent way of dealing with life's daily stresses and strains. In addition, such specialized equipment as massage tables, recliner/massage chairs, foot massagers, and flotation tanks are specifically designed to relieve stress.

You should bear in mind that physical exercise by itself may not be enough to take care of your stress symptoms. Although exercise is therapeutic, it does cause tension and soreness in the muscles. How much tension it causes depends on several factors, including your normal degree of muscular tension caused by posture, job stress, and so on.

We recommend massage as an additional way to relieve stress and contribute to total fitness (and because it's fun and makes you feel great). According to trainers and therapists, massage does the following things for you:

- It aids in preventing and treating injuries.
- It facilitates metabolism.
- It prepares the muscles for maximum exertion.
- It improves the circulation of blood and lymphatic fluid by causing your blood vessels to dilate reflexively.

Professional relaxation therapists often follow the pattern below to make sure that their clients experience maximum muscular response:

1. Preliminary warming	dry heat (sauna) wet heat (steam bath, Jacuzzi)
2. Tepid shower	
3. Rest	15 minutes, covered by a blanket or towel
4. Direct massage	stroking (toward heart) kneading shaking stretching friction (to work local muscle nodules) stroking

You should *never* massage an acutely injured muscle, because you can damage the muscle fibers by filling them up with too much blood too quickly. It's safe to massage a muscle when both active and passive movements are painless.

This section will introduce you to relaxation and stress reduction equipment, tell you how it works, and give you an idea how it fits into your personal fitness program.

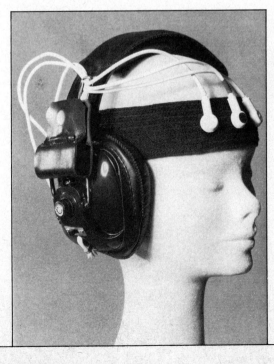

BIOSIG INSTRUMENTS, INC. ANTENSE™ BIOFEEDBACK HEADSET

The Antense converts minute levels of muscular tension into an audio tone. The higher the tone, the greater your level of tension and stress. You can't ordinarily control your tension, because you have no objective way to measure how tense you are. But by wearing the Antense for 15 minutes a day for two weeks, you'll learn to lower the tone by subconsciously relaxing tense muscles. After the first two weeks, you'll need to wear the unit only occasionally.

The Antense is light and easy to use (just put it on). The earpads are made of comfortable leather, and the headband itself (but not the electrodes) is washable. You can adjust the volume of the tone. It comes with detailed instructions and a biofeedback book.

WEIGHT:	10 oz.
SIZE:	9″ × 6″ × 4″
BATTERY:	one 9-volt
APPROXIMATE COST:	$99

SANYO® DA 2500 ELECTRIC MASSAGER

This flashlight-size unit is the most powerful hand-held massager we've seen. It will help increase circulation and relax tired muscles, thereby reducing stress whether you're at home or in the office. It has a two-speed motor and is sufficiently heavy-duty for professional use. It seems to have a more penetrating effect than most hand-held units. It comes with a polyurethane pressure-point attachment and a molded plastic foam footpad (not shown) to help you massage your back, neck, feet, and calf muscles.

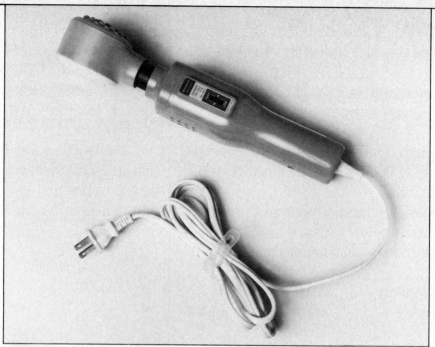
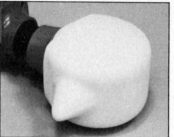

WEIGHT: 2 lbs.
SIZE: 2¼″ × 2¼″ × 11½″
APPROXIMATE COST: $100; up to $200 with attachments

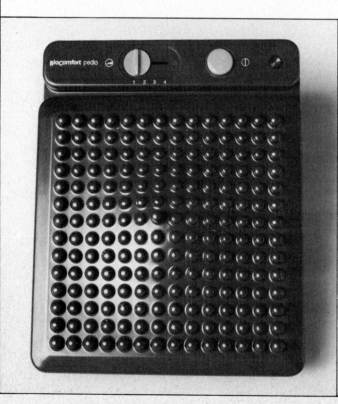

PEDIO® MASSAGER

This compact, well-built machine from Germany spreads relief throughout the body by massaging reflex points on your feet. You can also use it on your back by lying on it or having someone hold it in place. It comes in olive green and has four speeds. Options include a number of massage plates for different textures against your skin. Don't confuse the Pedio Massager with similar-looking cheaper models.

WEIGHT: 19 lbs.
SIZE: 17″ × 13″ × 8½″
HOUSE CURRENT
APPROXIMATE COST: $230

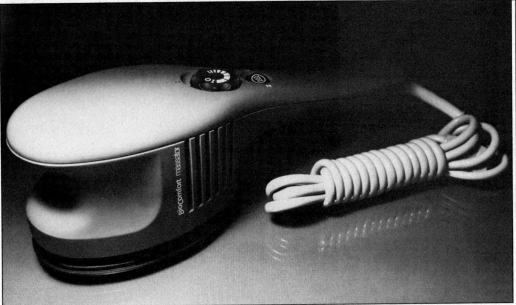

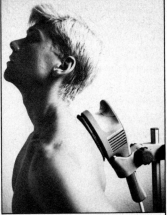

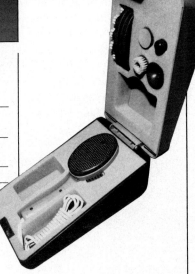

TRILEEN MASSATOR HAND MASSAGE SYSTEM

This is probably the best hand massage system on the market. Its range of vibration settings is virtually infinite. Press a separate button, and the Massator heats up to give you the combined benefits of massage and heat therapy. And it comes with a variety of standard accessories including a heatable base plate, a carrying case, a rubber scalp brush, a nap plate for thighs and feet, two cosmetic care brushes, a suction cup for the face, neck and breasts, and a "finger" unit for reflex zones and acupressure. There's even an optional wall bracket to let you massage your back without anyone's help. The unit is tan, with a 9-foot cord.

WEIGHT: shipping, 10 lbs.; unit alone, 6.5 lbs.

HOUSE CURRENT: 110 volts, 55 watts

SIZE OF CASE: 15″ × 9″ × 6″

APPROXIMATE COST: $275; wall bracket, $45 extra

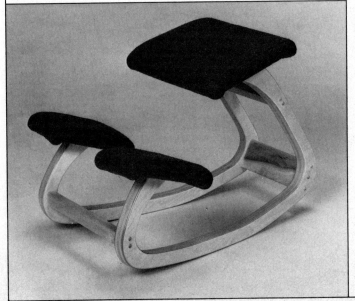

BACKSAVER™ CHAIR

There are several good chairs with this innovative design on the market. We've found the BackSaver to be very comfortable and reasonably priced.

In a conventional chair, your torso and thighs are at approximately a 90° angle. Ergonomic studies have shown that a 60° angle is more suited to the design of the human body. That's why people slouch in chairs—they're unconsciously moving toward that more relaxed 60° posture.

The BackSaver is designed to let you sit at 60°. Your knees rest against pads, thus sparing your lower back from carrying the full weight of your body. This rocker comes in kit form, with pads in eight colors, including navy, brown, burgundy, and Haitian cotton (off-white).

WEIGHT: 11½ lbs

SIZE: 20½″ × 28″ × 21″h

APPROXIMATE COST: $149

GET-A-WAY™ CHAIR

This black massage recliner chair gives you everything you want (and a few things you probably haven't thought of) in a massage unit. You can recline at any angle up to 165°. Dual massage rollers in the chair back travel from your head to the base of your spine. You can select short (3-inch) or long (6-inch) massage strokes. There's a vibrating motor with two settings for your mid-back. The footrest has its own two-speed vibrator for your calves. A detachable computer control that attaches magnetically to the chair's side lets you set speeds and time (10-, 20- or 30-minute cycles). An AM/FM radio and cassette player lets you listen to your favorite music through 4-inch wraparound speakers mounted in the headrest. The Get-A-Way chair comes with its own cassette of relaxing natural sound effects, plus a blackout visor to let you block out visible light. The problem with this unit is that you may never want to get up again.

WEIGHT: 100 lbs.	
SIZE: 30″ × 36″ × 40″h	
HOUSE CURRENT	
APPROXIMATE COST: $1,495	

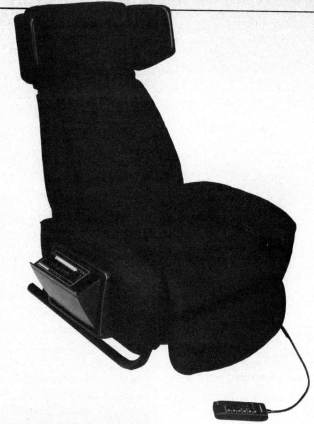

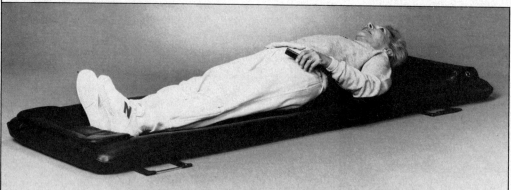

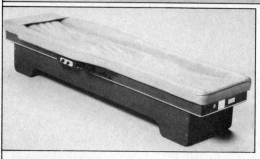

H.W.E. ACU-MASSAGE TABLE

The innovative rollers on this freestanding massage unit provide deep, penetrating massage. There are two sets of rollers, and their specially ribbed nobs are designed to simulate the pressure of a masseur's fingers. They roll along your spine's acupressure points to relieve stress and tension. A control lever on the unit's timer box lets you select upper-body, lower-body, or full-body (head to heel) massage.

The Acu-Massage table comes in two designs. Model B has a wood base; model FL has folding legs. Both have a brown Naugahyde cushion.

In addition, there's a portable table in black Naugahyde (shown here), which has all the features of the stationary models, and more. The portable unit has a hand-held remote control that lets you set the time of your massage, adjust the rollers to any position along the length of your body, and control the built-in heating pad. It folds in half for easy storage.

MODELS B AND FL	
WEIGHT: 100 lbs.	
SIZE: 24″ × 78″ × 6″h	
HOUSE CURRENT	
APPROXIMATE COST: $1,600	

PORTABLE MODEL	
WEIGHT: 35 lbs.	
SIZE: 24″ × 76″ × 6″h	
HOUSE CURRENT	
APPROXIMATE COST: $1,500	

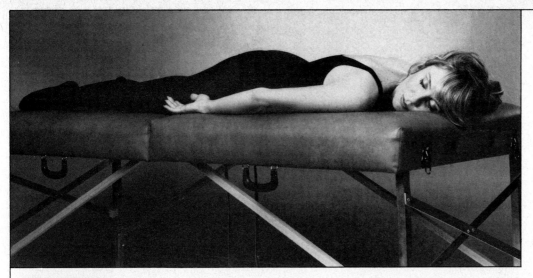

LOTUS FIRE™ MASSAGE TABLE

A good massage is one of the most sensual and relaxing of life's legal pleasures. If you're lucky enough to have a professional masseur/masseuse come to your home, or if you can talk a willing friend into giving you a complete body massage (perhaps on a *quid pro quo* basis), you'll want a good, solid massage table.

The Lotus Fire was designed with the professional masseur in mind. It's heavily padded, with strong steel supports so the masseur can put his whole body into each stroke. Masseur or not, it's a great surface to lie down and relax on. Collapsible for easy transport, it comes upholstered in chamois, vinyl, or suede in nine assorted colors.

WEIGHT: 40 lbs.

SIZE: 26″ to 38″ × 72″ × 24″ to 36″h

APPROXIMATE COST: $320 to $420, depending on upholstery; face cradle, $45

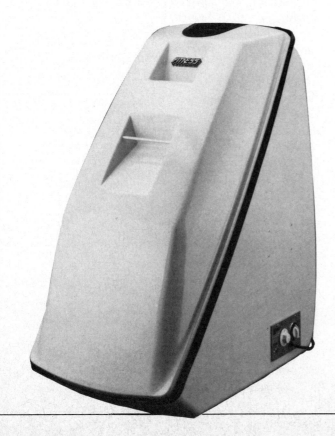

FITNESS™ F310 MOIST SAUNA

This lightweight fiberglass unit is the kind of device that used to be known as a steam cabinet. By exposing your body to hot steam, the F310 opens your pores, allows you to eliminate impurities, and leaves you feeling clean and refreshed. The seat adjusts to five different positions. The safety door needs no latch to seal in the steam, so you can't get locked in. No plumbing is necessary. There's a backrest pad, towel bar, and rear wheels for portability.

WEIGHT: 69 lbs.

SIZE: 27″ × 36″ × 45″h

HOUSE CURRENT

APPROXIMATE COST: $695

AMEREC DRY SAUNA

Since the Middle Ages, Swedes have relaxed by steaming themselves in wooden cabinet-like rooms called saunas, then running outdoors naked, jumping into snowbanks, and having themselves flogged with birch branches. Unlikely as it seems, this technique really does relax you. As proof, saunas have spread from Sweden all over the world.

If you've ever wanted to have a sauna in your own home, Amerec has a unit for you. The Amerec Dry Sauna operates a little differently from the traditional Swedish model, in which rocks are heated on a brazier, then water is poured on the hot rocks, creating steam. The Amerec Dry Sauna is basically a cedar cabinet with an electric heater. You put rocks on the heater to distribute the heat, and you may put water on the rocks if you wish. But if you do, use only a half cup—not, as the Swedes do, bucketsful. The idea behind the Dry Sauna is (as the name implies) that it uses *dry* heat. Because the heat is dry, the Dry Sauna gets hotter than the traditional Swedish kind. The ideal temperature for one of these units is between 160° and 180°F. Amerec's heater is a Finnish Metos® unit. Other good heaters are the Helo® brand from Finland, and the Tylo® brand from Sweden.

Sitting in a sauna can help you relax and un-

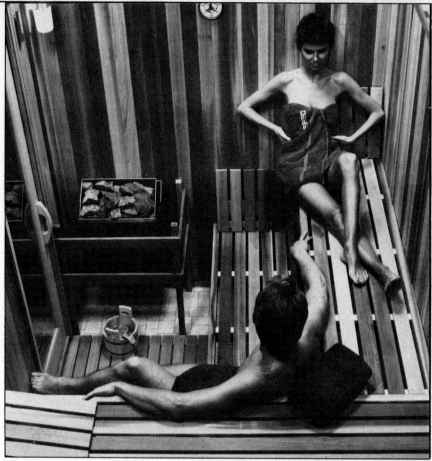

wind. Your pores open up and you perspire, thus giving your skin a thorough cleansing. If you like, you can invite friends over for a steamy social occasion. Here are a few tips to make your sauna experience safer and more enjoyable:

• If you have any health problems, consult your physician before using a sauna.

• It will take your sauna 20 to 30 minutes to warm up to the proper temperature.

• Excessive exposure to the sauna's high temperatures can be harmful. Don't sit inside one for more than 15 to 30 minutes at a stretch.

• Don't smoke or exercise in the sauna.

• Remove watches, jewelry, and anything else

made of metal before you enter the sauna. The temperature inside is high enough that metal objects can give you a nasty burn.

• You can repeat your sauna cycle two or three times, as the Swedes do. Between sessions, you'll want to give yourself a brief rest and take a cold shower (the equivalent of the Swedish snowbank). The shower will invigorate you and reduce your body temperature to a safe level for your next sauna session.

Amerec's Dry Saunas come in two configurations: modular (mostly preassembled) and precut (you put it together yourself). Both configurations feature insulated wall panels, head- and back-rests, and prehung doors. Both are made of cedar

and come with heaters and all necessary electrical connections. And both come in eight sizes.

MODULAR
WEIGHT: 500 to 1,250 lbs.
SIZE: 4' × 4' to 8' × 12'
ASSEMBLY TIME: one man, 8 hrs.
APPROXIMATE COST: $2,280 to $5,690
REQUIRED ELECTRICAL HOOKUP: residential, 240-volt single-phase current; commercial, 208-volt three-phase current

PRECUT
WEIGHT: 230 to 780 lb.
SIZE: 4' × 4' to 8' × 12'
ASSEMBLY TIME: one carpenter, a few days
APPROXIMATE COST: $1,520 to $4,120
REQUIRED ELECTRICAL HOOKUP: residential, 240-volt single-phase current; commercial, 208-volt three-phase current

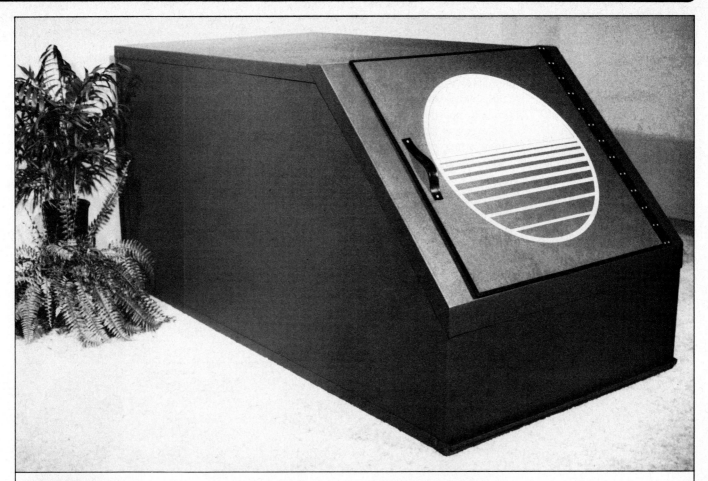

SAMADHI TANK

You've seen these water-filled isolation tanks in *Altered States* and, twenty years earlier, in *The Mind-Benders*. Although most people think it's the latest thing from California, the isolation tank actually dates back to 1954, when John Lilly developed the first one at the National Institute of Mental Health.

The principle behind the isolation tank is simple and well tested. It provides total relaxation by screening out all light and sound, and allowing the user to float with his weight supported by water heated to body temperature. The tank thus comes as close as possible to isolating the user from all external stimuli.

The Samadhi Tank Company has been producing these units for consumers since 1972. The current model, built entirely of plastic to reduce weight, was introduced in 1977. According to Samadhi's specs, it assembles in less than 15 minutes, although you need 2 to 4 hours to complete all the connections and fill it with water. Those who've used this device swear by it.

WEIGHT: shipping, 200 lbs.; filled, 1,800 lbs.

SIZE: 48″ × 94″ × 44½″h

HOUSE CURRENT

APPROXIMATE COST: $3,300; up to $4,040 with extra options

OASIS RELAXATION TANK

This king-size isolation tank is manufactured in (where else?) Texas. It features condensation control, a solid-state heater accurate to within 0.5°F, and a Jacuzzi pump and heater.

But what makes the Oasis tank really special are the options. You can elect to have a stereo speaker system mounted at the factory, then lie back in water-logged comfort and listen to music or instructional tapes.

The Oasis can also be equipped with Tank-a-Vision: a 13-inch roof-mounted video screen (not shown) enables you to watch sports instruction tapes, or pastoral tapes to help you relax more completely.

WEIGHT: 350 lbs.; filled, 2,350 lbs.

SIZE: 54" × 96" × 48"h

HOUSE CURRENT

APPROXIMATE COST:
Standard: $3,595
With audio: $3,995
With audio & video: $4,495

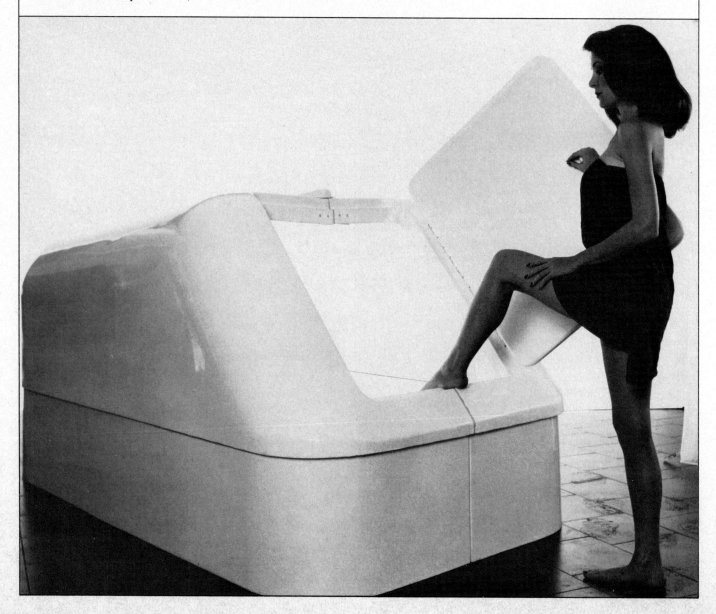

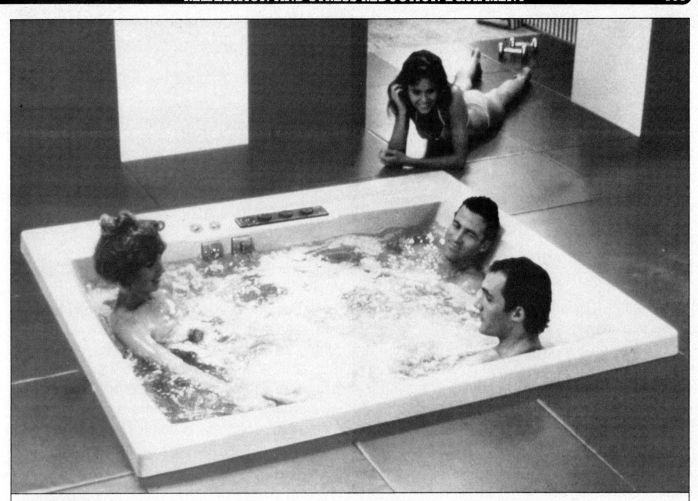

JACUZZI WHIRLPOOL BATH AVANZA™

The folks who invented the whirlpool bath have come up with this acrylic-and-fiberglass model that serves as both a bathtub and spa. For simple bathing, just fill the center well. For individual or group relaxation, fill it up completely.

The Avanza is completely preplumbed. You install it the same way you would a bathtub. A plumber hooks up the incoming hot and cold water lines to the water valve. The unit is self-enclosed with a four-inch rim and can be either top-mounted or flush-mounted. There are two separate pumps: a ¾-horsepower for spa mode, a ½-horsepower for bath mode. Both can be run simultaneously. The Avanza uses 220 volts of current, the same as for a clothes dryer.

The heating/filtration system keeps the water hot and clean. However, if you're going to use the unit as a spa (that is, if you're going to let water stand in it), you'll have to put pool chemicals, such as chlorine or bromine, into the water.

The Jacuzzi Whirlpool Bath Avanza comes with a full one-year warranty, including parts and labor. It's available in 13 colors.

SIZE: 72″ × 66″ × 30″ h
WEIGHT: 435 lbs.; filled, 1,800 lbs.
APPROXIMATE COST: $4,200

PORTABLE EQUIPMENT

Americans are traveling farther and more frequently than ever before. Whether you're a tourist, a movie star, a politician, or a business traveler, there's no need to get out of shape while you're on the road. A wide variety of portable exercise equipment, including dumbbells, jump ropes, and "mini-gyms," let you maintain cardiovascular fitness and even keep up weight and strength training wherever you go. Much of this portable equipment involves working against resistance—and all of it is equally useful in your own home, especially if your space or budget is limited.

When you're looking at portable fitness equipment, you want to make sure that it's light and easy to carry—in short, that it's really por-table. You should also keep an eye on quality of construction. Make sure whatever you're buying has seams that won't split, welds that won't separate, buckles that really buckle.

On the following pages you'll find a representative sample of the best of the many kinds of portable gym equipment on the market. When you're away from home, there's no longer any need to leave fitness behind.

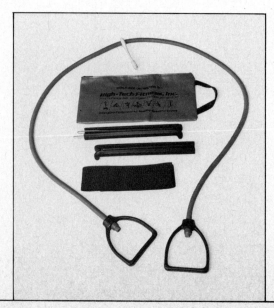

LIFELINE® GYM

The best known of all the portable gyms consists of a collapsible bar, a 7-foot rubber cable, foot and hand stirrups, a door attachment, an instruction book, and a carrying case. It even has a jogging treadmill belt, which you insert in the door hinge, that lets you run against resistance without covering ground. The heart of this system is the rubber cable. It comes in five different strengths, from easy to quite difficult, and provides resistance when you anchor the stirrups to your feet, your hands, or a stationary object. (Most people prefer the medium resistance.) The Lifeline Gym thus gives you the benefits of weight training without your having to carry barbell plates around.

WEIGHT: 2 lbs.
APPROXIMATE COST: $39.95

LATERAL RAISES

STARTING POSITION: Stand erect, with your arms at your sides and your hands grasping the stirrups of the Lifeline Gym cable. Secure the cable to the ground by standing on it, with your feet placed shoulder-width apart.

MOTION: Raise your arms laterally as far as possible, keeping the elbows locked. Return to the starting position by slowly lowering your arms to your sides.

PRECAUTIONS: Try to keep your elbows locked; bending them will reduce the value of the exercise. Exhale as you raise your arms, inhale as you lower them.

AREAS STRENGTHENED: Upper back, shoulders.

MUSCLES STRENGTHENED: Trapezius, deltoids.

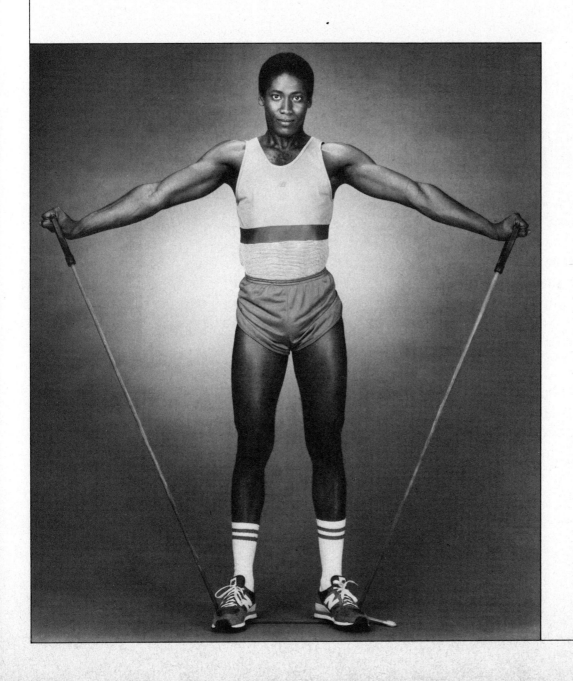

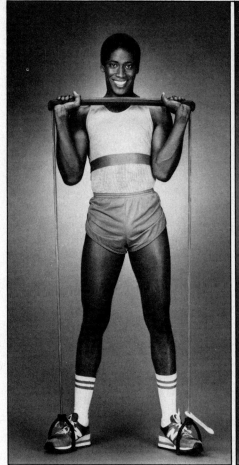
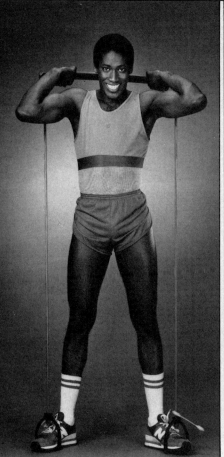
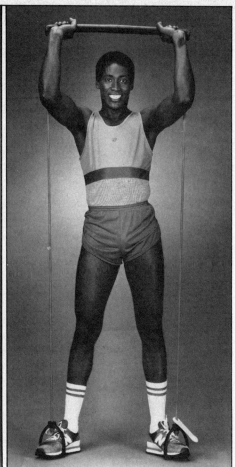

OVERHEAD PRESS

STARTING POSITION: Stand erect with your feet in the stirrups, shoulder-width apart, and grasp the Lifeline Gym bar with your hands, also shoulder-width apart. Rest the bar either on your collarbones or on your shoulders behind your head.

MOTION: Press the bar directly upward to full arm extension, or as far as possible. Return to the starting position by slowly lowering the bar.

PRECAUTIONS: Stabilize your body as much as possible during this exercise, in order to effectively isolate the working muscles. Especially avoid leaning your torso backward, to prevent lower back strain. You may want to wear a weight belt for lower back support. Exhale when pressing upward, inhale when returning to the starting position.

AREAS STRENGTHENED: Upper back, shoulders, back of upper arms.

MUSCLES STRENGTHENED: Trapezius, deltoids, triceps.

BICEPS CURLS

STARTING POSITION: With your feet in the stirrups, shoulder-width apart, stand erect with your arms straight down or with your elbows slightly bent. Grasp the Lifeline Gym bar with your hands, palms up and shoulder-width apart.

MOTION: By bending your elbows, bring the bar as close to your shoulders as possible. Slowly return to the starting position.

PRECAUTIONS: Stabilize your body as much as possible during this exercise in order to effectively isolate the working muscle groups. The only parts of your body that should move are your lower arms. Avoid arching your lower back (a weight belt might help), and don't move your upper arms or torso. Exhale as you raise your arms, inhale as you lower them.

AREAS STRENGTHENED: Front of upper arms, forearms.

MUSCLES STRENGTHENED: Biceps, brachialis, brachioradialis, flexor carpi ulnaris, flexor carpi radialis.

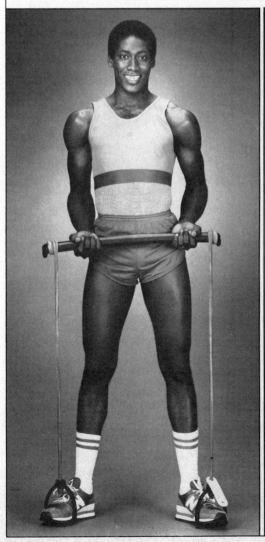
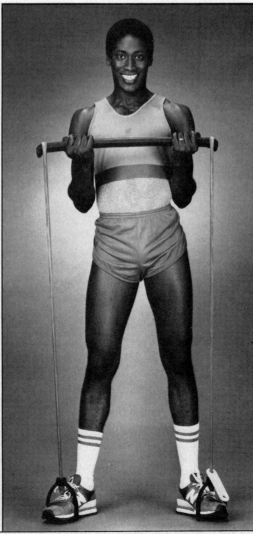

EXER-BARS™

This compact and inexpensive system can be used by either beginners or advanced gymnasts. Exer-Bars help you work on balance, coordination, and general strengthening of the body.

Each set includes a pair of curled chrome bars with comfortable black handgrips, an adjustable door bracket (not shown) for doing sit-ups, and a complete wall chart that illustrates 14 different exercises.

WEIGHT: 3 lbs. each
APPROXIMATE COST: $19.95

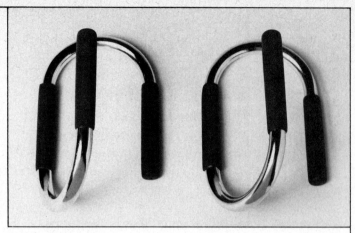

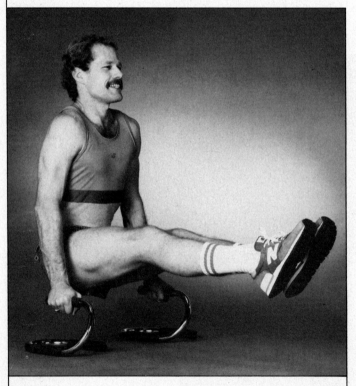

L-SEAT

STARTING POSITION: Sit on the floor and place the Exer-Bars on either side of your body, close to your hips. With slightly bent elbows, grasp the handgrips. Sit up straight, legs extended in front of you.

MOTION: Lift your body off the ground by pushing down with your arms until you've achieved full arm extension. Your basic position should remain unchanged: legs fully extended and perpendicular to the torso. Return to the starting position by slowly bending your elbows and lowering your body.

PRECAUTIONS: Exhale when pushing your body upward, inhale when returning to the starting position. It may be difficult for novices or beginners to hold the legs in the proper position.

AREAS STRENGTHENED: Back of upper arms, abdomen, hips.

MUSCLES STRENGTHENED: Triceps, rectus abdominis, internal and external obliques, quadriceps.

PUSH-UPS

You can work different muscles by varying your hand position for this exercise: A narrow handgrip, using one Exer-Bar, works the backs of the upper arms more. A wider grip, using two Exer-Bars, places greater stress on the chest and shoulders.

STARTING POSITION: Grip a single Exer-Bar with both hands, or grip two Exer-Bars. Your body should be prone and extended, your weight supported on your toes and hands. Your elbows are bent, and your shoulders, hips, and ankles should form a straight line.

MOTION: Push your body upward by straightening your elbows to full arm extension, while maintaining a straight body position. Return to the starting position by *slowly* bending your elbows and lowering your body.

PRECAUTIONS: Don't let your hips sag while performing this exercise. Keep your head in a neutral position; don't allow it to arch or drop down. Exhale when pushing upward; inhale when returning to the starting position.

AREAS STRENGTHENED: Front of shoulders, back of upper arms, chest.

MUSCLES STRENGTHENED: Anterior deltoids, pectoralis majors, triceps.

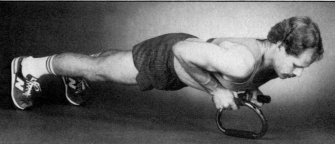
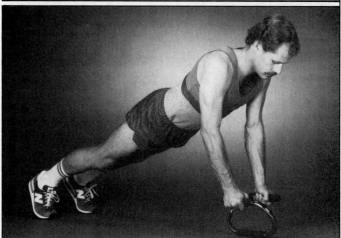
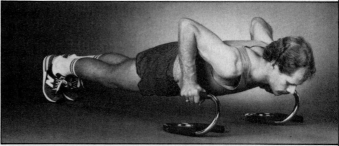
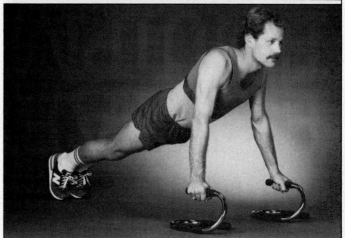

MAXISPORTS MAXIPOWER™

The MaxiPower lets you strengthen arm and shoulder muscles by pushing against the air pressure in its 23-inch cylinder. The red "power ring" is easily adjustable, and it gives a reading of the tension level you're working against (1 to 80 pounds of resistance). This device comes with a brochure detailing a MaxiPower fitness program.

WEIGHT: 12 oz.
APPROXIMATE COST: $39.95

PECTORAL SQUEEZE

You may hold the MaxiPower at various positions in front of your body for this exercise, from abdomen to shoulder height.

STARTING POSITION: Set the MaxiPower to the desired resistance. Stand erect, with your feet shoulder-width apart, and hold the Maxi-Power in front of your body, hands grasping the ends.

MOTION: Press against the ends of the MaxiPower so as to bring your hands as close together as possible. Slowly release the tension to return to the starting position.

PRECAUTIONS: Keep your arms as fully extended as possible during this exercise. Exhale when squeezing, inhale when releasing tension.

AREAS STRENGTHENED: Chest, shoulders.

MUSCLES STRENGTHENED: Pectoralis majors, anterior deltoids.

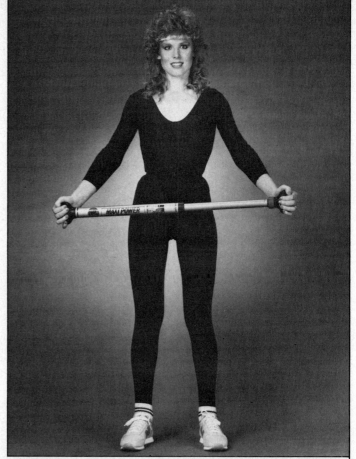

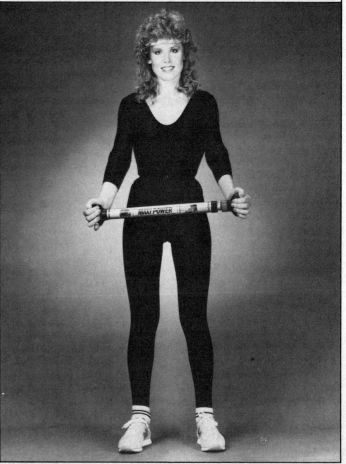

WORKOUT BAR™

This portable system comes with 20 pounds of weights, including a 1-pound modular bar that screws into a 5-foot unit or can be taken apart and turned into two dumbbells. The chrome weights and the black foam-handled bar collapse into a package that measures 4 × 4 × 12 inches. Easy to assemble with set screws.

WEIGHT: 20 lbs. (includes 6 2½-lb. weights)

APPROXIMATE COST: $100

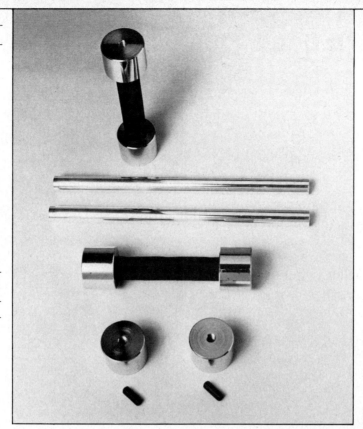

UPRIGHT ROW

STARTING POSITION: Stand with your knees slightly bent, feet shoulder-width apart, and grasp the middle of the Workout Bar with your hands 1 to 2 inches apart. Let your arms hang down straight in front of your body.

MOTION: Pull the bar straight up until your hands come to within 1 or 2 inches of your chin. Slowly lower the bar back to the starting position.

PRECAUTIONS: Keep your elbows above the bar during this exercise. Exhale as you raise the bar, inhale as you lower it.

AREAS STRENGTHENED: Shoulders, upper back, front of upper arms.

MUSCLES STRENGTHENED: Trapezius, deltoids, biceps.

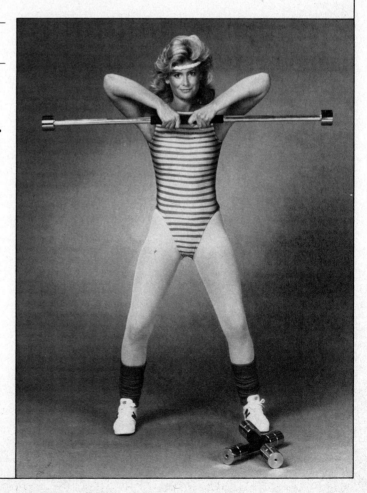

BENT-OVER TWIST

STARTING POSITION: With your feet shoulder-width apart, bend at the waist until your torso is parallel to the ground. Grasp the Workout Bar near the ends, and place it on the back of your shoulders.

MOTION: Twist at the waist from side to side, bringing the bar perpendicular to the floor at the end of each twist.

PRECAUTIONS: Although you can utilize some momentum in performing this exercise, avoid any excessively fast or violent twisting motion. Don't twist beyond the point where the bar is perpendicular to the ground. Breathe normally.

AREAS STRENGTHENED: Back of thighs, buttocks, lower back, abdomen, sides of torso.

MUSCLES STRENGTHENED: Hamstrings, gluteals, erector spinae, internal and external obliques.

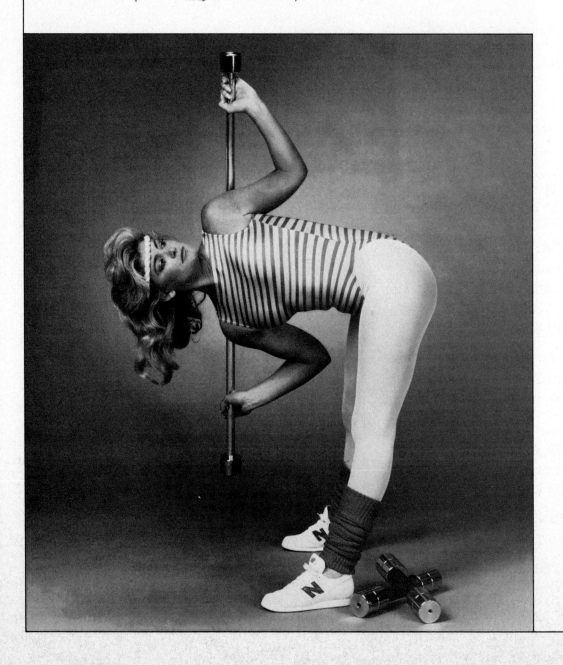

GYRO-JUMP®

The Gyro-Jump represents a technological advance in jump-rope design, although it comes in only one length and doesn't have a stroke counter. Its long handles (the manufacturers call this feature the Flex Shaft) create an upswing and a downswing, forcing the jumper's arms to work to reverse the handles' directions. And because the handles are made of flexible plastic, they create an extra oscillation, thereby increasing the leverage required to perform the movement. Consequently, the upper body gets a better workout. As complicated as all this sounds, the basic process is still good, old-fashioned jumping rope.

WEIGHT: 2½ lbs.
APPROXIMATE COST: $29.95

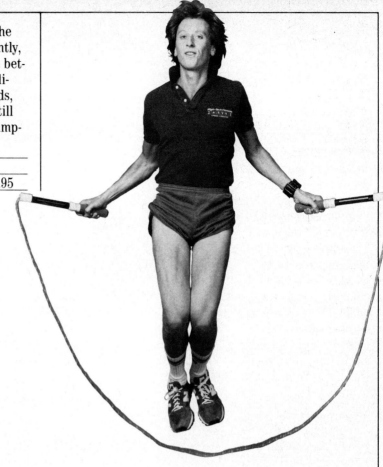

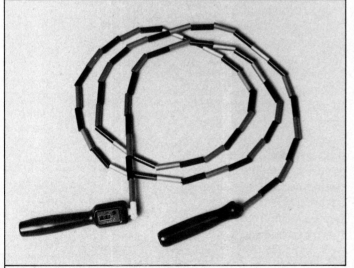

LIFELINE® JUMP ROPE

The Lifeline features a nylon cord inside light 1-inch long plastic cylinders. The handle contains a built-in digital stroke counter, and the rope's length is adjustable to suit all heights. An instruction book is included. This is one of the best lightweight jump ropes around.

WEIGHT: 1 lb.
APPROXIMATE COST: $15

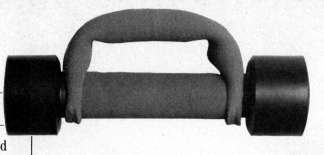

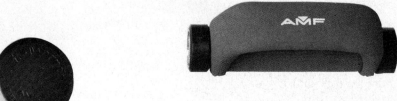

AMF AMERICAN HEAVYHANDS™

It's an old concept: Add weights to an aerobic exercise, and you'll exercise more in less time. AMF "perfected" this concept. These attractive and durable one-pound hand weights are cushioned for comfort, easy to hold, and adaptable to almost any aerobic activity. They come in regular and large sizes, and with add-on weights go from 2 to 10 pounds.

APPROXIMATE COST: $19.95; add-on weights, $7.99 to $39.99

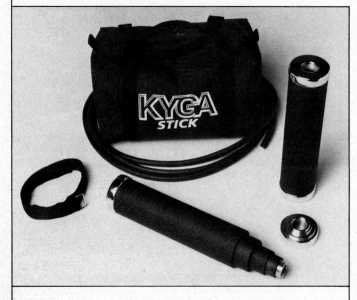

KYGA™ STICK

The KYGA system includes an extension bar, a rubber cable, stirrups, and a pair of hand weights and connectors. It lets you create two hand weights in 1-pound increments, from 1 to 10 pounds each. The cable attaches to the hand weights and can be used as a jump rope. The principle of working against your own resistance is the same as with other portable gym systems. The KYGA system comes complete with its own carrying case.

WEIGHT: 21 lbs.

APPROXIMATE COST: $120

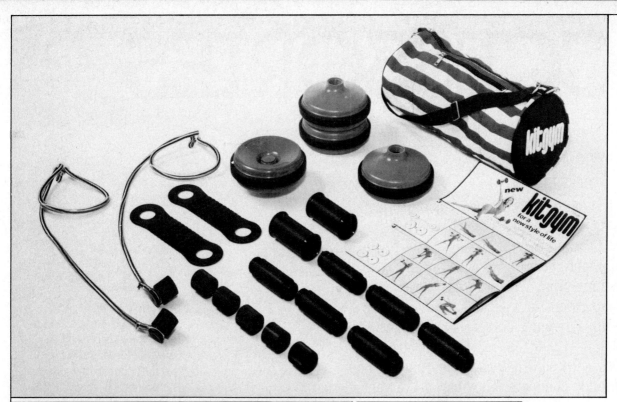

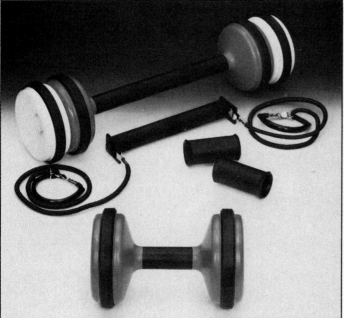

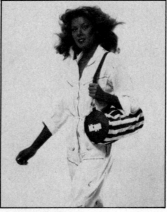

KITGYM™

The Kitgym includes a pair of dumbbells, a bar, resistance cables, foot straps, and an exercise mat. The special feature here is that the plastic bells (which can be connected to the bar to form a barbell) are hollow. Filling a dumbbell with water increases its weight to 3.5 pounds; with sand, to 6 pounds; and with number 8 lead shot, to 23 pounds.

You may not want to travel around with 23 pounds of shot in your suitcase, but the principle of increasing weight resistance by filling a hollow dumbbell is a sound one, and the Kitgym is a very portable unit.

WEIGHT: 5½ lbs.
APPROXIMATE COST: $50

ACCESSORIES

In the clothing business, "accessories" means shoes, scarves, ties—the things that can give an outfit a put-together look. In the home gym equipment business, "accessories" can mean anything from weight-lifting gloves and padded seat covers to a $2,000 electric pump that sets up a rushing current in your swimming pool.

Fitness accessories help make your exercise experience complete. They can make your workout more efficient, more effective, and more fun. And the ones you'll read about in this section are, we believe, the very best available today.

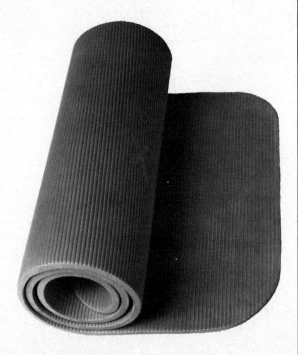

TORIN, INC., AIREX® MATS

Torin's Airex products are clearly one of the best lines of exercise mats available. Made of high-quality pure vinyl closed-cell foam, they are ultra-thin, but they absorb as much pressure as open-cell mats four times as thick. They feel amazingly warm and soft to the touch, and they're impervious to dirt and odors. Airex mats are space-efficient, light, easy to roll up, easily portable, and specially sanitized. They lie flat, they don't slide, and you can use them indoors and out. They're ideal for physical therapy, massage, gymnastics, and aerobics. They're available in various sizes in green, red, or black, and you can even order them with securing straps and carrying cases.

Sizes:	Weights:
$23'' \times 72'' \times 5/8''$	4 lbs.
$39'' \times 72'' \times 5/8''$	6 lbs.
$48'' \times 78'' \times 5/8''$	8 lbs.
$24'' \times 78'' \times 1''$	7 lbs.
$30'' \times 78'' \times 1''$	9 lbs.
$48'' \times 78'' \times 1''$	13 lbs.

APPROXIMATE COST:
$39 to $139

JOE WEIDER'S EZ-ON CLIP COLLARS

These quick and easy spring collars to hold weight plates on barbells and dumbbells are sold by the Joe Weider Company, a big name in the weight-training and fitness business since the 1930s. Other collars must be put on and removed by a screw mechanism; some even require an Allen wrench. But these Weider collars snap on and off by means of a steel spring. They are ideal for light weights or specialty bars.

WEIGHT: 6 oz.

APPROXIMATE COST: $4.95 per pair

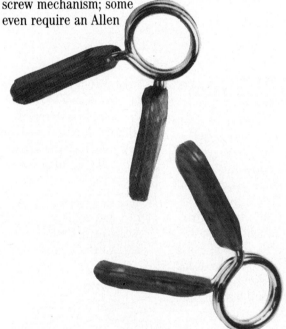

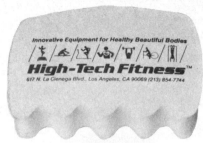

MAXISPORTS MAXIGRIP™

Here's a low-tech device that's hard to improve on. MaxiGrip's natural rubber ring develops your grip muscles. All you have to do is hold it in your hand and squeeze. It's great for golfers, players of racquet sports, and all others who rely on their grip strength. Note that a strong grip can help your elbow, too. The MaxiGrip is a very inexpensive way to help prevent painful golf and tennis elbow.

WEIGHT: 12 oz.

APPROXIMATE COST: $3

TRIANGLE™ GRIPPER

This dense vinyl foam gripper, designed for High-Tech Fitness by Triangle Manufacturing, is contoured to fit your hand. It comes in two sizes, for small/medium and medium/large hands.

WEIGHT: 6 oz.

APPROXIMATE COST: $1.50

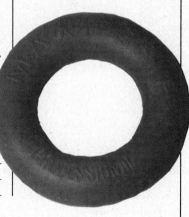

CEMCO OLYMPIC SPRING LOCK COLLARS

This is a safe, quick-release collar that snaps on and off. Like the Weider collars, they are used to keep plates from shifting or falling, but the Cemco collars are used on Olympic-size barbells.

WEIGHT: 8 oz.

APPROXIMATE COST: $4.95

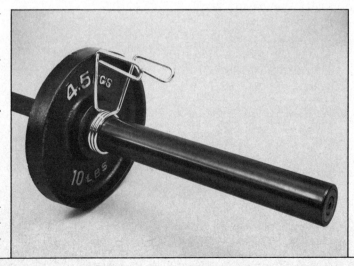

DALBERG WEIGHT-LIFTING BELTS

Weight-lifting belts help stabilize and support your lower back and pelvis. We think they're an absolute necessity for lunges, squats, and some presses.

Dalberg's belts have an innovative plastic core that is as flexible and durable as leather. They come in five moisture-repellent colors or a black leather finish. Dalberg makes their belts in both men's and women's sizes (S, M, L), and you have the option of customized printing and color combinations.

STYLES AND COLORS: 4″ power-lifting belt, royal blue and black; 4″ training belt, red and yellow; 6″ backed competition belt, green

APPROXIMATE COST: $50

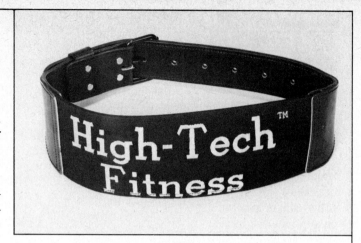

TRIANGLE BAND™

Wrist and ankle weights let you exercise more strenuously by making you work against the added resistance of gravity. And the Triangle Band is the most comfortable wrist/ankle weight system we've found. It's made of white plastic with red lettering, and one size fits all. After about a half-hour of wear, the Triangle actually starts to mold itself around your ankle or wrist. When you're not using it, you should store the band in a wrapped (that is, circular) position. You can clean the Triangle with mild soap and lukewarm water.

AVAILABLE WEIGHT: 1.1 lbs., 1.65 lbs., 2.2 lbs.

APPROXIMATE COST: $15 to $20 per pair

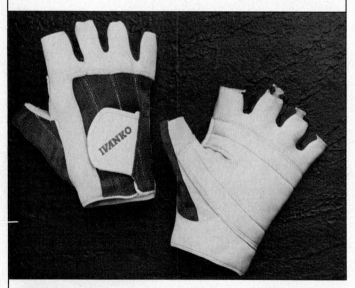

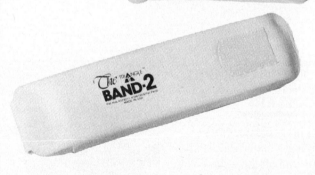

IVANKO® WEIGHT LIFTING GLOVES

If you've ever lifted free weights, you know why gloves are a good idea. They help you grip the weights even when your palms are sweating, and they prevent the calluses and blisters you're sure to get if you don't use them. Ivanko's gloves are well designed and sturdily made of leather and plastic. They can be cleaned with leather cleaner. Available in men's sizes S, M, L, and XL. And they come in an assortment of colors that can be coordinated with your active wear.

WEIGHT: 2 oz. per pair

APPROXIMATE COST: $15

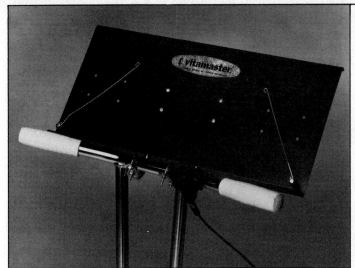

VITAMASTER® READING RACK

This black metal rack lets you read as you pedal your stationary bike. It comes in one flat piece and is easy to install, with a U-clamp that attaches it to the handlebars. The Vitamaster's two page-holders ensure that whatever you're reading stays flat. Just don't try to use it on a *real* bicycle.

WEIGHT: 4 lbs.
SIZE: 9″ × 18″
APPROXIMATE COST: $29.95

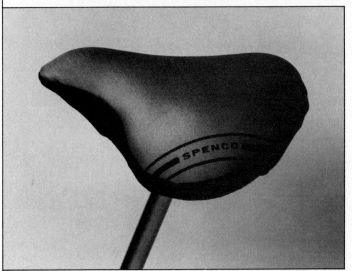

SPENCO® SADDLE PAD

The Spenco seat pad is made of plastic that absorbs pressure and shock to prevent soreness and numbness. It's durable, washable, and covered with weatherproof polypropylene.

The Spenco comes in three colors (black, blue, and red) and three sizes, to fit all saddles from racing bikes to extra-wide stationary exercise machine seats. It is the best seat cushion we've found.

WEIGHT: 1½ lbs.
APPROXIMATE COST: $25

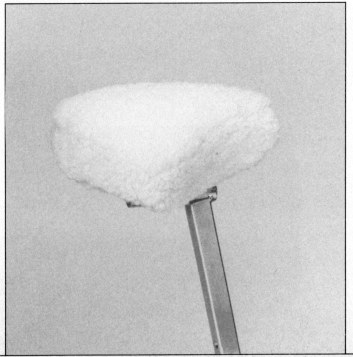

R & R SALES FANCY FURRY SEAT COVERS

At High-Tech Fitness, we call this seat cover the "Furry Fuzzy" because, well, it *is*. The synthetic fiber of the R & R is soft as sheepskin, but it's machine washable and fits most stationary and non-stationary bicycles. Available in eggshell white.

WEIGHT: 4 oz.
APPROXIMATE COST: $12.95

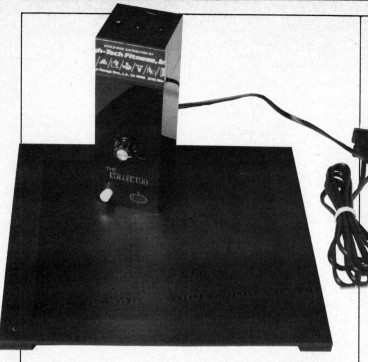

THE COLLECTOR BY ZESTRON, INC.

Negative ions help clean the air by precipitating out microscopic pollutants. Some people believe that negative ions in the air make people feel fresher and more alert. One way to increase the number of negative ions in your home's air is to use an ionizer.

Zestron's indoor air ionizer (shown here with the High-Tech Fitness label) has several things to recommend it. It has one of the highest negative ion outputs of any unit on the market, and it's one of the few ionizers that allow you to vary the ion level. Its solid-state circuitry has no moving parts, so there's nothing to wear out or replace. It comes with an easy-to-clean collector panel that sits on top of the unit and attracts most airborne pollutants. Finally, The Collector will operate anywhere in your home or office on household current for just pennies a month.

If you're living in a heavily polluted area, be forewarned: As The Collector cleans the air, it sometimes deposits a black film of pollutants (smog, dust, dirt, etc.) on the nearest wall or window.

SIZE: unit, 2¼″ × 2¼″ × 6¼″; collector panel, 10″ × 10″
APPROXIMATE COST: $139.95

NORELCO® CLEAN AIR HB5000

The Norelco air machine sucks air into its unique activated-charcoal filtration system, which rapidly removes odor-containing airborne particles. This compact unit runs on household current, and it will clear the air in a 24′ × 25′ room. It has a three-position switch, maxi air flow control, adjustable louver grill, washable foam layer, replaceable filters—even a special citrus scent pack to perfume the newly cleaned air.

SIZE: 7″ × 7″ × 7½″
APPROXIMATE COST: $54.95

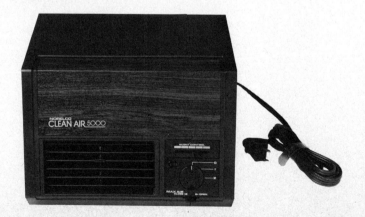

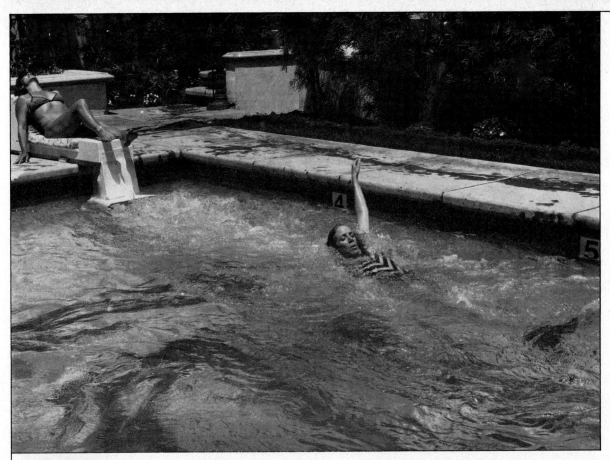

SWIM GYM™

The Swim Gym lets you turn your pool into a giant "swimming treadmill." This electric pump sets up a fast, smooth current in your pool, enabling you to work out by swimming in place instead of doing laps. The manufacturer says that by eliminating the slowing and turning necessary in doing laps, the Swim Gym increases the level of exercise by about 50 percent. The moving water is also an aid for hydrotherapy; and, because your heart rate accelerates faster, it's good for aerobics too. Last (and maybe least), your kids will have a great time with this unique device.

The pump is driven by a 3-horsepower motor that pulls approximately 15 amps (that's about 50¢ an hour on your electric bill) and provides a flow of over 2,000 gallons a minute. That's enough of a water current to satisfy anyone, from a beginner to a Mark Spitz. The farther away you are from the pump, the easier it will be to swim against the current.

This device is a permanent installation, like your pool pump. It's a one-piece unit, with the pump extending approximately 2½ feet underwater. The Swim Gym gives you the experience of ocean swimming, without the rip tides and stinging jellyfish.

SIZE: underwater pump 12″ ×30″; chassis 5½′×1′×16″

APPROXIMATE COST: $2,000 to $3,000 (still in prototype at printing)

HOW TO SET UP YOUR HOME GYM

Your home gym is the one place where your quest for fitness won't be impaired by distance, bad weather, or lack of time. It's the place to go to rehabilitate an injury or to sweat out a temporary depression. Imagine how much easier losing weight would be if, instead of turning left toward the kitchen, you could turn right into your home gym and ride a mile on your stationary bike!

By now, you're thinking seriously (we hope) about putting together your own home gym. But before you reach for your check book, you'll want to turn your attention toward what kind of equipment you want and where you're going to put it.

The best way to begin is by asking yourself some questions. In fact, these are the same questions the High-Tech Fitness staff asked our 25,000-plus clients to help them decide what's best.

Who's Going to Use Your Gym?

This question bears on both the size of your home gym and the equipment you'll want to put in it. Are you the only person who's going to be working out? Will your entire family be using your gym, or only certain family members? What about your friends? It's fun to socialize while working out. Unlike your health club or local "Y", your home gym lets you pick your exercise partners. You don't have to worry about being held back by someone who's hopelessly out of shape—or about being intimidated by someone who's in terrifyingly good condition.

Be sure you evaluate not just your family's present needs, but its future needs, as well. Your 10-year-old son is too young for strength training now. But in four or five years, he may want to start building himself up for high-school sports.

Take into account any physical or medical limitations you (or anyone who uses your gym) may have. Should you buy equipment that can be used for rehabilitation?

What Are Your Goals?

Your choice of equipment will be largely dictated by your personal fitness goals. What do you want to do with your body? You may want to accomplish some or all of the following goals: improve muscle tone and build strength; increase endurance; enhance cardiovascular fitness; increase flexibility; alleviate stress or depression; improve balance and coordination; rehabilitate the back, heart, or an injured joint; lose weight; gain weight.

How Much Money Can You Afford to Spend?

We were bound to get to this one sooner or later. You can outfit a home gym for virtually any amount from $250 to a million. This latter figure will get you a serviceable set of solid gold dumbbells, along with a platinum weight machine and diamond-studded bench cover.

Assuming for the moment that you're not the owner of a Persian Gulf oil emirate, you'll want to shop with an eye for value. "Value" is not synonymous with "cheapness." "You get what you pay for" may be a cliché, but, like most clichés, there's a peanut of truth hidden within its chocolate coating and its hard candy shell.

The important thing about any high-tech equipment you buy is that *it should be of sufficiently high quality to do what it's designed to do.* Shoddily-made equipment is usually less expensive than the good stuff—but not always. The people who make it can cut prices because they cut corners on materials and construction.

As a result, it's often not capable of standing up to the kind of beating it's going to get from being used in a vigorous fitness program.

Cut-rate fitness equipment can leave you with a feeling of frustration when it breaks down. You'll be raring to go, and your "Sleaze-Right Multi-Station Weight Machine and Facial Sauna" will be in the shop for repairs. You'll feel even more frustrated if the thing breaks down with you in it.

If you're serious about fitness, you should look at your equipment as an investment. You'll want to use it hard and often, and you'll want it to stand up to such use. If you're just going to buy, say, a rowing machine to assuage your guilt, and then let it stand in the closet and gather cobwebs, it's okay to go out and get the cheapest one you can find.

Once you've decided how much you can afford to spend on your home gym, a related question arises: What percentage of my total budget should I spend for each of the various types of fitness equipment?

You'll be relieved to know that the answer to this one is easy. *You should spend the most money on the equipment that corresponds to the aspect(s) of fitness you're most interested in.* If you want to become a professional body-builder and you don't care much about aerobics, it's foolish to spend $4,000 on a treadmill while scrimping on weight equipment.

How Much Time Will You Spend in Your Gym?

The more time you have to exercise, the more kinds of conditioning you'll be able to work at. And that means the more different types of equipment you're going to want.

Different kinds of physical training require different schedules. Aerobic fitness requires a minimum of three workouts per week (better five or six). Each workout must last at least 15 minutes (preferably more), and you must work at your target heart rate for the entire time. (In other words, warm-ups, stretches and cool-downs don't count against the required time.) Weight training, on the other hand, may require a longer work-out. But it's vitally important that you give each muscle group at least a full day's rest before working on it again.

We've divided the routines in our personal fitness programs into basic, intermediate, and advanced levels. Generally speaking, the basic workouts last 30 minutes; the intermediates, 60; and the advanced, 90.

Try not to let too many days go by without doing *something* for your body. It's all too easy to slide into bad habits, and even on the busiest of days, you can sneak into your home gym for five or ten minutes of vigorous activity that will relax you and keep your body in tone.

How Much Room Should You Use for Your Gym?

The more space the better, of course. You're going to be working out hard, and you'll want to be as unconfined as possible. The ideal is to devote an entire room to fitness. But if your house or apartment doesn't happen to have a spacious vacant room, the den or sewing room, an enclosed patio, part of the garage or basement, a walk-in closet, or even a section of the living room or bedroom should do nicely.

An added bonus: Much of the new high-tech equipment is easily portable and can be folded up and stored when not in use.

What Else Can You Do to Make Your Workout More Enjoyable?

Exercise is, of necessity, dull—in order to be effective, movements must be repeated again and again. So try to make the time pass as agreeably as possible.

The most fundamental form of diversion is music. It's also a powerful stimulus, as shown by the success of the many fitness programs combining aerobics with dance. If you don't want to invest in special workout tapes, your transistor, Walkman or cassette player will do. Stay away from mood music—it's *too relaxing.* Sustained rhythmic music, like disco and certain rock 'n roll, is invigorating and will help you establish a cadence to repetitive movements.

Television can also be a positive influence while you're working out, particularly if you're exercising on an aerobic device, such as a rower or treadmill or stationary bike. Watch stimulating programs, the kind that will evoke an emotional response and get you charged up. The news is an effective energizer for most people. Stay away from sitcoms. The eye-candy that passes for entertainment is conducive to relaxation, not stimulation. In fact, sitcoms have been shown to induce Alpha waves in the brain, the same sort of waves characteristic of relaxation, meditation, and sleep.

Listening to motivational fitness program tapes, reading, or listening to cassettes of recorded books are other diversions that can make working out more fun and more productive.

What Special Features Should Your Gym Have?

The décor of your home gym should be as enticing as your taste and pocketbook allows. The room should be light and airy, well-ventilated (there may be odors that won't remind you of Chanel #5), and accessible—this is important, because if it is dingy or cluttered or over in the west wing, you'll find excuses not to exercise. Keep the room cool—you're going to build up a lot of body heat. But stay away from rooms that have too much moisture, because of equipment rusting problems.

Install at least one full-length mirror to give you positive feedback as your body changes. A mirror also allows you to observe the movements of your body and prevent sloppiness and "cheating."

Glued-down industrial or indoor/outdoor carpeting is ideal. It's attractive and resilient, and it prevents equipment from sliding around. If you use thickly padded indoor carpeting, you run the risk of equipment sliding or making indentations that won't go away.

Unless you're seven feet tall and want to jump rope on your rebounder, the standard 8-foot ceiling will accommodate almost all equipment.

Before selecting your equipment, consider the structural soundness of your floor (though virtually any floor in a well-built house or apartment will support a complete home gym, downstairs neighbors notwithstanding); the capacity of your electrical wiring (some heavy-duty motorized equipment requires 220-volt wiring, but most run on standard 110, like your toaster); and your plumbing (some whirlpool units may require special plumbing work).

SHOULD YOU HAVE A PERSONAL FITNESS TRAINER?

The newest wrinkle in Hollywood is the personal fitness trainer—an individual coach who comes to your door and helps you work out at home in a one-to-one situation. Personal trainers can be expensive. Their services generally cost from $25 to $100 per 45- to 120-minute session. Are they worth it?

I've worked out with personal trainers for several years now. They've helped me exercise more efficiently and effectively. I've made faster gains than I would have without them, and I've been able to maintain those gains. The fact that personal fitness trainers can be pricey means they aren't for everybody. But I'm delighted with the improvements I've made.

How do you look for a personal fitness trainer? There is yet *no national certification* for personal fitness trainers. That means it's up to you to find one who has a strong, basic knowledge of exercise physiology.

It's entirely possible to find a trainer who has an M.S. or Ph.D. in exercise physiology, or equivalent credentials. Referrals are probably the most dependable way to do this. Do your friends have personal fitness trainers? Are they happy with them? You can also call up the Exercise Physiology department of your local college or university and ask them to refer you to a graduate student who might act as your trainer. It's an iron-clad rule of life that grad students always need money, and they'll be glad to have the work.

Three recognized organizations can be of help: the American College of Sports Medicine (ACSM) in Indianapolis, Indiana, the International Dance Exercise Association (IDEA) in San Diego, California, and the American Home Fitness Association (AHFA) in Cincinnati, Ohio. The ACSM membership includes virtually every kind of professional in sports medicine, fitness, cardiology, physical therapy, and related fields. IDEA is a nonpartisan organization for aerobics companies, aerobics instructors, and students. IDEA is currently working with the ACSM on setting up national standards for the certification of fitness instructors. AHFA is a non-profit association researching the area of personal fitness trainers.

How to
MAKE YOUR HOME GYM FIT YOUR LIFESTYLE

Each one of us leads his or her own, unique life. So it's no surprise that each of us will have different requirements and needs for home gym equipment.

However, we all need to make the very best use of whatever space we have. We need, whenever possible, to exercise efficiently, combining fitness with other activities to save time. (You can catch up on the TV news or use a Dictaphone while rowing or treadmill walking.) And we all want equipment that will give us the best value for our dollar.

In this chapter we've described 12 common lifestyles and situations, we've detailed the special fitness requirements of each, and we've made suggestions about what equipment to buy. In each case, you should pick the most important equipment first, then include enough other fitness gear (as time and/or money allows) to give yourself a complete workout. We've left out some accessories and monitoring devices because, although they're important, their selection depends in large part on the specific exercises you want to do. You should, however, have an accurate pulse monitor no matter what kind of gym you choose.

Sedentary Worker

Sedentary jobs are the kinds of jobs most of us have. They feature lots of sitting and not much moving around, and they lead to common ailments like typist's cramps, secretary's spread, and office worker's paunch.

If you have such a job, you'll want to do some sort of aerobic activity that keeps you vertical. That means your first equipment purchase should probably be a rebounder or treadmill. You'll want either free weights or a weight machine for strength, an inversion gym to help you relax and keep the blood flowing away from the feet (and not into the seat), and a slant board to help you work out from a different angle.

Footworker

Footworkers are people whose jobs require them to be on their feet a lot. Nurses, waitresses, mailmen, and retail clerks fall into this category, as do millions of others.

If you have one of these jobs, the last thing you want is to come home after a long day and get back on your feet. For this reason, your first big equipment buy should be a stationary bike or a rower—something that'll give you a workout while letting you take a load off your feet. Gravity boots and a bar, or better, a complete inversion gym will help your circulation and your relaxation. Free weights or a weight machine will help you keep up the strength you need. (You may prefer a machine, just because it offers you the chance to do more exercises while sitting or lying down.) And with any left-over money, you may want to treat yourself to a foot or back massager.

Budget Conscious

Where there's a will ... there's a way. Lack of a long lost billionaire uncle leaving you $9/10$ of his estate shouldn't keep you from having your own personal home workout area. For under $250.00 (less than a year's membership to a typically good health club), you can put together a solid (albeit basic) home gym, with most of the components you'll need to get and stay in shape. And one you can always add to, making it even more complete.

Start with a mat for stretching, a jump rope for aerobics (use mat to cushion shock when jumping), a barbell and 100 pounds of iron plates for strength training, and boots and a bar for hanging, doing chin-ups and pull-ups.

As budget permits, add a weight belt if you're adding weights, or if into aerobics, a rebounder or bike, then a pulse monitor.

Space Saver

Here's the excuse we hear most often: "Patrick, a home gym sounds great. It would certainly solve my fitness needs and problems, but I just don't have the room!" The solution is simple. Pick equipment that is portable, collapsible, easy-to-store and doesn't take up a lot of room even when you are exercising. All the following equipment meet these criteria:
- Rowing machine, rebounder, or collapsible bike.
- Pulse monitor

- Adjustable dumbbell set for portable strength training
- Chin-up bar and gravity boots
- Jump rope and mat

People in the Spotlight

People in the spotlight are actors, models, dancers, entertainers—people who have to look good to earn a living. If you're one of these, you undoubtedly already work out—a lot—to keep yourself looking trim and gorgeous. Just think how much easier life would be if you could work out at home.

Because body sculpturing is very important to visible people, you'll need free weights and benches or a multi-station weight machine that will let you perform a wide variety of exercises. A slant board or a stomach conditioner is a good idea, and you'll want a barre, or some other aid to help you keep limber. A rebounder will maintain your coordination and your cardiovascular fitness. Gravity boots and a chin-up bar will let you stretch and do bending and hanging exercises.

Surrounding your home gym with mirrors is a particularly good idea if you're a glamour person in a glamour job. Then again, mirrors are something that glamorous people often already have plenty of. While you're at it, don't forget some portable gym equipment. Those weeks on location without working out can take their toll.

Executive

Executives need, more than anything else, to save time. That means that you may want to work while working out. You can do this with a certain degree of organization. Fortunately, organization is what executives are best at.

You'll probably want to start with an aerobic exercise device such as a stationary bicycle. Get a reading rack, so you can read *The Wall Street Journal* or the trades as you pedal. You may want some office accessories, such as a dictating machine and a speaker phone. Don't, however, use these when you're doing stress reduction activities.

A pulse monitor is an absolute necessity. You'll want a weight set or single-station weight machine for strength training, and a gravity inversion device. A TV with a video player will let you watch videotapes and catch the news. An audio tape player will allow you to listen to motivational tapes, cassette books, and business reviews—or just relax with music.

A Get-A-Way chair or another stress reduction device is an especially good idea. Turn the phone off while you're using it, or you won't reduce your stress level by much. Finally, a treadmill or any other second aerobic device will be useful. Of course, you can always add any other equipment that strikes your fancy—and that you have the space for.

Weekend or Serious Athlete

You want to train yourself for the sports you enjoy, and you want to stay limber and fit to protect yourself from injury. If you're a serious athlete, you'll be using (and reusing) your home gym equipment more than a weekend jock will. Obviously, the more you use your fitness gear, the heavier-duty you'll want it to be.

Start with a rower or rebounder for total-body aerobic exercise. Since all sports require strength in one or more major muscle groups, you'll need some kind of weight set: either free weights (dumbbells, barbells, benches) or a multi-station weight machine or its equivalent (such as a Total Gym).

If you're using heavy weights, you'll need a strong floor. The ground floor is better than an upper floor, and your garage floor is better still.

It's a good idea to have the Rack, the Nu-Barre, or some device that will let you perform stretching and flexibility exercises. Finally, you'll want a simple chin-up bar, and gravity boots or some other inversion device.

Families

Your name doesn't have to be Jackson or Osmond or Kennedy for you to require a family gym. If your gym is going to be used by more than one person, you'll want enough equipment so you and your family (or friends) can work out together. If you do have a large family, the evening workout might be one of those increasingly rare occasions when everybody gets together in the same room at once. Here's where having more than one unit of the same equipment (especially pulse monitors) makes sense.

You'll want to start with a multi-station weight machine, one at which three or more people can exercise at once. You should have some combination of rebounders, rowers, and/ or stationary bikes for cardiovascular fitness. Free weights and benches are useful; the larger your group, the more likely you are to find that you can never have too many weights. Gravity boots and a bar or a complete inversion gym are a good thing to have, and if your family is big enough, you may want a sauna or spa that seats several people at a time. Finally, you should stock your gym with plenty of light-weight accessories such as jump ropes, sandbags and other portable gym equipment. These are especially good for children.

Senior Home Gym

Many older people find themselves staying home more than they used to. They're concerned for their safety on the streets, and some may worry about incurring sudden health problems even while walking around the block (an excellent form of exercise, by the way). A space-saving home gym could be just what the doctor ordered if you're over 65. After checking with him, you might want to start with a stationary bike (the best aerobic device for older people), treadmill, or rebounder.

A pulse monitor is especially important for seniors; in fact, you might want to buy a combined pulse and blood pressure monitor. A light set of dumbbells will help you maintain your strength and keep your joints padded with muscles. That way, you'll be less vulnerable to painful fractures and hip injuries that seem to become more of a problem with age. Finally, you'll want a floor mat so you can do those all-important stretching and flexibility exercises.

Manual Laborers

"I work hard all day long. The *last* thing I need is more physical exercise." Many people who have physical jobs, such as movers, telephone linemen, and construction workers, believe this. The problem is that most physical jobs, no matter how tough they are, don't work your entire body. Many of them involve lifting; that is, they require short bursts of anaerobic activity. If you have such a job, you'll need to develop cardiovascular fitness—something your work won't provide. Your gym should start, then, with a stationary bike, rower, or treadmill—and perhaps a jump rope, just to give yourself a little variety.

A slant board will help you condition your back (all-important if your job involves lifting) and your stomach (all-important if you drink beer after work). Gravity boots and a chinning bar or a complete inversion gym will help you literally unbend at the end of a hard day. You'll certainly want free weights and a bench, or some form of weight machine. After all, there's no sense ignoring the aspect of fitness that can help you most on the job. Finally, spending a little money on massage equipment might turn out to be the best investment you'll ever make.

You Already Belong to a Health Club

Many of High-Tech Fitness's clients already belong to gyms or health clubs. But, like most of us, they can't go to the club to work out every single day. So they use their home gyms as a back-up system, a place to exercise when they can't make it to their away-from-home gyms.

If you're such a person, it's a good idea not to try to duplicate the equipment at your club. Instead, supplement it. You probably already know the equipment you enjoy using. If your interest is weight training, for instance, you probably don't need a full-line Universal or Nautilus system at home. But you might want to buy a set of free weights and a multi-purpose bench for the house. A rower, stationary bike, or other aerobic device is a good idea. Many gyms don't have rowing machines. Most gyms don't have inversion devices, either, so a set of gravity boots and a bar will give you something else to come home to. Some relaxation equipment may help assuage your feelings of guilt about not being down at the gym, getting your money's worth from your monthly dues.

In any case, remember to choose equipment that doesn't duplicate the gear at your club, but that lets you do the exercises you like. That way, you'll work out harder and more often.

Your Dream Gym

Maybe you're the sort of discriminating person who won't settle for less than the best. Maybe you're status-conscious and want to impress your friends and neighbors. Maybe you're just plain *rich*. Whatever the case, your home gym is a great place to show off.

At High-Tech Fitness, we've set up some rather snazzy gyms for celebrities and others who are simply wealthy without being famous. Most exercise devices come with a selection of options that rival the extras you can buy for your car. You can chrome-plate almost all metal parts these days, and you can even cover your weight benches in real leather. And after that, there's the wonderful world of custom-built equipment: saunas, hot tubs, and virtually any kind of strength equipment, all designed, built, and installed to *your* specifications. If your home already has all the fitness equipment you could possibly want, what about your yacht? And your Lear jet?

It's entirely possible to turn your home gym into the kind of palatial health center that would embarrass even J. R. Ewing. And the money you spend on your home gym is not money wasted. What healthier investment could you make?

PERSONALIZED GYMS

Home gyms are more than a passing fad. They're more, even, than a stationary fad. They're here to stay, a feature of the American cultural landscape.

The gym owners shown on these pages come from various walks of life, and they use their gyms to achieve various fitness goals. Don't be deterred if you don't have as much space as some of the gyms we illustrate take up (although one is in a closet), or if you can't afford much equipment (although one has only two pieces). These are only examples, illustrations of what you *can* do, not what you *must* do.

The important thing is that all these owners use their gyms to keep fit at home, with maximum privacy and convenience, and that any piece of equipment you own helps you do the same.

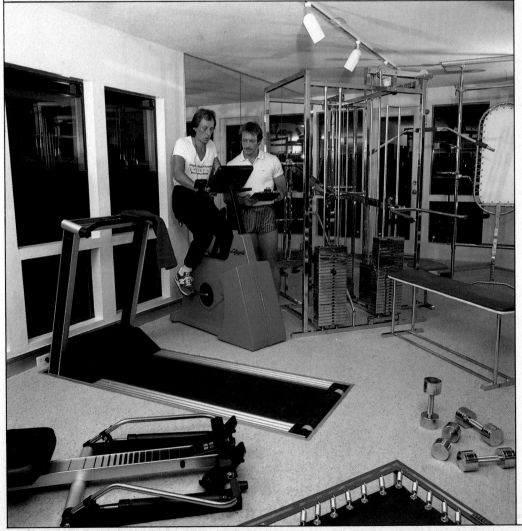

This is my personal gym. The guy with the moustache is my trainer, Bill Prihoda. I work out here at least three times a week. Sometimes I have friends over. My schedule is fairly hectic, so it became apparent early on that a health club wasn't going to meet my fitness needs completely. I wanted a home gym that would let me do it all. A high-tech, clean décor was important. I made sure I had good ventilation, two walls of mirrors (you can only see one), glued-down industrial carpeting, music, and plenty of natural light. What does my home gym do for me? Three things: It lets me blow off steam. It keeps me looking and feeling great. And it gives order to my physical life.

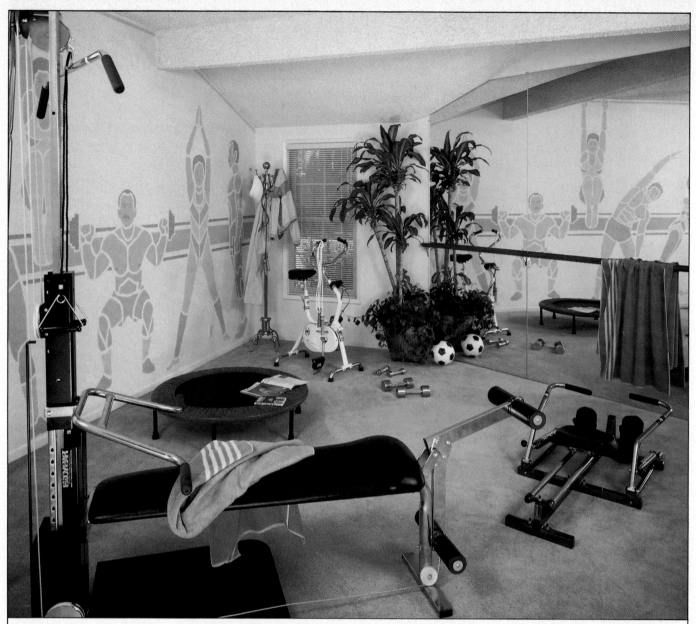

Above: It's easy to see that Bobby Powell is a designer. Her home gym, designed for a complete family workout, reflects her sense of taste and artist's flair. Note the use of wall graphics for color and motivation. The plants provide a pleasing stopping point for the eye, and mirrors make

the room look larger. "I didn't spend a fortune on my equipment," she says. "My primary goal was to create a sporty and fun environment that was in harmony with the rest of the house."

Right: Dan Zimmerman is a single interior designer. Because he's a partner in his own firm, he works long and irregular hours. His home gym allows him to work out three times a week for 90 minutes per workout. Here he's shown hanging from a chrome A-frame inversion system. "I've always wanted to be in top shape," he says. "By avoiding the social aspects of a gym, you can really get a workout."

Dan makes the most of the space in his condo by equipping his loft-gym with the aforementioned inversion machine, a rower, a stationary bike, and a set of free weights (not shown). "My business is fast-paced," says Zimmerman. "I need something to let out frustration. By working out, I find I have a better outlook, and I look and feel healthier."

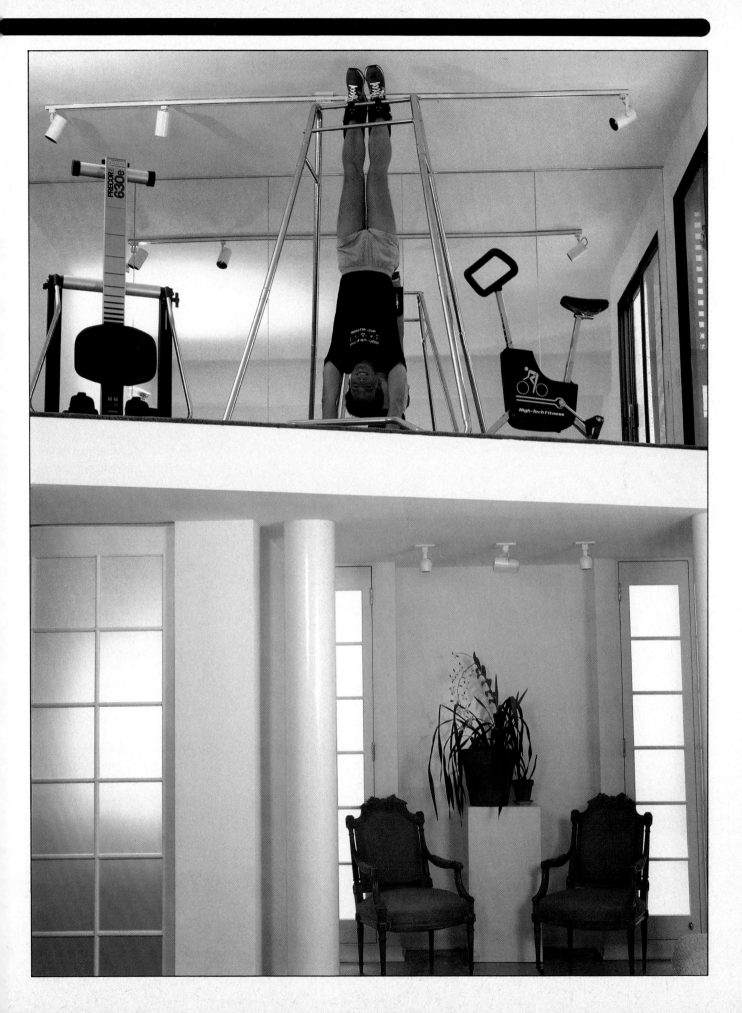

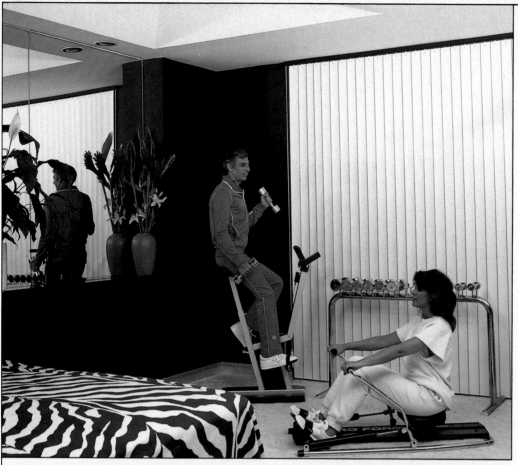

Left: Paul Schwartz is a marketing executive; his wife Sheila is the office manager of a medical office. They usually exercise three or four times a week, for 20 to 40 minutes per workout. "Neither of us particularly wants to grow up to be Lou Ferrigno," says Paul. "We use the chrome-plated dumbbells mostly to stay trim and toned and to supplement our aerobics." With space at a premium, Paul and Sheila can easily fit their home gym into a corner of the bedroom. "Our room décor is black and white, very simple," says Sheila. "So we picked cleanly designed equipment. The chrome plating on the dumbbells, for example, is strictly for looks."

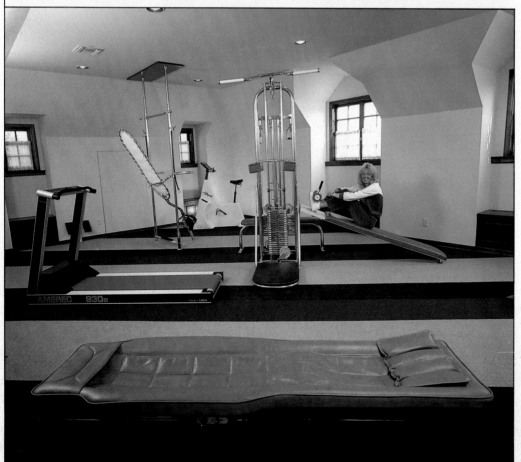

Left: Real-estate executive Tony Brent, his wife Tisha, and their teenage sons Jason and Jeremy can all work out at the same time in their family fitness center. The Brents designed and built this room specifically to house their gym, which is a relatively complete one. The Brents feel their investment has been worth it. "We've always enjoyed exercising," says Tisha, "and now we're no longer inconvenienced by having to go out to a gym. We feel that working out with friends at home is a nice, wholesome activity." Jason, the older of the two Brent boys, adds, "I like using the whole thing—usually before golf, to warm up."

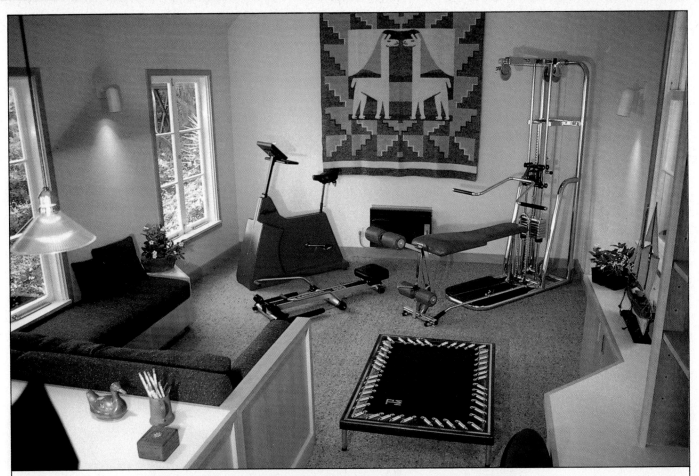

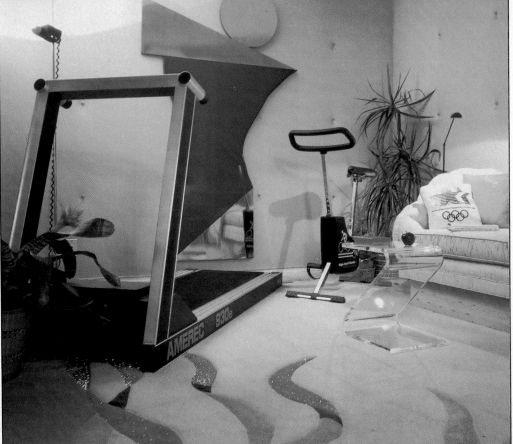

Above: "When I decided to convert an unused room into a home gym," says Sharon M. Rosenberg, owner of several manufacturing firms, "I wanted to make it look as homey and un-gym-like as possible. I added a desk, so I can both work and work out *there*. I'm thrilled that I've been able to take off pounds and inches without leaving home."

Left: A living room may be an unorthodox place for a gym, but designer Edna O'Brien, ASID, wanted to make a statement: Good design and practicality can coexist happily. "The house's interior is ultracontemporary, so I wanted the most futuristic-looking fitness equipment on the market."

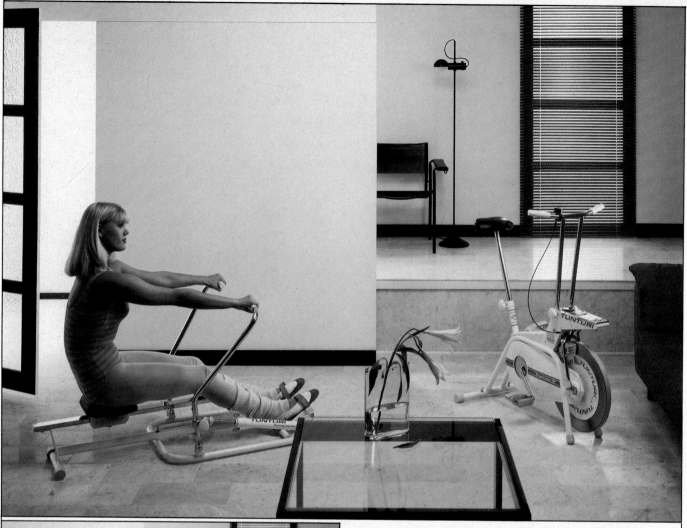

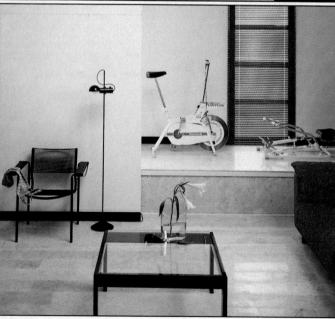

Above: This apartment gym is located in Europe, where the apartments are even smaller than in New York City. Two pieces of equipment, a rower and a stationary bike, are all that's really needed for a vigorous yet varied fitness routine. After you're through using them, they can be stored unobtrusively—as has been done at left.

Right: Composers Burt Bacharach and Carole Bayer Sager have always considered fitness an important part of their lives. As two of the most successful contemporary composers of popular music, they've been able to pick a complete array of the very best equipment, including a rowing machine that will leave them in shape to row all the way from "the moon to New York City." "Our interior designer purposely created a beautiful room where we'd want to come often to work out," says Bacharach. "As a result," adds Sager, "we use it often."

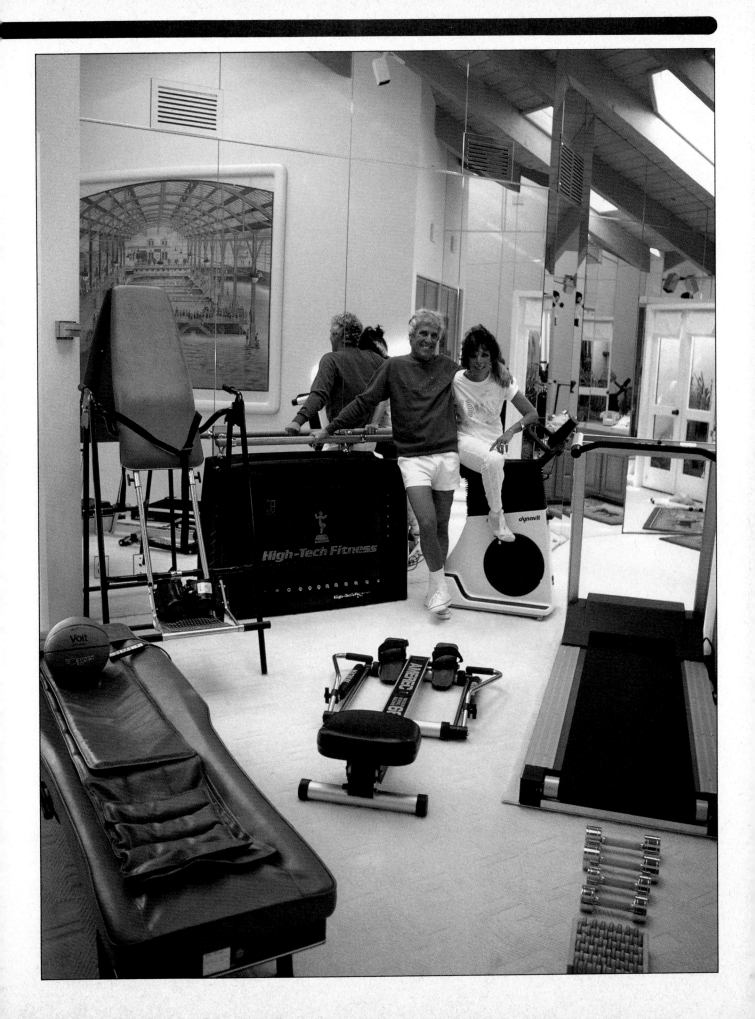

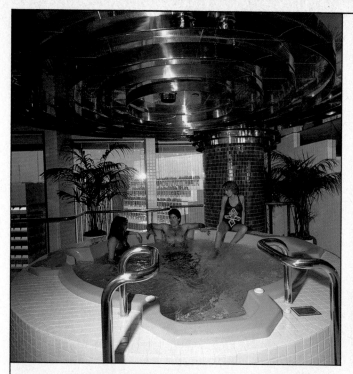

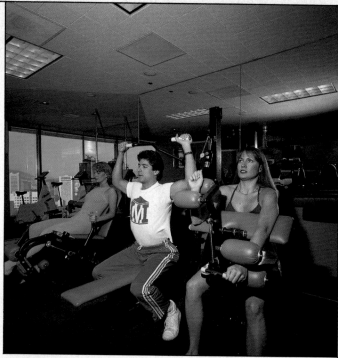

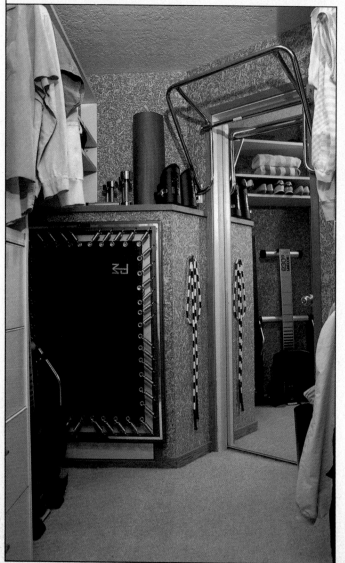

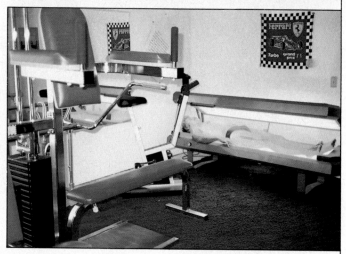

Top, right: A mortgage banking company has put a full line of equipment into this 500-square-foot space. As a bonus, employees can enjoy a soothing hot tub (top, left) after they work out.

Left: "I used to belong to a crowded health club," says secretary Bonnie Marché, "but I always ended up waiting in line to use the machines." When she's through exercising, she stores her space-saver gym in a closet.

Above: Executive John Johnson converted his unused garage into a compact and functional home health club twelve years ago. He started with a set of free weights and is still updating his gym. Johnson says, "Having this kind of equipment and being able to fit my workouts into my lunch hour really has kept me looking and feeling great."

CORPORATE FITNESS

More and more chief executives have discovered that setting up a corporate gym is a good, sound business investment. They've found that such facilities offer a strong dose of preventive medicine, keeping employees happier and healthier and cutting down on corporate medical insurance premiums.

Today, over 50,000 U.S. and 1,000 Canadian firms are involved in some aspect of corporate fitness. They recognize the indisputable correlation between fitness programs and health improvements, reduced absenteeism, fewer job turnovers, improved attitudes, increased energy, and decreased fatigue. Employees and management alike have been able to lose weight, manage stress, lower cholesterol and blood pressure levels, and reduce or prevent back problems. Employees frequently develop a camaraderie and group spirit, encouraging and motivating one another—even visiting one another's home gyms to work out together.

Take a look at these facts and figures:

• Between 1977 and 1983, the cost of corporate health insurance premiums skyrocketed from $30 billion to $78 billion.

• After studying 1,125 employees of two large Toronto insurance companies, researchers projected that a business with 1,400 employees would save 3,500 lost days per year through a fitness program. That translated into about $175,000 in employee/days saved annually.

• General Telephone of Florida started a corporate fitness program. Four months later, GTE found that participants exhibited a 70 percent decrease in stress symptoms.

• NASA found out the following things about fitness program participants: 62% reported better job performance; 89% had improved stamina; 40% slept more soundly; more than 60% lost weight; there was no reduction in productivity due to time taken off to work out.

• Control Data Corporation found that employees with poor health habits were 86% likelier to miss work than their healthier colleagues.

• Participants in Johnson and Johnson's "Live for Life" fitness program reduced sick days by 13%. Sick days among nonparticipants *increased* by 9%.

• Thirty-six major insurance companies indicate that they would reduce life insurance premiums to hypertensives who control their blood pressure. Typical savings are 28% for a whole life policy, and over 50% for term insurance.

As so many corporate officers have learned, a physically fit work force is a productive work force.

WARM-UP FLEXIBILITY EXERCISES

Warm-up flexibility exercises are an important part of any type of fitness routine. The sedentary and repetitious ways we move our bodies in daily life differ greatly from how we move them when exercising. It is this "difference" that indicates our need to prepare (via warm-up) the muscles, joints, and delivery systems of the body for an exercise session.

In general, warm-up preparation increases the elasticity of the muscles by increasing local circulation and temperature of the soft tissue and fluids in the working area. In addition, warm-up "sets" the excitability of the nervous (electrical) system to a level which is appropriate to activity rather than rest. Since all physiological systems of the body must operate in precise concert with each other, all of them must be adequately "informed" of the coming activity. This insures that you will experience maximum performance as well as minimum injury. Warm-ups must always be done smoothly and gradually. Intense, bouncing, ballistic, or stressful warm-up movements will tighten the body and do exactly what we are trying to avoid.

If you are warming up prior to a sports performance, there are some additional benefits. Since warmed-up muscles can be stretched further, contracted faster, and have a greater range of motion, your warmed-up performance will include better reaction times and faster acceleration. Sports enthusiasts should also go through some sports specific movements after their general warm-up movements. In other words, do some "mimic" slow motion movements that are taken exactly from your sport. Pitch a hypothetical ball, swing an imaginary bat, or jump and slam dunk a pretend basketball to help focus both mind and muscles on the contest to come.

To help you achieve a well-informed warm-up, keep the following points in mind:

• STRETCHING SHOULD NOT BE PAINFUL. When doing flexibility exercises, you should move the body part being stretched to a point just below the pain threshold. Try to hold the position for a time in a relaxed fashion. Then, before repeating the stretch, totally relax and remove all tension from the muscles involved. Never attempt to stretch the muscle further by bouncing or yanking into a position.

• DON'T GO OVERBOARD WITH FLEXIBILITY. Although it is true that flexibility is needed to balance the forces around individual joints, and that achieving this balance will prevent injury, it is also true that anything can be overdone. If the body is too flexible, joints can be injury prone due to being unstable. Often people who are naturally flexible tend to overdo in this area because it is one in which they can excel. Unfortunately the body may suffer at the hand of a satisfied ego!

• DON'T COMPETE WITH ANOTHER'S FLEXIBILITY. Comparing yourself with others in terms of flexibility (as well as other fitness capabilities) is not advised. Degrees of flexibility vary from person to person, joint to joint, side to side, from age to age, with the time of day, and between the sexes. Elasticity of ligaments, tendons, and fasciae, as well as inherent joint construction, is an individual matter.

• DON'T LOOK FOR RESULTS IN LARGE QUANTITIES. Flexibility seems to be achieved more slowly and in smaller increments than other fitness areas (strength, for instance). Because the rewards are smaller and slower, flexibility exercises often get discounted and overlooked. Realize their importance and anticipate your possible disenchantment with them—*and do them.*

The following list of exercises will stretch all the major muscle groups. We have ordered them in the traditional warm-up manner from sitting to standing, from head to feet. Although there is no heavy-duty physiological reason to validate this order, it is usually followed simply because one's main workout session is done standing. The basic number and approach to repetitions and length of time to perform each movement can be found in the individual fitness programs on pages 238–279.

BODY AREA	EXERCISES
Neck and shoulders	Neck Bend
Torso and upper hips	Waist Stretch
Entire back and back of legs	Full Forward Bend
Entire back and back of legs	Full Forward Bend Variation
Entire back and back of legs	Waist Hang
Upper back and back of legs	Triangle
Shoulders, chest, and neck	Fish
Neck, shoulders, lower back, and legs	Shoulder Stand
Back of legs and upper back	Bend and Reach
Back of legs and inner thighs	Hamstring Stretch
Front and back of legs and hips	Suspended Stretch
Inner thighs and back of legs	Standing Split

Annette Annechild, a member of the High-Tech Fitness Team, demonstrates her flexibility routine.

THE NECK BEND. Sit in a comfortable, cross-legged position, with your arms extended straight out from your shoulders, palms down. Bring your ear toward your shoulder, gently stretching your neck. Relax and breathe. Hold the position for a few seconds. Then return your head to the upright position, rest, and repeat on the other side.

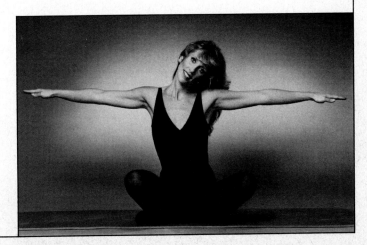

THE WAIST STRETCH. Sit with your legs tucked under your buttocks, toes pointed. Extend your arms overhead, palms facing in, arms in line with your ears. Shift your weight so that you sit on one hip, stretching your arms in the opposite direction. Inhale when you are sitting upright; exhale as you stretch.

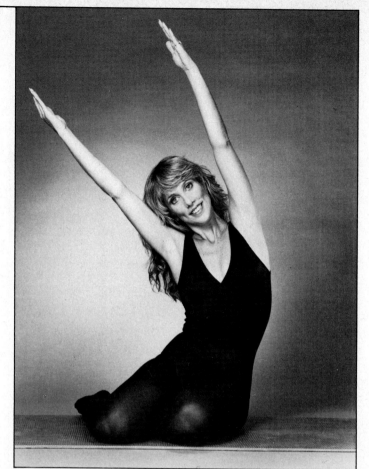

Lift your torso, inhale, and shift your weight to sit on the other hip, stretching your arms in the opposite direction and exhaling.

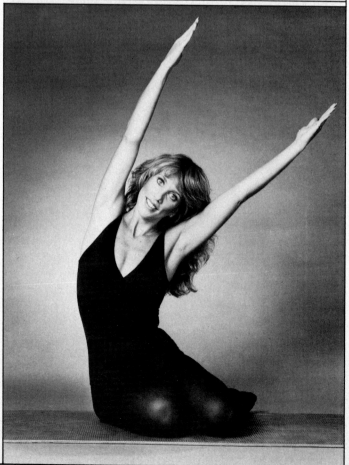

THE FULL FORWARD BEND. Sit with your legs straight and together, back straight, your feet flexed. Stretch your arms over your head and inhale.

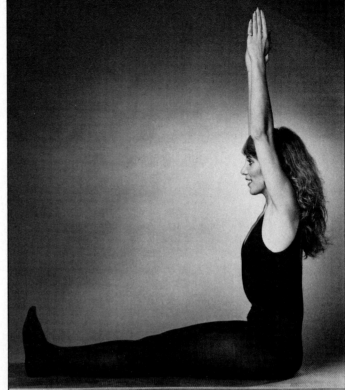

Exhale as you bend forward. Try to hold on to your toes or ankles. Drop your head and shoulders and breathe deeply. Relax. Don't push or bounce. Slowly return to the starting position. The Full Forward Bend should be relaxed and steady for optimum results. Do this exercise daily.

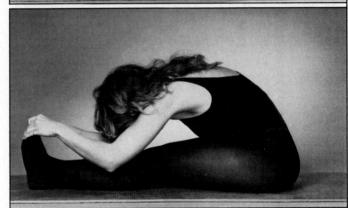

THE FULL FORWARD BEND VARIATION. Sit with your legs straight and together, your feet flexed. Grasp your toes or ankles. Keep your head up and your back straight. Breathe deeply and don't bounce.

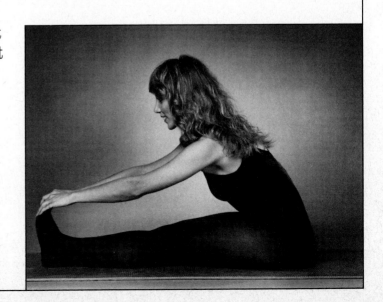

THE FISH. Lie flat on your back, feet flexed. Raise your torso to a 45° angle, using your elbows for support and keeping your legs straight. Drop your head back until the crown of the head rests on the floor. Your weight should be on your head, elbows, and buttocks, with your back deeply arched. Breathe deeply. To return to the starting position, slowly raise your head and then lower your torso to the floor.

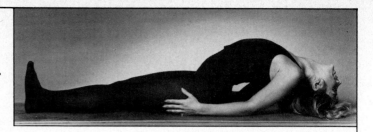

THE SHOULDER STAND. Do this exercise after The Fish to stretch out your back muscles. Lie on your back. Lift your legs and torso off the floor so that your body rests on your shoulders. Place your hands under your hips for support and to help lift your body. Keep your elbows as close together as possible, with your hands side by side, fingers together and pointing toward your buttocks. Keep your fingers on your back. Close your eyes and breathe.

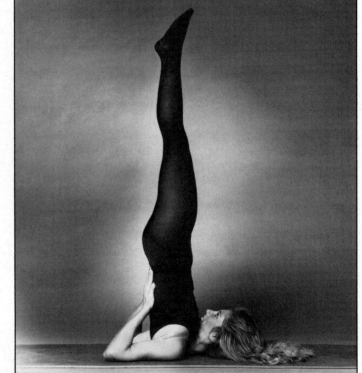

To come down from the shoulder stand, bring your legs over your head until your toes rest on the floor, if possible. Place your hands on the floor, palms down. Then bend your knees slightly, and using your hands as brakes, lower your torso *slowly*. When your buttocks touch the floor, straighten your legs and lower them, using your stomach muscles. Then rest, breathing deeply. Try to do this exercise every day.

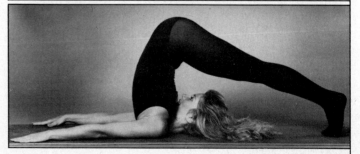

THE WAIST HANG. Stand straight with your feet together and your arms stretched overhead. Inhale.

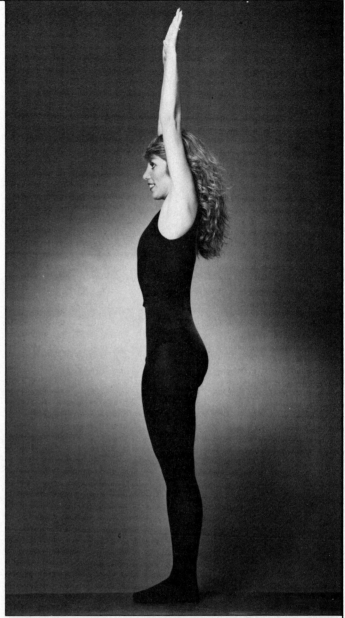

Gently bring your upper body forward. Exhale as you lower your arms and torso. Let your neck and shoulders relax as you stretch toward the floor. At the beginning you may not be able to touch the floor. Stretch only as far as is comfortable. Breathe deeply and relax.

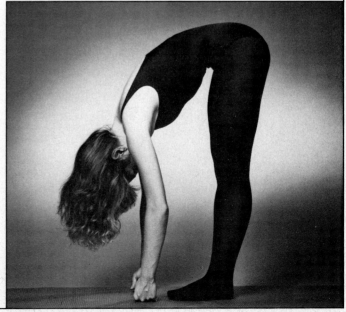

THE TRIANGLE. From a kneeling position, hands on the floor, straighten your legs, torso, and arms so that your body forms a triangle with the floor. Inhale and lift onto your toes. Exhale as you lower your heels slowly to the floor to stretch your calves. Hold the position for a few seconds before repeating. Bend your knees and return to the kneeling position.

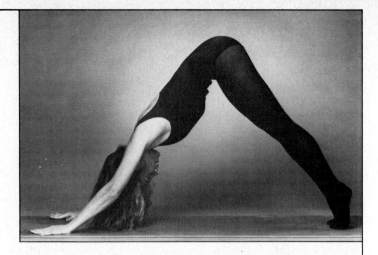

THE BEND AND REACH. Stand to the side of the barre with your legs and feet together. Grasp the barre for support. Hold your free arm over your head. Bend forward at the waist, keeping your back flat, legs straight, and your head up. Stretch as far as possible. Breathe deeply and relax. Bend your knees slightly and slowly return to the starting position.

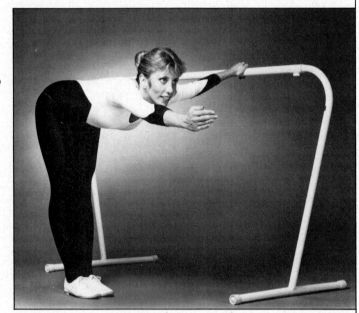

THE HAMSTRING STRETCH. Face the barre at a 45° angle. Place the heel of your outside foot on top of the barre. Bending at the waist, stretch forward over the elevated leg. Reach toward your toes and hold the position. Keep both legs straight and do not bounce. Repeat with the other leg.

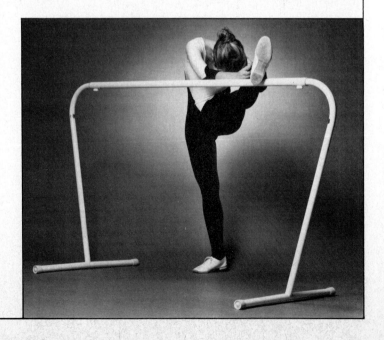

THE SUSPENDED STRETCH. Face away from the barre at a 45° angle. Place the instep of your near leg on the barre behind you. Keeping both legs straight, stretch down over your outside foot. Reach for your toes. Keep your back flat and your legs straight. Repeat with the other leg.

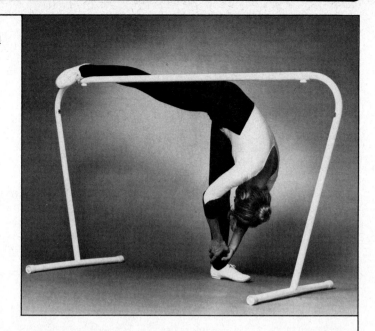

THE STANDING SPLIT. Stand to the side of the barre, and grasp it for support. Facing straight ahead, keep your back flat and your body erect. Raise your outside leg and grab the heel. As you pull the foot higher and higher, straighten your leg. (If you cannot straighten your leg while holding your foot, grab the back of your calf and straighten and lift as far as you are able.) Repeat with the other leg.

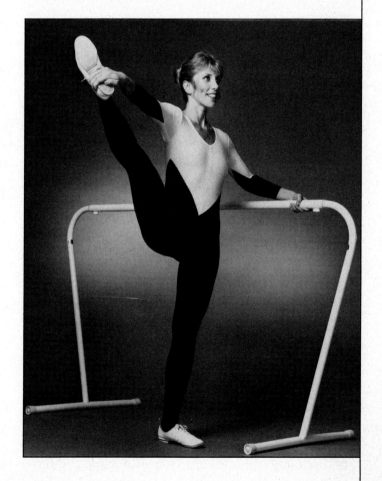

COOLING DOWN/ STRETCHING EXERCISES

Doing stretching exercises ("cooling down") at the end of your workout is a way to focus on problem-solving, rehabilitation, and relaxation rather than body preparation. You'll notice, however, that the movements are similar to the ones you do when warming up.

At the end of a workout, your muscles are pliable, warm, and unusually receptive to the effects of stretching. Because they're so ready to stretch, spending time at workout's end to stretch out the kinks caused by your exercises, your daily posture (standing, sitting, walking, etc.), or your innate structural deviations can have a more permanent effect on your muscles. This effect is especially needed to counteract the inflexibility we all develop over the years.

In its extreme form, this inflexibility can show itself as arthritis and/or calcification in and around the tissues near the joints. Some medical studies suggest that poor flexibility can be responsible for bad posture, compression of peripheral nerves, dysmenorrhea (painful menstruation), and other ailments.

In addition, sports medicine specialists believe that every time you exercise, the stress on your muscles produces multiple, very slight injuries. (Dr. William Southmayd, in his book *Sportshealth,* calls them "microinjuries.") When these small injuries heal, they leave tiny areas of scar tissue on the muscles, thus making the muscles a little bit shorter than they were before. So you must stretch to balance your newly strengthened musculature and to keep your now-strong muscles pliable, efficient, and comfortable for exercise as well as for daily living.

On the following pages, you'll see some common stretches that you can do to cool down after a workout. These stretches will increase the flexibility of each area of your body and allow your muscles to relax after a workout. Here's a list of these stretches, as well as the body areas each one benefits. We recommend that you do them in this order:

BODY AREA	EXERCISES
Ankle	Point and Flex
Calf	Push
Hamstrings	Straddle Stretch
	Hurdler's Stretch
	Sit and Reach
Quadriceps	Kneeling Stretch
	Standing Ankle Grab
Hips	Knee Tuck and Hip Twist
Back	Back Roll
Shoulders	Cat Stretch
Neck	Four-Corner Neck Stretch

THE POINT AND FLEX. Sit with your legs straight ahead, your back flat, and your head in a neutral position. Inhale, point your toes and hold; then exhale, flex your foot, and hold.

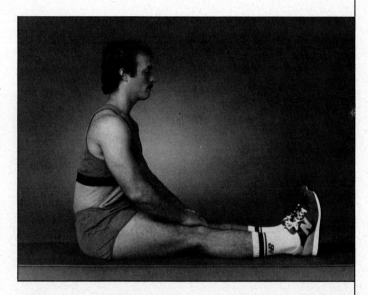

THE PUSH. This exercise may be done with your hands against a wall or on the floor. Start with your feet in a forward stride position, your front leg bent, toes pointed straight ahead. Lean as far forward as possible, supporting your body with your hands flat on the floor or wall. Push the heel of your straight leg down to the floor and exhale. Repeat with the other leg.

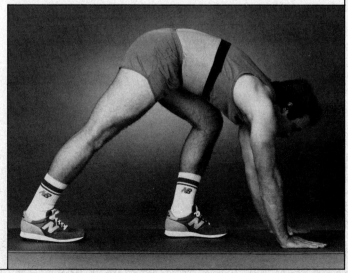

THE STRADDLE STRETCH . Sit in a comfortable straddle position, with legs straight and toes pointed toward the ceiling. Keeping your back flat, inhale and stretch to one side, pulling your opposite arm over your head. Exhale and stretch straight to the side. Do not turn your waist or bounce. Repeat on the other side.

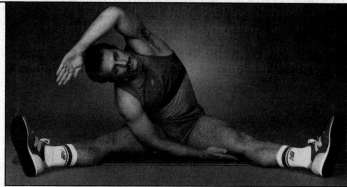

Sit in a straddle position with your legs straight, feet flexed. Keeping your back flat and head up, bend toward one leg and hold on to your ankle or toes with both hands. Exhale, hold the position, and don't bounce. Repeat on the other side.

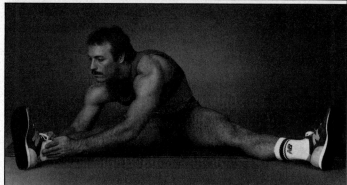

THE HURDLER'S STRETCH. Sit with your legs straight in front, your back flat, and your head in a neutral position. Bend one knee and place the sole of your foot on the inside of the opposite thigh. Lean forward over your straight leg and reach for your toes. Hold the position and exhale; then repeat with the other leg.

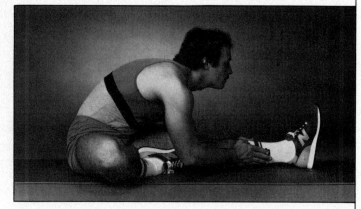

THE SIT AND REACH. Sit with your back flat, head in a neutral position, and your legs straight in front of you. Keeping your back flat, reach for your ankles and lean over your legs. Exhale and hold. Do not bounce.

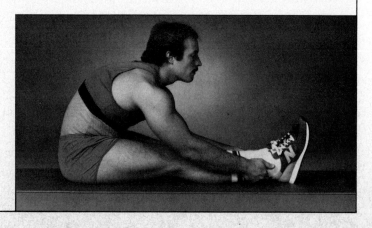

THE KNEELING STRETCH. Kneel on a mat or carpet, with your heels directly under your buttocks, toes pointed. Lean back, placing your hands on the mat behind you. Keeping your arms straight and your stomach tucked in, push your hips forward until the body forms a straight line from knee to shoulder. Exhale and hold.

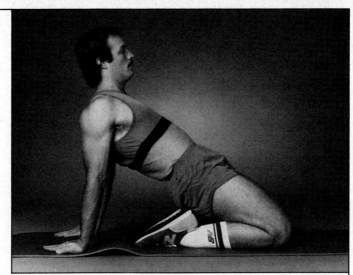

THE STANDING ANKLE GRAB. Stand up straight, toes straight ahead. Balance on one leg while bending the other knee. Keeping both legs in alignment, pull the ankle of your bent leg toward your buttocks and exhale. Don't let the bent knee come forward. Repeat with the other leg.

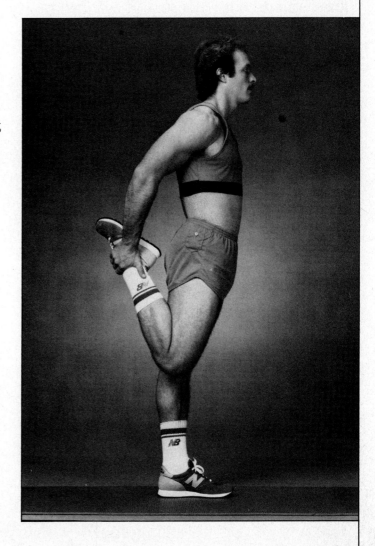

THE KNEE TUCK AND HIP TWIST. Sit with your back flat, your head in a neutral position, and both legs straight in front of you. Bend one leg and cross it over the other. Place your foot on the floor next to the outer side of the straight leg. Grab the front of your bent leg with both hands and tuck it into your chest. Exhale and hold.

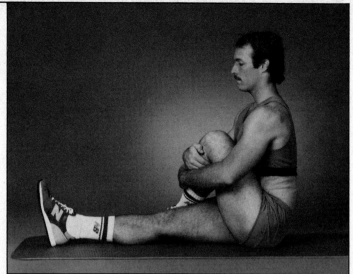

Place the opposite elbow on your bent knee, with the other arm straight and slightly to the back of your torso. Turn toward your straight arm, pushing against your knee with your elbow to help you twist at the waist. Keep your back as straight as possible as you twist, and turn your head toward your straight arm. Repeat on the other side.

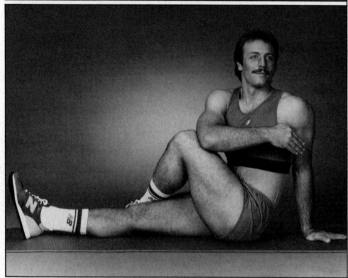

THE BACK ROLL. Sit on the floor with your legs straight in front of you. Lift your legs and roll back onto your shoulders. Support yourself with your arms. Let your knees drop as close to your ears as possible. Relax and breathe very deeply. Return to the starting position by slowly uncurling your torso, while you support your weight on your arms. Keep your knees bent until your legs reach the floor.

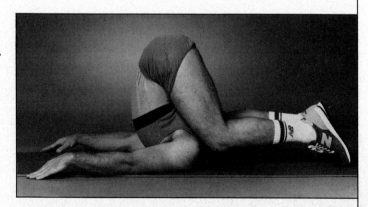

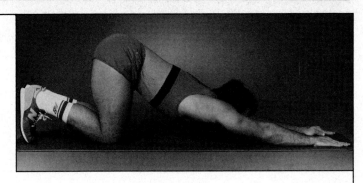

THE CAT STRETCH. From a kneeling position, feet flexed, lower your shoulders and stretch your arms out in front of you. Keeping your arms straight, your knees *behind* your hips, and your head looking forward, reach as far as you can. Exhale and hold. To release the position, slowly move your hips behind your knees and slide your hands toward your knees.

THE FOUR-CORNER NECK STRETCH. Imagine that your head is encased in a cube. Slowly roll your head in a circle, stretching your neck, not just down or sideways, but *into* each of the cube's four corners in turn. Breathe deeply and relax. Repeat, circling in the other direction.

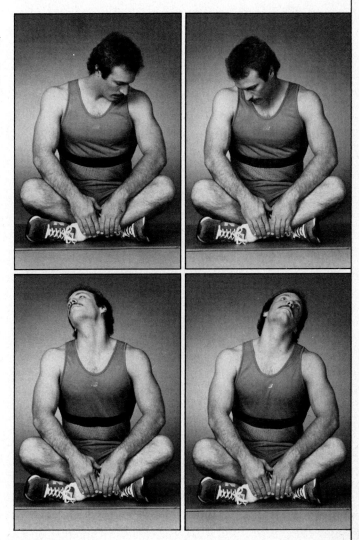

LIGHT WEIGHT TRAINING PROGRAM

A great way to tone, trim and define your muscles is to use light weights and high reps. If you follow this program faithfully, you'll get stronger, firmer, and bring your muscles into greater definition. It's efficiently designed so there's no functional duplication of muscle groups. In other words, each exercise develops the muscle groups differently. Best of all, you can work out by using 2- to 5-pound weights. So even when you travel, you can take your portable weight set with you to keep fit and feeling alive on the road.

If you are just starting out on your exercise program, we suggest beginning with 2-pound dumbbells. Work for three sessions per week on alternating days. For best results try to isolate body movement to only the exercising body part. Do one set of 20 repetitions of each exercise for two weeks (6 workouts). Then accelerate to two sets of 20 repetitions at the same weight. After another two weeks (6 workouts), increase your weight to 3 pounds, and decrease the repetitions back to one set of 20. Continue this pattern until you achieve the contours you desire (1 set of 20 ... 2 sets of 20 ... add weight, reduce sets, etc.). If you are feeling any strain at the end of the 6-workout segment, do not increase your workload. Wait until your muscles and body feel comfortable. When you do increase the weights, do not exceed an increment of 2 pounds.

In general, remember to exhale when you are lifting the weight against gravity, and inhale when you are lowering it with the aid of gravity. There is no reason to breathe unusually deeply or heavily when lifting light weights, but it is always a good idea to develop the good breathing habits of exhaling and inhaling at the proper points in the exercises.

BODY AREA	EXERCISES
Lower arms	Wrist Curls
Upper arms	Arm Curls
Shoulders	Dumbbell Flys
Back and shoulders	Bent-Waist Arm Lifts
Arms	Kickbacks
Pectoral muscles (For men, chest strength and firmness; for women, lift and definition to the breasts.)	Flys
Stomach and thighs	The Walk
Inner and outer thighs	Single-Leg Lift
Inner and front thighs	Bent-Knee Leg Lift
Legs and buttocks	Hip Swing

Annette Annechild, a member of the High-Tech Fitness Team, demonstrates her *Five-Pound Workout* routine.

WRIST CURLS. Sit in a comfortable cross-legged position. Place your wrists on your knees and let your hands fall over your knees, palms up, grasping the dumbbells.

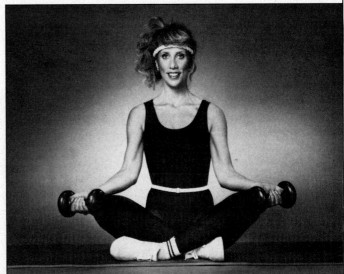

Moving only your wrists, lift the dumbbells up and toward you, then lower them slowly. Work your arms alternately or together, and keep your waist lifted and your back straight. Exhale as the weights come up, inhale as you lower them.

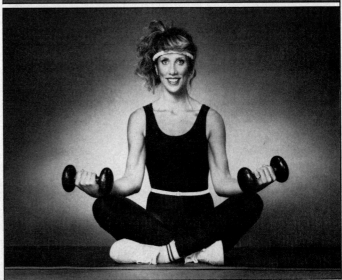

ARM CURLS. Stand with your feet shoulder-width apart. Hold the dumbbells in your hands, palms up. Bend your arm at the elbow and bring the weight slowly up toward your shoulder, then slowly lower it to the starting position. Try not to move your upper arm. Alternate arms, and keep your back straight.

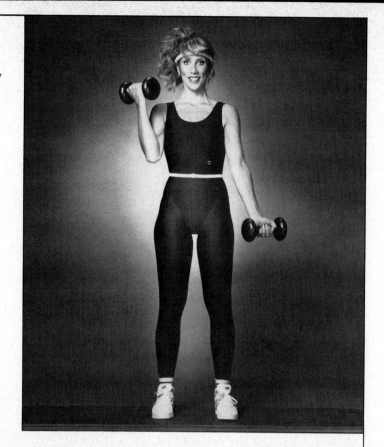

DUMBBELL FLYS. Grasp the dumbbells with your arms at your sides, palms facing in. Lift your arms straight out to shoulder height, then lower them slowly. Keep your elbows locked during the entire movement. Exhale as you lift your arms, inhale as you lower them. Keep your back straight.

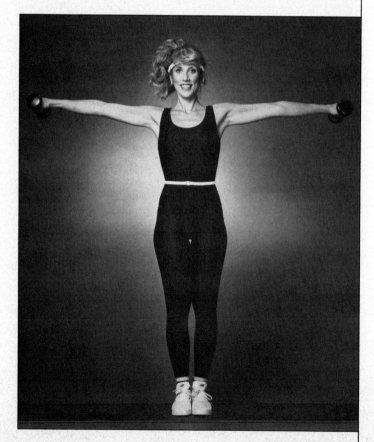

BENT-WAIST ARM LIFTS. Bend forward at a 90° angle, keeping your back flat, with your arms straight down, palms facing, grasping the dumbbells. Raise your arms slowly to shoulder height, then lower them. Exhale as you raise your arms, inhale as you lower them. (If you feel any strain on your back, bend your knees slightly.)

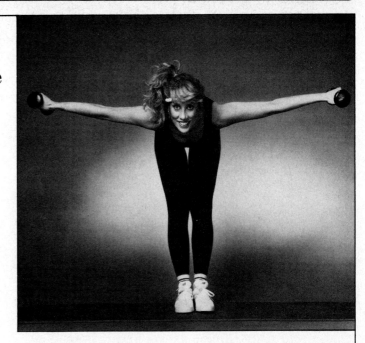

TRICEPS EXTENSION. Kneel with your knees shoulder-width apart. Place your hands on the floor directly under your shoulders. Grasp a dumbbell with one hand. Bend and lift your arm as you lock your elbow against your waist.

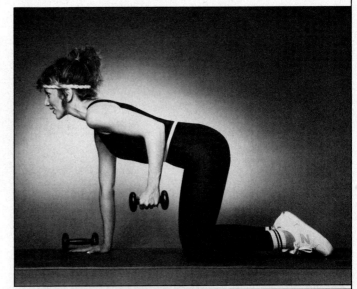

Keeping your working arm firmly against your side, slowly straighten the arm to the back, until it's fully extended from the elbow. Then lower your arm. Exhale as you extend your arm, inhale as you lower it. Repeat with the other arm.

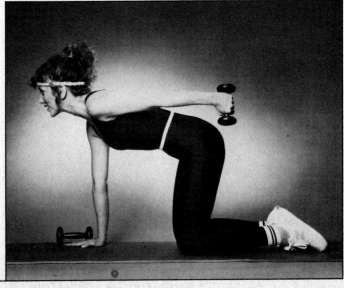

FLYS. Lie on your back with your knees bent and your feet shoulder-width apart. Place the dumbbells about a foot away from your hips and grasp them with your palms up.

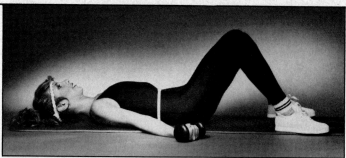

Keeping your back flat on the floor and your arms straight, bring the dumbbells up together over your pelvic area. Do this movement slowly and with good concentration for the best results. You can also do this exercise by stretching your arms straight out from the shoulder along the floor, palms up, and then raising the weights directly over your face. Exhale as you raise your arms, inhale as you lower them.

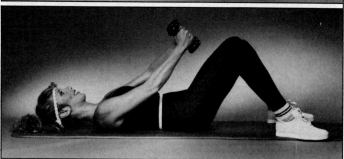

THE WALK. This exercise is especially effective with ankle weights. Lean back on your elbows, with your hands close to your body, palms down. Raise your legs, and begin a slow "walk" with your toes pointed. Keep your legs low and fully extended. Alternate your legs when you "walk." Breathe deeply in rhythm as you move your legs. Do as many of these as you can, as often as you can. Increase the number of repeats with each workout.

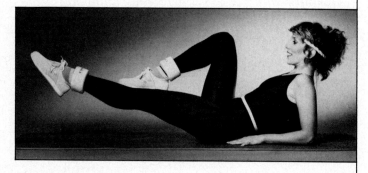

THE SINGLE-LEG LIFT. This is done wearing a weight on only the upper (working) leg. Lie on your side, legs straight, with your legs and torso forming a straight line. Bend your elbow and support your head on your hand. Place the other hand in front of your chest, palm down.

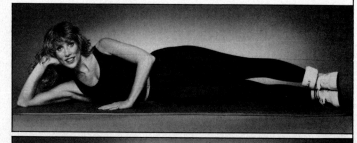

Raise the top leg about 12 inches off the lower leg. Be sure the lower leg doesn't move. Exhale as you raise your leg, inhale as you lower it. Repeat on the other side.

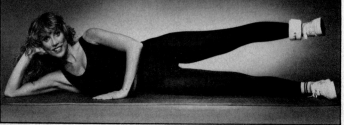

THE BENT-KNEE LEG LIFT. Lie on your side in the same position as for the Single-Leg Lift, ankle weight in place. Keeping your leg straight, raise it as high as you can, toes to the ceiling.

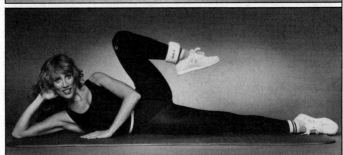

Bend your knee and point your foot. Do not allow your knee to drop forward. Then straighten your leg and lower it slowly back to the starting position. Exhale as you bend your knee and as you lower your leg, inhale as you raise your leg the first and second times. Repeat on the other side.

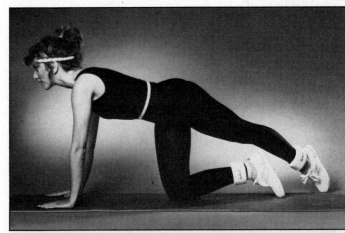

THE HIP SWING. This is a very effective and strenuous exercise. Kneel with your hands and legs shoulder-width apart. Extend one leg, keeping the knee locked and the foot pointed.

Swing the leg out horizontally as far as you can, toward your head. At the same time, bend at the waist and turn your head sideways to meet your foot. Keep your leg raised to at least shoulder height. Return to the starting position. Exhale as you move your leg forward, inhale as you straighten out. Repeat with the other leg.

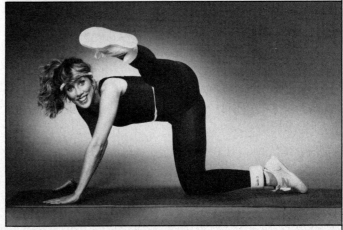

PERSONAL FITNESS PROGRAMS DESIGNED FOR YOU

The High-Tech Fitness Team of personal trainers, physicians, and exercise physiologists has come up with personal fitness programs designed just for you. We've taken into account your age, your physical condition, and your goals. We've formulated these programs to help you achieve the degree of fitness you want.

Because we think your body is serious business, we give you a few words of caution.

Don't start an exercise program without assessing your current state of health. We know we've said this before, but it's important enough for us to repeat. The best way to find out how healthy you are is to go to a physician or other health care specialist and take a physical. Ideally, the physical should include a stress EKG. If you're over 35, a smoker, have a family history of heart disease, or if you've been inactive for a long time, a stress EKG is a must.

Get yourself a reliable pulse monitor. Without one, it'll be hard to know whether you're getting aerobic benefits from your workouts. And, of course, a pulse monitor will show if you're working too hard and pushing your heart toward the danger zone.

The following exercise programs were prepared by High-Tech Fitness Team members Mario Pace, Ph.D., Steven Arnold, M.D., Joy Grau, M.S., and Bill Prihoda, M.S. A good program is not a magic one, but rather well-rounded, and designed for a specific purpose or audience. If these or other good programs are followed regularly, you *will* get positive results. Your body has no choice, it will just happen!

Each program has a special focus (age, sex, specific sport group). All include segments for flexibility, warm-up, aerobic work, cooldown, strength training, and stretching. Since the average person's life seems to be organized around *non*-exercise, the High-Tech Fitness Team feels most of us need *all* of these exercise segments. If your life is more active, however, you may wish to focus on only one or two aspects, since you may be getting the other activities elsewhere.

We have conveniently outlined three progressive levels of involvement, which allows you to proceed modestly from a motivational as well as safety standpoint. Too much, too soon, too fast invariably results in physical injury or mental burnout. So remember, even though we have outlined for you what we feel to be a sound format, each of us is an individual and we perform unpredictably for reasons often felt only by ourselves. Don't follow anyone else's program or formula as "the law." When exercising, it is necessary to listen and learn from your own body's instructions. This may mean, for example:

• Doing a little less overall if your energy is low.

• Modifying, deleting, or reducing the weight on an exercise that seems to be causing a problem.

• When it comes time to progress, augmenting only those exercises you have become adapted to and are comfortable with ... not those you still find straining or fatiguing.

• Changing your aerobic work from outdoor to indoor (due to weather), or from weight-bearing to non-weight-bearing (because of injury).

• Performing strength work before aerobic work because it seems to correlate best with how your body expends energy. (Some people are so exhausted after aerobics, they have nothing left for strength work. Some even do the workouts for each on separate days.)

Although we haven't included any prescribed regimen of exercises for children, we'd like to address the topic briefly. Physical fitness helps youngsters develop coordination, self-confidence, and lifelong good habits. When parents and children participate in physical activity together, the children learn a very important lesson: We must continue to move and exercise through our whole lives. Too many children see exercise only as play. When they grow up and begin to play in different ways (hobbies, work, other non-active pastimes), they cease to exercise and they gain weight. Letting your child see you take the time to exercise deliberately and take care of yourself may be the most valuable health-care technique you can pass on. CAUTION: *No* child in this age bracket is ready for strength training using weights.

As for the sports-specific programs, bear in mind that the best way to train for any sport is to play it regularly. However, since most of us are only recreational athletes indulging on the weekend rather than week-long, we can only do the next best thing. We can move, stretch, and strengthen the muscles used in our sport as part of our personal High-Tech Fitness program. You will notice that these programs have been grouped according to similar requirements in terms of muscular endurance, muscular strength, cardiovascular endurance, and in some cases similar movement patterns. These programs are not designed for the professional athlete. Obviously, training for the professional or semi-professional athlete would require a more detailed analysis of both the specifics of the sport and the athlete's specific body mechanics, movement style, and body physiology.

Before embarking on the program which best suits you, it is important that you understand a few basic definitions and concepts.

Aerobics—Aerobic literally means "with oxygen," and incorporates any of a group of partial- or total-body movements that are somewhat repetitive in nature. They should be performed so that your heart rate is elevated to a predetermined range for 15 to 35 minutes, or even longer. As you become more fit, you will need to increase the vigor of the movements in order to reach your target heart rate range. Remember, the *type* or *style* of your movements does not constitute aerobics. Your achievement of target heart rate is what makes an activity aerobic. Many people take classes they think are aerobic, but may or may not be. If you don't monitor what the movements are doing to your heart rate, you *cannot* know what is aerobic for you and what is not. You could very easily be doing too little or too much.

Antagonists—Pairs of muscle groups which oppose each other (biceps and triceps, hamstrings and quadriceps) are called antagonists. Developing one member of one of these pairs but not another upsets your muscular equilibrium. As one muscle becomes stronger than its antagonist, it decreases the flexibility of the joint controlled by the pair. The result: Both muscles and the affected joint become more susceptible to injury.

It's easy to exercise yourself into muscular imbalance. You can work your quads by riding your bike or running over hills and ignore your hamstrings. You'll lose flexibility and strength in your hamstrings, and eventually you may experience a painful hamstring pull.

The solution is to make sure you work not only the muscles you want to develop, but also their antagonists. All exercise programs in this book were developed with an eye toward exercising both members of antagonistic pairs.

Cool-Down—A segment of activity that mimics your aerobic workout in style (like warm-up) but is done at a much slower pace. It has been pointed out by Dr. Kenneth H. Cooper, author of the best sellers *Aerobics* and *The New Aerobics,* that a majority of cardiovascular irregularities occur during recovery after exercise. It is important to cool down, because stopping vigorous activity abruptly can cause as much as 60 percent of your blood to pool suddenly below the waist, depriving your heart and brain. This may cause nausea, light-headedness, or more serious reactions. After a five-minute cool-down, take your heart rate. If it is well below 120 beats per minute, then you have exercised within your capacity. If it is higher than this, your cardiovascular workload (percentage of maximum heart rate) should be lowered.

Flexibility—A segment near the beginning of an exercise program directed at joint mobility. By moving all the joints through their various movements and ranges of motion, the tendons, ligaments, and other soft tissues are prepared for the work to come. This preparation means no surprises and therefore fewer injuries.

4 × 4—Stands for four sets of four reps. You place a weight on the bar that you can handle for four reps. Then you do four sets of four reps at this weight. Warm up and cool down by doing ten reps at 40% of your 1 r.m. each time.

One Repetition Maximum—(1 r.m.) The maximum amount of weight you can lift in just one repetition of an exercise. This value needs to be determined by trial and error with a spotter. Once determined for each exercise, you will use it to calculate, by percentage, the amount of weight in a given set of a given exercise. This is the same principle as using a percentage of your maximum heart rate when doing your aerobic workout.

Positive and Negative Work—When you raise a weight, your muscles contract. They're doing positive work. When you lower the weight, they lengthen. They're doing negative work.

Because negative work is easier (it's aided by gravity), we have a tendency to ignore it, and to pay less attention to proper exercise form. In fact, both parts are important since the same muscles are being worked during both movements.

It's a common mistake to jerk a weight upward, using body momentum to help you raise it, then let it slip down. (This happens most often during leg extensions.) If you do this, you're not only depriving yourself of the intended benefits of the exercise you're performing, you're also risking injury.

Raise and lower your weights smoothly and slowly enough to stop the movement during any stage of an exercise. A good rule to follow is that it should take nearly twice as long to lower a weight as it does to raise it.

Pyramiding—(△) Pyramiding is a strength training term that means sequentially increasing your weight and decreasing your reps. You start at 40 to 50 percent of your 1 r.m. for ten reps, and you wind up at 85 to 90 percent of your 1 r.m. for one rep. Then you do another rep at 85 to 90 percent, rest, repeat this one rep, then finish with 10 more at 40 to 50 percent. You decrease or increase your reps by two each set. Here's what a typical pyramid chart* looks like:

Weight	Reps
90	10
115	8
130	6
145	4
160	2
175	1
175	1
90	10

Repetition—(rep) One completed movement of any given exercise: up and down, back and forth, out and in, etc.

Set—A group of repetitions done continuously with little or no rest between each one. When several sets are performed with the same or different amounts of weight, the rest time between sets is typically 45 to 90 seconds.

Strength Training—A series of exercises designed to work certain muscle groups at certain angles and at certain paces, against gradually increasing levels of resistance. The angles and paces and sets and repetitions chosen by trainers are focused on an individual's needs. These needs may concern a sport, rehabilitation, general toning, or achieving muscular balance around a particular joint. The average person would benefit immensely from a well-balanced strength program that worked oppos-

1 r.m. would be 200 pounds in this example.

ing major functional muscle groups. In simple terms, these would include pushing and pulling movements at each joint in all of its possible movement directions.

Stretching—A group of exercises to be done after all the muscles are moved, warm, pliable, and perhaps a bit fatigued. The major focus is on lengthening the posture muscles, which bear unrelenting work day after day, whether you're exercising or merely living. Sometimes other musculature is included if a specific sport or activity done on the job, for example, is producing an imbalance.

Visual Imaging—Mentally focusing and isolating in your mind the specific muscle or muscle group being used in an exercise. This has been shown to place greater stress on the area, and therefore produces more intense muscular contraction and better results in the form of tone, shape, and strength.

Warm-Up—A warm-up segment of movement should always precede your aerobic workout (regardless of where it is placed in your overall format). It should basically be a slower version of whatever aerobic activity you are going to perform. This begins to gradually elevate the heart rate and body temperature and also readies many complicated electrical/chemical/physiological processes within the body.

A word about proper breathing. If you're exercising aerobically—jogging, bike riding, rebounding, working on a treadmill, or whatever—you should breathe regularly, deeply, and as normally as you can. When you're pumping iron, doing push-ups, leg lifts, general calisthenics—any kind of exercise that consists of a weight-bearing movement followed by a return movement—you exhale when the weight or resistance is going *against* the pull of gravity (up), and you inhale when the resistance is slowly going *with* the pull of gravity (down). Thus, when you do a push-up, you exhale as you push yourself up by straightening your arms, and you inhale as you lower yourself by flexing them. When you're bench pressing, exhale as you push the weight up, and inhale as you lower it toward your chest.

Something About Our
CHARTS

What would a fitness book be without charts? The difference is, you fill out *these* charts yourself.

Progress Chart I will help you keep track of your weight and aerobic fitness. Once a week, you write down the date (same day and time each week), then weigh yourself, write down your weight, and record the percent of difference in either direction, gain or loss.

Take your pulse when you wake up that morning, and write down the result. Then, after you finish working out, wait two minutes and take your pulse. The more aerobically fit you are, the closer these two readings become. Again, write it down.

Progress Chart II helps you monitor the progress you're making with your measurements and is self-explanatory. Measure yourself once a week—try to measure on the same day each week. Write down the date, then record the measurements of your chest/bust, waist, hip, thigh, upper arm, and calf.

The High-Tech Fitness Personal Workout Chart logs your exercise program. Across the top row of boxes, you can write 13 separate dates. The dates correspond to each of your workouts. Down the left hand side, you write the name of each exercise in your workout routine. Each little box at the intersection of an exercise column and a date column is divided into thirds. That allows you to write three items of information in each box. For example, my first day (April 21) of doing the shoulder press, I did three sets of 10 reps at a weight of 30 pounds. So I wrote a "3" in the upper-left-hand corner, a "10" in the upper-right-hand corner, and a "30" in the bottom triangle.

This system works for aerobics, too. On April 21, I ran two (upper left) miles (upper right) in 19 minutes and 49 seconds.

Why three compartments instead of four? Four wouldn't have left you enough space to write anything in, and two didn't seem to leave you enough categories to write about. Actually, neither does three. On flexibility and stretching, for example, you could be doing six exercises in each category. So instead, we're suggesting that you just check off each of these two categories when you've finished.

You can see that I actually did a few pyramids and 4×4's with weights. (You'll find these two terms defined in the introduction to this chapter.) Those three rows of big boxes on the bottom should leave you enough space to write down your results. If they don't, I'm really sorry. They are absolutely the biggest squares we could fit in this book format.

By the way, even though we worked very hard to develop these charts, we're not going to stick up one of those "reproduction is punishable by law" notices. Feel free to reproduce the charts as much as you want. Think of them as *your* charts.

PROGRESS CHART I

	DATE	WEIGHT	+/− DIFFERENCE	RESTING PULSE (UPON ARISING)	RECOVERY PULSE 2 MINUTES AFTER AEROBICS
1st Week					
2nd Week					
3rd Week					
4th Week					
5th Week					
6th Week					
7th Week					
8th Week					
9th Week					
10th Week					

*Generally, weight loss should not exceed 2 to 3 pounds per week. It's best to weigh yourself first thing in the morning.

PROGRESS CHART II

	DATE	CHEST/ BUST	WAIST	HIP	THIGH	UPPER ARM	CALF
1st Week							
2nd Week							
3rd Week							
4th Week							
5th Week							
6th Week							
7th Week							
8th Week							
9th Week							
10th Week							

HIGH-TECH FITNESS PERSONAL WORKOUT CHART

PATRICK HEITER'S WORKOUT 4/21/84 – 5/31/84

(Key: SETS | REPS / WEIGHT)

	4/21	4/24	4/26	5/1	5/3	5/8	5/11
SHOULDER PRESS	3 / 10 / 30	3 / 10 / 30	3 / 10 / 30	3 / 10 / 35	3 / 10 / 35	3 / 8 / 40	1, 2 / 10, 8 / 40
LAT PULLDOWNS	3 / 10 / 80	3 / 10 / 80	3 / 10 / 80	3 / 10 / 80	1, 3 / 10, 10 / 60, 80	1, 3 / 10, 10 / 60, 80	1, 3 / 10, 10 / 80, 90
ARM CURLS	3 / 10 / 25	3 / 10 / 25	3 / 10 / 25	3 / 10 / 25	3 / 10 / 30	3 / 10 / 30	3 / 10 / 35
TRIECEPS EXTENSIONS	3 / 10 / 30	3 / 10 / 30	3 / 10 / 30	2, 1 / 10, 8 / 40	2, 1 / 10, 8 / 40	3 / 10 / 40	3 / 10 / 40
SQUATS	2 / 10 / 75	2 / 10 / 75	2 / 10 / 75	3 / 10 / 75	3 / 10 / 85	3 / 10 / 85	3 / 10 / 85
SIT-UPS	2 / 20 / ∅	2 / 20 / ∅	2 / 20 / ∅	2 / 20 / 10	2 / 20 / 10	2 / 25 / 10	2 / 25 / 10
CURLS	2 / 50 / ∅	2 / 50 / ∅	1 / 100 / ∅	1 / 100 / ∅	1 / 110 / ∅	1 / 110 / ∅	1 / 110 / ∅
FLEXIBILITY	✓	✓	✓	✓	✓	✓	✓
AEROBICS	2 / MI / 19:49	2 / MI / 22:05	2 / MI / 20:38	2 / MI / 19:45	2½ / MI / 21:19	2½ / MI / 22:21	BIKE / L 4 / 20:00
STRETCHING	✓	✓	✓	✓	✓	✓	✓

	5/13	5/15	5/19	5/22	5/29	5/31
SHOULDER PRESS	1, 2 / 10, 8 / 40	3 / 10 / 40	3 / 10 / 40	3 / 10 / 40	3 / 10 / 40	3 / 10 / 40
LAT PULLDOWNS	1, 3 / 10, 10 / 80, 90	1, 3 / 10, 10 / 80, 90	1, 3 / 10, 10 / 80, 90	1, 3 / 10, 10 / 80, 90	1, 3 / 10, 10 / 80, 90	1, 3 / 10, 10 / 80, 90
ARM CURLS	3 / 10 / 35	3 / 10 / 35	3 / 10 / 40	3 / 10 / 40	3 / 10 / 40	3 / 10 / 40
TRIECEPS EXTENSIONS	3 / 10 / 40	3 / 10 / 40	3 / 10 / 40	3 / 10 / 40	3 / 10 / 40	3 / 10 / 40
SQUATS	2 / 10 / 95	2 / 10 / 95	3 / 10 / 95	3 / 10 / 95	3 / 10 / 95	3 / 10 / 95
SIT-UPS	2 / 25 / 10	2 / 25 / 10	3 / 25 / 10	3 / 25 / 10	3 / 25 / 10	3 / 25 / 10
CURLS	1 / 120 / ∅	1 / 120 / ∅	1 / 120 / ∅	1 / 120 / ∅	1 / 120 / ∅	1 / 120 / ∅
FLEXIBILITY	✓	✓	✓	✓	✓	✓
AEROBICS	TRED / 5-9 MPH / 20:00	2½ / MI / 19:45	2½ / MI / 20:06	BIKE / L 4 / 20:00	BIKE / L 4 / 20:00	TRED / 5-9 MPH / 20:00
STRETCHING	✓	✓	✓	✓	✓	✓

Use below for weight reps.

	Δ*	Δ	Δ	4x4**	4x4	4x4	Δ
BENCH PRESS	10-70 8-90 6-110 4-130 1-150 10-70	10-70 8-90 6-110 4-130 1-150 10-70	10-70 8-90 6-110 4-140 1-160 10-70	10-70 4-90 4-110 4-140 4-160 10-70	10-80 4-160 4-160 4-160 4-160 10-80	10-80 4-160 4-160 4-160 4-160 10-80	10-80 8-110 6-130 4-140 1-170 10-80

	Δ	Δ	Δ	Δ	Δ	Δ
BENCH PRESS	10-80 8-120 6-140 4-160 1-180 10-80	10-80 8-120 6-140 4-160 1-180 10-80	10-80 8-120 6-140 4-160 1-180 10-80	10-80 8-120 6-140 4-160 1-180 10-80	10-80 8-120 6-140 4-160 1-180 10-80	10-80 8-120 6-140 4-160 1-180 10-80
						REPS WEIGHT

*Δ = PYRAMID **4x4 = 4 SETS OF 4 REPS AT PRESCRIBED WEIGHT

HIGH-TECH FITNESS PERSONAL WORKOUT CHART

Use below for weight reps.

Exercise Program for
OVERWEIGHT MEN AND WOMEN

You've heard it before, but we'll say it again, anyway. A short-term approach to fitness is not enough. Dieting is not enough. You need a *complete* change of lifestyle, including regular exercise and better eating habits. Exercising at low levels of energy expenditure for progressively longer periods of time has been shown to be the most effective procedure for people with lots of weight to lose. Consequently, we've incorporated a circuit design into the strength training program. That means you should perform the entire series of exercises in numerical order twice, then three times.

BASIC

Flexibility

GOAL
Perform each exercise 2 times for 15 seconds

EXERCISES
1. neck bend
2. waist hang
3. triangle
4. full forward bend

Warm-Up for Aerobics

GOAL
Perform any of these activities for 2 to 5 minutes at minimum resistance, setting, or speed.

EXERCISES
row, or
treadmill walk, or
bicycle, or
rebound

Aerobics

GOAL
Work for 10 minutes at target heart rate.

EXERCISES
row, or
treadmill walk, or
bicycle, or
rebound

Cool-Down from Aerobics

GOAL
Gradually reduce intensity of exercise until heart rate drops below 100 beats per minute.

Strength Training

GOAL
Sets: 1. $10 \times 40\%$ 1 r.m.
     2. $10 \times 50\%$ 1 r.m.

EXERCISES
1. bench press
2. upright row
3. lat pull-downs
4. flys
5. leg press
6. inner thigh pull
7. outer thigh pull
8. sit-ups $(10 \times)$
9. back extensions $(10 \times)$

Stretching

GOAL
Perform each exercise 2 times for 15 seconds.

EXERCISES
1. sit and reach
2. knee tuck and hip twist
3. standing ankle grab
4. four-corner neck stretch

INTERMEDIATE

Flexibility

GOAL
Perform each exercise 3 times for 30 seconds.

EXERCISES
Same

Warm-Up for Aerobics

GOAL
Same

EXERCISES
Same

Aerobics

GOAL
Work for 20 minutes at target heart rate.

EXERCISES
Same

Cool-Down from Aerobics

GOAL
Same

Strength Training

GOAL
Sets: 1. $10 \times 40\%$ 1 r.m.
     2. $10 \times 50\%$ 1 r.m.
     3. $10 \times 60\%$ 1 r.m.

Gradually increase to two complete circuits.

EXERCISES
1 through 7, plus
8. sit-ups ($20 \times$)
9. back extensions ($20 \times$)

Stretching

GOAL
Perform each exercise 3 times for 30 seconds.

EXERCISES
Same

ADVANCED

Flexibility

GOAL
Perform each exercise 4 times for 45 seconds.

EXERCISES
Same

Warm-Up for Aerobics

GOAL
Same

EXERCISES
Same

Aerobics

GOAL
Work for 30 minutes at target heart rate.

EXERCISES
Same

Cool-Down from Aerobics

GOAL
Same

Strength Training

GOAL
Sets: 1. $10 \times 40\%$ 1 r.m.
     2. $10 \times 50\%$ 1 r.m.
     3. $10 \times 60\%$ 1 r.m.

Gradually increase to three complete circuits.

EXERCISES
1 through 7, plus
8. sit-ups ($30 \times$)
9. back extensions ($30 \times$)

Stretching

GOAL
Perform each exercise 4 times for 45 seconds.

EXERCISES
Same

Exercise Program for
UNDERWEIGHT MEN AND WOMEN

You need to eat more and better. You should balance complex carbohydrates (for energy) with proteins (to build lean muscle mass), then consolidate your muscle gains by exercise. It's important to remember that people become underweight and undernourished for many reasons: medical problems, psychological problems, bad living habits, chronic disease, poverty. Usually, whatever underlying reasons that exist must be remedied before normal weight can be attained. Once they are remedied, you should start to eat more, but very gradually. Frequently, an undernourished person's system can't handle a large metabolic load. For this reason, we recommend small, frequent, high-calorie feedings. (Protein shakes are a good choice.) To gain weight, your caloric intake should be one-third to one-half more than you need to maintain a constant weight. Since you're exercising while trying to gain, remember to include the calories you burn during every workout when you calculate your maintenance figure.

BASIC

Flexibility

GOAL
Perform each exercise 2 times for 15 seconds.

EXERCISES
1. neck bend
2. waist stretch
3. triangle

Warm-Up for Aerobics

GOAL
Perform any of these activities for 2 to 5 minutes at minimum resistance, setting, or speed.

EXERCISES
row, or treadmill, or bicycle, or rebound

Aerobics

GOAL
Work for 15 minutes at target heart rate.

EXERCISES
row, or treadmill, or bicycle, or rebound

Cool-Down from Aerobics

GOAL
Gradually reduce intensity of exercise until heart rate drops below 100 beats per minute.

Strength Training

GOAL
Sets: 1. $10 \times 50\%$ 1 r.m.
2. $10 \times 60\%$ 1 r.m.
3. $10 \times 70\%$ 1 r.m.

EXERCISES
1. bench press
2. shoulder press
3. squats
4. arm curls
5. leg curls
6. lat pull-downs
7. upright row
8. pull-overs
9. sit-ups ($10 \times$)
10. back extensions ($10 \times$)

Stretching

GOAL
Perform each exercise 2 times for 15 seconds.

EXERCISES
1. sit and reach
2. knee tuck and hip twist
3. standing ankle grab
4. four-corner neck stretch

INTERMEDIATE

Flexibility

GOAL	EXERCISES
Perform each exercise 3 times for 30 seconds.	1 through 3, plus 4. full forward bend 5. waist hang

Warm-Up for Aerobics

GOAL	EXERCISES
Same	Same

Aerobics

GOAL	EXERCISES
Work for 20 minutes at target heart rate.	Same

Cool-Down from Aerobics

GOAL
Same

Strength Training

GOAL	EXERCISES
Sets: 1. $10 \times 50\%$ 1 r.m. 2. $8 \times 70\%$ 1 r.m. 3. $6 \times 80\%$ 1 r.m.	1 through 8, plus 9. sit-ups $(20 \times)$ 10. back extensions $(20 \times)$

Stretching

GOAL	EXERCISES
Perform each exercise 3 times for 30 seconds.	Same

ADVANCED

Flexibility

GOAL	EXERCISES
Perform each exercise 4 times for 45 seconds.	1 through 5, plus 6. fish

Warm-Up for Aerobics

GOAL	EXERCISES
Same	Same

Aerobics

GOAL	EXERCISES
Work for 30 minutes at target heart rate.	Same

Cool-Down from Aerobics

GOAL
Same

Strength Training

GOAL	EXERCISES
Sets: 1. $10 \times 50\%$ 1 r.m. 2. $8 \times 70\%$ 1 r.m. 3. $6 \times 80\%$ 1 r.m.	1 through 8, plus 9. sit-ups $(30 \times)$ 10. back extensions $(30 \times)$

Stretching

GOAL	EXERCISES
Perform each exercise 4 times for 45 seconds.	Same

Exercise Program for
WOMEN 20–35

Many women in this age bracket are concerned with looking good and performing well in sports which are currently popular and social for co-ed groups. Now is the time to contour your body. Exercise to control fat on the hips, inner and outer thighs, back of upper arms, and lower stomach. Increasing circulation from aerobics benefits the cardiovascular system and helps prevent cellulite and wrinkles later on.

BASIC

Flexibility

GOAL
Perform each exercise 2 times for 15 seconds.

EXERCISES
1. neck bend
2. waist stretch
3. triangle
4. fish

Warm-Up for Aerobics

GOAL
Perform any of these activities for 2 to 5 minutes at minimum resistance, setting, or speed.

EXERCISES
row, or
treadmill, or
bicycle, or
rebound

Aerobics

GOAL
Work for 15 minutes at target heart rate.

EXERCISES
row, or
treadmill, or
bicycle, or
rebound

Cool-Down from Aerobics

GOAL
Gradually reduce intensity of exercise until heart rate drops below 110 beats per minute.

Strength Training

GOALS
Sets: 1. $10 \times 50\%$ 1 r.m.
　　　2. $10 \times 60\%$ 1 r.m.
　　　3. $10 \times 70\%$ 1 r.m.

EXERCISES
1. incline press
2. pull-overs
3. pulley row
4. lat pull-downs
5. leg press
6. sit-ups $(30 \times)$
7. back extensions $(10 \times)$

Stretching

GOAL
Perform each exercise 2 times for 15 seconds.

EXERCISES
1. sit and reach
2. knee tuck and hip twist
3. standing ankle grab
4. the push

INTERMEDIATE

Flexibility
GOAL
Perform each exercise 4 times for 30 seconds.

EXERCISES
1 through 4, plus
5. full forward bend

Warm-Up for Aerobics
GOAL
Same

EXERCISES
Same

Aerobics
GOAL
Work for 20 minutes at target heart rate.

EXERCISES
Same

Cool-Down from Aerobics
GOAL
Same

Strength Training
GOAL
Same

EXERCISES
1 through 5, plus
6. sit-ups (60×)
7. back extensions (20×)
8. inner thigh pull
9. outer thigh pull
10. buttocks pull
11. leg curls
12. calf raises

Stretching
GOAL
Perform each exercise 4 times for 30 seconds.

EXERCISES
1 through 4, plus
5. straddle stretch
6. four-corner neck stretch

ADVANCED

Flexibility
GOAL
Perform each exercise 6 times for 60 seconds.

EXERCISES
1 through 5, plus
6. waist hang

Warm-Up for Aerobics
GOAL
Same

EXERCISES
Same

Aerobics
GOAL
Work for 5 minutes at target heart rate.

EXERCISES
Same

Cool-Down from Aerobics
GOAL
Same

Strength Training
GOAL
Same

Gradually increase to two complete circuits.

EXERCISES
1 through 12, except for
6. sit-ups (75×)
7. back extensions (40×)

Stretching
GOAL
Perform each exercise 6 times for 60 seconds.

EXERCISES
1 through 6

Exercise Program for
WOMEN 35–50

Gravity begins to take its toll at this age, especially if you haven't been on an exercise program before. There's a noticeable droop from the cheekbones to the kneecaps. Fatty deposits between the knees and on the hips, abdomen, and back of upper arms become more obvious. Your body's metabolism is slowing, and calories don't come off as easily as they did in the previous decade. You may also need to lose extra pounds that crept up on you during your child-bearing years. So you must not only work out, you must work out more regularly now. It's also important to exercise to help stave off the tendency toward osteoporosis (brittle bones), which begins around this age. Mild muscular work has been shown to help reverse osteoporotic tendencies that seem more pronounced as women approach menopause.

BASIC

Flexibility

GOAL
Perform each exercise 3 times for 15 seconds.

EXERCISES
1. neck bend
2. waist stretch
3. triangle

Warm-Up for Aerobics

GOAL
Perform any of these activities for 2 to 5 minutes at minimum resistance, setting, or speed.

EXERCISES
row, or
treadmill, or
bicycle, or
rebound

Aerobics

GOAL
Work for 15 minutes at target heart rate.

EXERCISES
row, or
treadmill, or
bicycle, or
rebound

Cool-Down from Aerobics

GOAL
Gradually reduce intensity of exercise until heart rate drops below 100 beats per minute.

Strength Training

GOAL
Sets: 1. $10 \times 60\%$ 1 r.m.
     2. $10 \times 70\%$ 1 r.m.

EXERCISES
1. bench press
2. upright row
3. leg press
4. back extensions ($5 \times$)
5. sit-ups ($10 \times$)

Stretching

GOAL
Perform each exercise 3 times for 15 seconds.

EXERCISES
1. sit and reach
2. knee tuck and hip twist
3. standing ankle grab
4. the push

INTERMEDIATE

Flexibility

GOAL
Perform each exercise 4 times
for 30 seconds.

EXERCISES
1 through 3, plus
4. full forward bend
5. waist hang

Warm-Up for Aerobics

GOAL
Same

EXERCISES
Same

Aerobics

GOAL
Work for 20 minutes at target
heart rate.

EXERCISES
Same

Cool-Down from Aerobics

GOAL
Same

Strength Training

GOAL
Sets: 1. $15 \times 60\%$ 1 r.m.
      2. $15 \times 70\%$ 1 r.m.

EXERCISES
1 through 3, plus
4. back extensions ($10 \times$)
5. sit-ups ($20 \times$)
6. arm curls
7. triceps extensions
8. calf raises

Stretching

GOAL
Perform each exercise 4 times
for 30 seconds.

EXERCISES
1 through 4, plus
5. straddle stretch

ADVANCED

Flexibility

GOAL
Perform each exercise 5 times
for 45 seconds.

EXERCISES
1 through 5, plus
6. fish

Warm-Up for Aerobics

GOAL
Same

EXERCISES
Same

Aerobics

GOAL
Work for 40 minutes at target
heart rate.

EXERCISES
Same

Cool-Down from Aerobics

GOAL
Same

Strength Training

GOAL
Sets: 1. $20 \times 60\%$ 1 r.m.
      2. $20 \times 70\%$ 1 r.m.

If you have weight to lose,
gradually increase to two
complete circuits.

EXERCISES
1 through 3, plus
4. back extensions ($20 \times$)
5. sit-ups ($40 \times$)
6 through 8, plus
9. inner thigh pull
10. outer thigh pull
11. buttocks pull

Stretching

GOAL
Perform each exercise 5 times
for 45 seconds.

EXERCISES
1 through 5, plus
6. four-corner neck stretch

Exercise Program for WOMEN 50–65

At this age, women must pay attention to cardiovascular fitness. Exercise will maintain muscle tone and shape, continue to help protect you from osteoporosis (brittle bones), and keep weight under control. If you have built up to it, you can still work out quite hard at this age. The only noticeable difference may be some restriction of movement in certain joints. If you haven't been exercising, it is still not too late to start. A 1973 study done on female subjects between the ages of 52 and 79 showed that the relative improvements that can be made at this age (in physical work capacity) are of the same order of magnitude as often reported for younger people. So don't put it off!

BASIC

Flexibility

GOAL
Perform each exercise 3 times for 15 seconds.

EXERCISES
1. neck bend
2. waist stretch
3. triangle

Warm-Up for Aerobics

GOAL
Perform any of these activities for 2 to 5 minutes at minimum resistance, setting, or speed.

EXERCISES
row, or
treadmill, or
bicycle, or
rebound

Aerobics

GOAL
Work for 15 minutes at target heart rate.

EXERCISES
row, or
treadmill, or
bicycle, or
rebound

Cool-Down from Aerobics

GOAL
Gradually reduce intensity of exercise until heart rate drops below 90 beats per minute.

Strength Training

GOAL
Sets: 1. $10 \times 40\%$ 1 r.m.
2. $10 \times 50\%$ 1 r.m.
3. $10 \times 60\%$ 1 r.m.

EXERCISES
1. bench press
2. upright row
3. leg press
4. leg extensions
5. sit-ups ($10 \times$)
6. back extensions ($3 \times$)

Stretching

GOAL
Perform each exercise 3 times for 15 seconds.

EXERCISES
1. sit and reach
2. knee tuck and hip twist
3. standing ankle grab
4. the push

INTERMEDIATE

Flexibility
GOAL
Perform each exercise 4 times for 30 seconds.

EXERCISES
1 through 3, plus
4. full forward bend

Warm-Up for Aerobics
GOAL
Same

EXERCISES
Same

Aerobics
GOAL
Work for 20 minutes at target heart rate.

EXERCISES
Same

Cool-Down from Aerobics
GOAL
Same

Strength Training
GOAL
Same

EXERCISES
1 through 4, plus
5. sit-ups (15×)
6. back extensions (6×)

Stretching
GOAL
Perform each exercise 4 times for 30 seconds.

EXERCISES
1 through 4, plus
5. straddle stretch

ADVANCED

Flexibility
GOAL
Perform each exercise 5 times for 45 seconds.

EXERCISES
1 through 4, plus
5. waist hang

Warm-Up for Aerobics
GOAL
Same

EXERCISES
Same

Aerobics
GOAL
Work for 30 minutes at target heart rate.

EXERCISES
Same

Cool-Down from Aerobics
GOAL
Same

Strength Training
GOAL
Same

If you have weight to lose, gradually increase to two complete circuits.

EXERCISES
1 through 4, plus
5. sit-ups (25×)
6. back extensions (12×)

Stretching
GOAL
Perform each exercise 5 times for 45 seconds.

EXERCISES
1 through 5, plus
6. four-corner neck stretch

Exercise Program for
MEN 20–35

Problem areas for men in this age bracket include oblique muscles and the upper stomach. Many are still participating in some form of competitive recreational sports, and they should be taking gym exercises to prepare their bodies for playing irregularly and on weekends. A program should focus on cardiovascular fitness as well as strength.

BASIC

Flexibility

GOAL
Perform each exercise 2 times for 15 seconds.

EXERCISES
1. neck bend
2. full forward bend
3. waist hang
4. waist stretch

Warm-Up for Aerobics

GOAL
Perform any of these activities for 2 to 5 minutes at minimum resistance, setting, or speed.

EXERCISES
row, or treadmill, or bicycle, or rebound

Aerobics

GOAL
Work for 15 minutes at target heart rate.

EXERCISES
row, or treadmill, or bicycle, or rebound

Cool-Down from Aerobics

GOAL
Gradually reduce intensity of exercise until heart rate drops below 110 beats per minute.

Strength Training

GOAL
Sets: 1. $10 \times 50\%$ 1 r.m.
      2. $10 \times 60\%$ 1 r.m.
      3. $10 \times 70\%$ 1 r.m.

EXERCISES
1. bench press
2. shoulder press
3. parallel squats
4. curls
5. lat pull-downs
6. leg curls
7. sit-ups ($25 \times$)
8. back extensions ($25 \times$)

Stretching

GOAL
Perform each exercise 2 times for 15 seconds.

EXERCISES
1. standing ankle grab
2. point and flex
3. knee tuck and hip twist
4. sit and reach

INTERMEDIATE

Flexibility

GOAL
Perform each exercise 4 times for 30 seconds.

EXERCISES
1 through 4, plus
5. triangle

Warm-Up for Aerobics

GOAL
Same

EXERCISES
Same

Aerobics

GOAL
Work for 20 minutes at target heart rate.

EXERCISES
Same

Cool-Down from Aerobics

GOAL
Same

Strength Training

GOAL
Sets: 1. $10 \times 50\%$ 1 r.m.
　　　2. $9 \times 60\%$ 1 r.m.
　　　3. $8 \times 70\%$ 1 r.m.
　　　4. $7 \times 80\%$ 1 r.m.

EXERCISES
1 through 6, plus
7. incline press
8. sit-ups ($50 \times$)
9. back extensions ($50 \times$)

Stretching

GOAL
Perform each exercise 4 times for 30 seconds.

EXERCISES
1 through 4, plus
5. the push

ADVANCED

Flexibility

GOAL
Perform each exercise 6 times for 60 seconds.

EXERCISES
1 through 5

Warm-Up for Aerobics

GOAL
Same

EXERCISES
Same

Aerobics

GOAL
Work for 40 minutes at target heart rate.

EXERCISES
Same

Cool-Down from Aerobics

GOAL
Same

Strength Training

GOAL
Sets: 1. $10 \times 50\%$ 1 r.m.
　　　2. $8 \times 60\%$ 1 r.m.
　　　3. $6 \times 70\%$ 1 r.m.
　　　4. $4 \times 80\%$ 1 r.m.
　　　5. $2 \times 90\%$ 1 r.m.

EXERCISES
1 through 6, plus
7. incline press
8. pull-overs
9. sit-ups ($75 \times$)
10. back extensions ($75 \times$)

Stretching

GOAL
Perform each exercise 6 times for 60 seconds.

EXERCISES
1 through 5, plus
6. straddle stretch

Exercise Program for
MEN 35–50

Although stomach and oblique muscles continue to be a problem, cardiovascular fitness is probably the most important focus for this age group. Stress tends to mount in career positions at this age, and there's not much we can do to reduce these pressures. But a physically healthy heart, lungs, and body can certainly withstand stress a lot better than a weak, inefficient, flimsy one. If stomach exercises are started or continued at this time, they will further prevent the debilitating effects of back problems that often occur at this age.

BASIC

Flexibility

GOAL
Perform each exercise 3 times for 15 seconds.

EXERCISES
1. neck bend
2. full forward bend
3. waist hang
4. waist stretch

Warm-Up for Aerobics

GOAL
Perform any of these activities for 2 to 5 minutes at minimum resistance, setting, or speed.

EXERCISES
row, or
treadmill, or
bicycle, or
rebound

Aerobics

GOAL
Work for 15 minutes at target heart rate.

EXERCISES
row, or
treadmill, or
bicycle, or
rebound

Cool-Down from Aerobics

GOAL
Gradually reduce intensity of exercise until heart rate drops below 100 beats per minute.

Strength Training

GOAL
Sets: 1. $10 \times 50\%$ 1 r.m.
       2. $10 \times 60\%$ 1 r.m.

EXERCISES
1. bench press
2. shoulder press
3. leg press
4. arm curls
5. lat pull-downs
6. leg curls
7. sit-ups ($20 \times$)
8. back extensions ($20 \times$)

Stretching

GOAL
Perform each exercise 3 times for 15 seconds.

EXERCISES
1. standing ankle grab
2. point and flex
3. knee tuck and hip twist
4. sit and reach

INTERMEDIATE

Flexibility

GOAL
Perform each exercise 4 times for 30 seconds.

EXERCISES
1 through 4, plus
5. triangle

Warm-Up for Aerobics

GOAL
Same

EXERCISES
Same

Aerobics

GOAL
Work for 20 minutes at target heart rate.

EXERCISES
Same

Cool-Down from Aerobics

GOAL
Same

Strength Training

GOAL
Sets: 1. 10 × 50% 1 r.m.
2. 8 × 60% 1 r.m.
3. 6 × 70% 1 r.m.

EXERCISES
1 through 6, plus
7. incline press
8. sit-ups (40 ×)
9. back extensions (40 ×)

Stretching

GOAL
Perform each exercise 4 times for 30 seconds.

EXERCISES
1 through 4, plus
5. the push

ADVANCED

Flexibility

GOAL
Perform each exercise 5 times for 45 seconds.

EXERCISES
1 through 5

Warm-Up for Aerobics

GOAL
Same

EXERCISES
Same

Aerobics

GOAL
Work for 40 minutes at target heart rate.

EXERCISES
Same

Cool-Down from Aerobics

GOAL
Same

Strength Training

GOAL
Sets: 1. 10 × 50% 1 r.m.
2. 8 × 60% 1 r.m.
3. 6 × 70% 1 r.m.

EXERCISES
1 through 6, plus
7. incline press
8. pull-overs
9. sit-ups (60 ×)
10. back extensions (60 ×)

Stretching

GOAL
Perform each exercise 5 times for 45 seconds.

EXERCISES
1 through 5, plus
6. straddle stretch

Exercise Program for
MEN 50–65

Cardiovascular fitness is still more important than anything else, but stiff joints and limited range of movement begin to be problems. Do aerobics for your heart and lungs, flexibility and stretching exercises for joint mobility, and follow a moderate weight program to maintain muscle shape and tone. Perform all activities in modest amounts. It seems that all the injuries, bad habits, and abuses of a lifetime begin to make themselves felt during this time of life.

BASIC

Flexibility

GOAL
Perform each exercise 3 times for 15 seconds.

EXERCISES
1. neck bend
2. full forward bend
3. waist hang
4. waist stretch

Warm-Up for Aerobics

GOAL
Perform any of these activities for 2 to 5 minutes at minimum resistance, setting or speed.

EXERCISES
row, or
treadmill, or
bicycle, or
rebound

Aerobics

GOAL
Work for 15 minutes at target heart rate.

EXERCISES
row, or
treadmill, or
bicycle, or
rebound

Cool-Down from Aerobics

GOAL
Gradually reduce intensity of exercise until heart rate drops below 90 beats per minute.

Strength Training

GOAL
Sets: 1. $10 \times 50\%$ 1 r.m.

EXERCISES
1. bench press
2. shoulder press
3. leg press
4. arm curls
5. lat pull-downs
6. leg curls
7. sit-ups ($15 \times$)
8. back extensions ($15 \times$)

Stretching

GOAL
Perform each exercise 3 times for 15 seconds.

EXERCISES
1. standing ankle grab
2. point and flex
3. knee tuck and hip twist
4. sit and reach

INTERMEDIATE

Flexibility

GOAL
Perform each exercise 4 times for 30 seconds.

EXERCISES
1 through 4, plus
5. triangle

Warm-Up for Aerobics

GOAL
Same

EXERCISES
Same

Aerobics

GOAL
Work for 20 minutes at target heart rate.

EXERCISES
Same

Cool-Down from Aerobics

GOAL
Same

Strength Training

GOAL
Sets: 1. 10 × 40% 1 r.m.
     2. 10 × 50% 1 r.m.

EXERCISES
1 through 6, plus
7. sit-ups (30 ×)
8. back extensions (30 ×)

Stretching

GOAL
Perform each exercise 4 times for 30 seconds.

EXERCISES
1 through 4, plus
5. the push

ADVANCED

Flexibility

GOAL
Perform each exercise 5 times for 45 seconds.

EXERCISES
1 through 5

Warm-Up for Aerobics

GOAL
Same

EXERCISES
Same

Aerobics

GOAL
Work for 30 minutes at target heart rate.

EXERCISES
Same

Cool-Down from Aerobics

GOAL
Same

Strength Training

GOAL
Sets: 1. 10 × 40% 1 r.m.
     2. 8 × 50% 1 r.m.
     3. 6 × 60% 1 r.m.

EXERCISES
1 through 6, plus
7. sit-ups (45 ×)
8. back extensions (45 ×)

Stretching

GOAL
Perform each exercise 5 times for 45 seconds.

EXERCISES
1 through 5, plus
6. straddle stretch

Exercise Program for
MEN AND
WOMEN OVER 65

Maintaining cardiovascular fitness is the overriding goal for both sexes. Well-toned muscles will make your body stable and nicely padded in case of a fall or accident. Exercise will help all your joints retain their range of motion, and good blood circulation will help keep your sex drive alive. This is the age when you'll appreciate the safety and convenience of being able to exercise at home.

BASIC

Flexibility

GOAL
Perform each exercise 3 times for 10 seconds.

EXERCISES
1. neck bend
2. waist stretch
3. full forward bend

Warm-Up for Aerobics

GOAL
Perform any of these activities for 2 to 5 minutes at minimum resistance, setting, or speed.

EXERCISES
treadmill, or
bicycle
rebound (next to solid object for balance support)

Aerobics

GOAL
Work for 15 minutes at target heart rate.

EXERCISES
treadmill, or
bicycle
rebound (next to solid object for balance support)

Cool-Down from Aerobics

GOAL
Gradually reduce intensity of exercise until heart rate drops below 90 beats per minute.

Strength Training

GOAL
Sets: 1. 10 × 30% 1 r.m.
     2. 10 × 40% 1 r.m.

EXERCISES
1. bench press
2. lat pull-downs
3. leg press
4. buttocks pull
5. sit-ups (10 ×)
6. back extensions (5 ×)

Stretching

GOAL
Perform each exercise 2 times for 10 seconds.

EXERCISES
1. standing ankle grab
2. point and flex
3. knee tuck and hip twist
4. sit and reach
5. calf stretches

INTERMEDIATE

Flexibility
GOAL
Perform each exercise 4 times
for 20 seconds.

EXERCISES
1 through 3, plus
4. waist hang

Warm-Up for Aerobics
GOAL
Same

EXERCISES
Same

Aerobics
GOAL
Work for 20 minutes at target
heart rate.

EXERCISES
Same

Cool-Down from Aerobics
GOAL
Same

Strength Training
GOAL
Sets: 1. $10 \times 40\%$ r.m.
     2. $10 \times 50\%$ 1 r.m.

EXERCISES
1 through 4, plus
5. sit-ups ($15 \times$)
6. back extensions ($10 \times$)
7. inner thigh pull
8. outer thigh pull

Stretching
GOAL
Perform each exercise 4 times
for 20 seconds.

EXERCISES
Same

ADVANCED

Flexibility
GOAL
Perform each exercise 5 times
for 30 seconds.

EXERCISES
1 through 4, plus
5. triangle

Warm-Up for Aerobics
GOAL
Same

EXERCISES
same

Aerobics
GOAL
Work for 30 minutes at target
heart rate.

EXERCISES
Same

Cool-Down from Aerobics
GOAL
Same

Strength Training
GOAL
Sets: 1. $15 \times 40\%$ 1 r.m.
     2. $15 \times 50\%$ 1 r.m.

If you have weight to lose,
gradually increase to two
complete circuits.

EXERCISES
1 through 4, plus
5. sit-ups ($20 \times$)
6. back extensions ($10 \times$)
7 through 8

Stretching
GOAL
Perform each exercise 6 times
for 30 seconds.

EXERCISES
Same

Exercise Program for TEENAGE GIRLS

Fitness develops shapely contours, grace, and poise. Increased blood circulation is good for the skin, and exercise can alleviate cramps and other menstrual symptoms. Physical activity can also prepare girls for competition in life. Esther Williams has said that the confidence she gained from being a teenage swimming champion helped her face challenges throughout the rest of her career.

Peer group pressure is intense among teenage girls and sometimes makes them feel powerless in matters of physical appearance. They may come to the false conclusion that they either are or aren't attractive, and that there's simply nothing to be done about it. This age is a good time for young women to become aware that they have control over their bodies, their health, and their appearance.

BASIC

Flexibility

GOAL
Perform each exercise 2 times for 10 seconds.

EXERCISES
1. neck bend
2. waist stretch
3. triangle
4. fish

Warm-Up for Aerobics

GOAL
Perform any of these activities for 2 to 5 minutes at minimum resistance, setting, or speed.

EXERCISES
row, or
treadmill, or
bicycle, or
rebound

Aerobics

GOAL
Work for 15 minutes at target heart rate.

EXERCISES
row, or
treadmill, or
bicycle, or
rebound

Cool-Down from Aerobics

GOAL
Gradually reduce intensity of exercise until heart rate drops below 115 beats per minute.

Strength Training

GOAL
Sets: 1. $10 \times 50\%$ 1 r.m.
　　　2. $15 \times 60\%$ 1 r.m.

EXERCISES
1. flys
2. incline press
3. upright row
4. lat pull-downs
5. inner thigh pull
6. outer thigh pull
7. buttocks pull
8. sit-ups $(20 \times)$
9. back extensions $(20 \times)$

Stretching

GOAL
Perform each exercise 2 times for 10 seconds.

EXERCISES
1. sit and reach
2. knee tuck and hip twist
3. standing ankle grab
4. the push

INTERMEDIATE

Flexibility

GOAL
Perform each exercise 3 times for 20 seconds.

EXERCISES
1 through 4, plus
5. full forward bend

Warm-Up for Aerobics

GOAL
Same

EXERCISES
Same

Aerobics

GOAL
Work for 30 minutes at target heart rate.

EXERCISES
Same

Cool-Down from Aerobics

GOAL
Same

Strength Training

GOAL
Sets: 1. 15 × 50% 1 r.m.
2. 20 × 60% 1 r.m.

EXERCISES
1 through 7, plus
8. sit-ups (40 ×)
9. back extensions (40 ×)
10. leg press
11. leg curls
12. calf raises

Stretching

GOAL
Perform each exercise 3 times for 20 seconds.

EXERCISES
1 through 4, plus
5. straddle stretch

ADVANCED

Flexibility

GOAL
Perform each exercise 4 times for 30 seconds.

EXERCISES
1 through 5, plus
6. waist hang

Warm-Up for Aerobics

GOAL
Same

EXERCISES
Same

Aerobics

GOAL
Work for 45 minutes at target heart rate.

EXERCISES
Same

Cool-Down from Aerobics

GOAL
Same

Strength Training

GOAL
Sets: 1. 15 × 50% 1 r.m.
2. 20 × 60% 1 r.m.

Gradually increase to two complete circuits.

EXERCISES
1 through 7, plus
8. sit-ups (60 ×)
9. back extensions (60 ×)
10 through 12

Stretching

GOAL
Perform each exercise 4 times for 30 seconds.

EXERCISES
1 through 5, plus
6. four-corner neck stretch

Exercise Program for
TEENAGE BOYS

Many teenage boys are interested in developing strength and coordination to prepare for school athletics. Male teens have traditionally been the most enthusiastic purchasers of Charles Atlas and Joe Weider mail-order bodybuilding courses. Physical gains made in the teen years come faster and are easier to maintain throughout life. Fat cells are developed early in life, so it's important to make weight gains in lean muscle tissue instead of fat. For this reason, aerobics should be emphasized. Also because team sports so often involve physical contact, a program of flexibility (which is often overlooked) will improve muscular balance and joint mobility, thereby reducing the risk of injuries. Injuries from contact sports can be especially damaging to younger athletes, since the ends of bones don't stop growing until around the age of 21.

BASIC

Flexibility

GOAL
Perform each exercise 2 times for 10 seconds

EXERCISES
1. full forward bend
2. fish
3. waist stretch

Warm-Up for Aerobics

GOAL
Perform any of these activities for 2 to 5 minutes at minimum resistance, setting, or speed.

EXERCISES
row, or
treadmill, or
bicycle, or
rebound

Aerobics

GOAL
Work for 15 minutes at target heart rate.

EXERCISES
row, or
treadmill, or
bicycle, or
rebound

Cool-Down from Aerobics

GOAL
Gradually reduce intensity of exercise until heart rate drops below 115 beats per minute.

Strength Training

GOAL
Sets: 1. $10 \times 50\%$ 1 r.m.
2. $10 \times 60\%$ 1 r.m.
3. $10 \times 70\%$ 1 r.m.

EXERCISES
1. bench press
2. shoulder press
3. parallel squats
4. arm curls
5. lat pull-downs
6. leg curls
7. sit-ups $(30 \times)$
8. back extensions $(30 \times)$

Stretching

GOAL
Perform each exercise 2 times for 15 seconds.

EXERCISES
1. standing ankle grab
2. point and flex
3. knee tuck and hip twist
4. sit and reach

INTERMEDIATE

Flexibility
GOAL
Perform each exercise 3 times for 20 seconds.

EXERCISES
1 through 3, plus
4. neck bend

Warm-Up for Aerobics
GOAL
Same

EXERCISES
Same

Aerobics
GOAL
Work for 30 minutes at target heart rate.

EXERCISES
Same

Cool-Down from Aerobics
GOAL
Same

Strength Training
GOAL
Sets: 1. $10 \times 50\%$ 1 r.m.
2. $8 \times 60\%$ 1 r.m.
3. $6 \times 70\%$ 1 r.m.
4. $4 \times 80\%$ 1 r.m.

EXERCISES
1 through 6, plus
7. incline press
8. sit-ups ($60 \times$)
9. back extensions ($60 \times$)

Stretching
GOAL
Perform each exercise 3 times for 30 seconds.

EXERCISES
1 through 4, plus
5. the push

ADVANCED

Flexibility
GOAL
Perform each exercise 4 times for 30 seconds.

EXERCISES
1 through 4

Warm-Up for Aerobics
GOAL
Same

EXERCISES
Same

Aerobics
GOAL
Work for 45 minutes at target heart rate.

EXERCISES
Same

Cool-Down from Aerobics
GOAL
Same

Strength Training
GOAL
Sets: 1. $10 \times 50\%$ 1 r.m.
2. $8 \times 60\%$ 1 r.m.
3. $6 \times 70\%$ 1 r.m.
4. $4 \times 80\%$ 1 r.m.
5. $6 \times 70\%$ 1 r.m.

EXERCISES
1 through 7, plus
8. dumbbell pull-overs
9. sit-ups ($90 \times$)
10. back extensions ($90 \times$)

Stretching
GOAL
Perform each exercise 4 times for 45 seconds.

EXERCISES
1 through 5, plus
6. straddle stretch

Exercise Program for
BASKETBALL VOLLEYBALL DOWNHILL SKIING

All of these sports require the highest levels of muscular strength and endurance, as well as high levels of cardiovascular endurance. Strength is needed in both upper and lower limbs, but muscle mass need not be as high as some of the contact sports. All involve jumping, agility, and the ability to change direction rapidly. Since movements are in response to a ball, an opponent, or an unpredictable terrain, you need good flexibility and joint durability in case of falls or collisions.

BASIC

Flexibility

GOAL
Perform each exercise 3 times for 15 seconds.

EXERCISES
1. neck bend
2. waist stretch
3. triangle
4. fish
5. suspended stretch
6. waist hang

Warm-Up for Aerobics

GOAL
Perform any of these activities for 2 to 5 minutes at minimum resistance, setting, or speed.

EXERCISES
row, or
treadmill, or
rebound

Aerobics

GOAL
Work for 15 minutes at target heart rate.

EXERCISES
row, or
treadmill, or
rebound with hand weights

Cool-Down from Aerobics

GOAL
Gradually reduce intensity of exercise until heart rate drops below 110 beats per minute.

Strength Training

GOAL
Sets: 1. $10 \times 50\%$ 1 r.m.
2. $10 \times 60\%$ 1 r.m.
3. $10 \times 70\%$ 1 r.m.

EXERCISES
1. bench press
2. upright row
3. squats
4. calf raises
5. sit-ups ($30 \times$)
6. back extensions ($15 \times$)

Stretching

GOAL
Perform each exercise 4 times for 20 seconds.

EXERCISES
1. knee tuck and hip twist
2. standing ankle grab
3. cat stretch
4. sit and reach

INTERMEDIATE

Flexibility

GOAL

Perform each exercise 6 times for 30 seconds.

EXERCISES

Same

Warm-Up for Aerobics

GOAL

Same

EXERCISES

Same

Aerobics

GOAL

Work for 30 minutes at target heart rate.

EXERCISES

Same

Cool-Down from Aerobics

GOAL

Same

Strength Training

GOAL

Sets: 1. 20 × 50% 1 r.m.
  2. 15 × 60% 1 r.m.
  3. 10 × 70% 1 r.m.

EXERCISES

1 through 4, plus
5. sit-ups (60 ×)
6. back extensions (30 ×)
7. incline press
8. lat pull-downs
9. wrist curls

Stretching

GOAL

Perform each exercise 8 times for 40 seconds.

EXERCISES

1 through 4, plus
5. back roll
6. hurdler's stretch

ADVANCED

Flexibility

GOAL

Perform each exercise 9 times for 45 seconds.

EXERCISES

Same

Warm-Up for Aerobics

GOAL

Same

EXERCISES

Same

Aerobics

GOAL

Work for 40 minutes at target heart rate.

EXERCISES

Same

Cool-Down from Aerobics

GOAL

Same

Strength Training

GOAL

Sets: 1. 20 × 50% 1 r.m.
  2. 15 × 60% 1 r.m.
  3. 10 × 70% 1 r.m.

Gradually increase to two complete circuits.

EXERCISES

1 through 4, plus
5. sit-ups (90 ×)
6. back extensions (60 ×)
7 through 9, plus
10. leg curls
11. leg extensions
12. bent-over twist

Stretching

GOAL

Perform each exercise 12 times for 60 seconds.

EXERCISES

1 through 6, plus
7. four-corner neck stretch

Exercise Program for
FOOTBALL HOCKEY LACROSSE WRESTLING

In general, these sports require a great deal of overall body strength, good muscular endurance, quickness and muscle mass. Cardiovascular endurance does not need to be as high as one might expect, due to the broken flow of activity which occurs because of position played or player substitution. Flexibility is very important in these and all contact sports, since injury probability is high. The more flexible and durable the joints, the lower the chance of problems, especially when complemented by good muscles for strength, padding, and stability.

BASIC

Flexibility

GOAL
Perform each exercise 3 times for 15 seconds

EXERCISES
1. neck bend
2. waist stretch
3. triangle
4. fish
5. suspended stretch
6. waist hang

Warm-Up for Aerobics

GOAL
Perform any of these activities for 2 to 5 minutes at minimum resistance, setting, or speed.

EXERCISES
row, or
treadmill, or
bicycle

Aerobics

GOAL
Work for 15 minutes at target heart rate.

EXERCISES
row, or
treadmill, or
bicycle

Cool-Down from Aerobics

GOAL
Gradually reduce intensity of exercise until heart rate drops below 110 beats per minute.

Strength Training

GOAL
Sets: 1. 10 × 60% 1 r.m.
      2. 10 × 70% 1 r.m.

EXERCISES
1. bench press
2. shoulder press
3. upright row
4. lat pull-downs
5. squats
6. sit-ups (30 ×)
7. back extensions (30 ×)

Stretching

GOAL
Perform each exercise 4 times for 20 seconds.

EXERCISES
1. knee tuck and hip twist
2. standing ankle grab
3. cat stretch
4. sit and reach

INTERMEDIATE

Flexibility
GOAL
Perform each exercise 6 times for 30 seconds

EXERCISES
Same

Warm-Up for Aerobics
GOAL
Same

EXERCISES
Same

Aerobics
GOAL
Work for 20 minutes at target heart rate.

EXERCISES
Same

Cool-Down from Aerobics
GOAL
Same

Strength Training
GOAL
Sets: 1. 10 × 60% 1 r.m.
     2. 8 × 70% 1 r.m.
     3. 6 × 80% 1 r.m.

EXERCISES
1 through 5, plus
6. sit-ups (60 ×)
7. back extensions (60 ×)
8. arm curls
9. triceps extensions
10. leg extensions
11. leg curls
12. calf raises

Stretching
GOAL
Perform each exercise 8 times for 40 seconds.

EXERCISES
1 through 4, plus
5. back roll
6. hurdler's stretch

ADVANCED

Flexibility
GOAL
Perform each exercise 9 times for 45 seconds.

EXERCISES
Same

Warm-Up for Aerobics
GOAL
Same

EXERCISES
Same

Aerobics
GOAL
Work for 30 minutes at target heart rate.

EXERCISES
Same

Cool-Down from Aerobics
GOAL
Same

Strength Training
GOAL
Sets: 1. 10 × 50% 1 r.m.
     2. 8 × 60% 1 r.m.
     3. 6 × 70% 1 r.m.
     4. 4 × 80% 1 r.m.

EXERCISES
1 through 12, except for
6. sit-ups (90 ×)
7. back extensions (90 ×)

Stretching
GOAL
Perform each exercise 12 times for 60 seconds.

EXERCISES
1 through 6, plus
7. four-corner neck stretch

Exercise Program for
RACQUETBALL HANDBALL TENNIS SQUASH

Programs for the racquet sports focus on a high degree of muscular and cardiovascular endurance. These sports require only moderate muscular strength in both the upper and lower body. They demand torso strength and stability to control rapid, unplanned changes of direction, which often occur over very short distances. They also demand intense concentration and good depth perception.

BASIC

Flexibility

GOAL
Perform each exercise 3 times for 15 seconds.

EXERCISES
1. neck bend
2. waist stretch
3. triangle
4. fish
5. suspended stretch
6. waist hang

Warm-Up for Aerobics

GOAL
Perform any of these activities for 2 to 5 minutes at minimum resistance, setting, or speed.

EXERCISES
row, or
treadmill, or
rebound

Aerobics

GOAL
Work for 15 minutes at target heart rate.

EXERCISES
row, or
treadmill, or
rebound with hand weights

Cool-Down from Aerobics

GOAL
Gradually reduce intensity of exercise until heart rate drops below 110 beats per minute.

Strength Training

GOAL
Sets: 1. $10 \times 50\%$ 1 r.m.
       2. $10 \times 60\%$ 1 r.m.

EXERCISES
1. flys
2. lat pull-downs
3. triceps extensions
4. arm curls
5. wrist curls
6. hand gripper squeeze
7. leg press

Stretching

GOAL
Perform each exercise 4 times for 20 seconds.

EXERCISES
1. knee tuck and hip twist
2. standing ankle grab
3. cat stretch
4. sit and reach

INTERMEDIATE

Flexibility

GOAL
Perform each exercise 6 times for 30 seconds

EXERCISES
Same

Warm-Up for Aerobics

GOAL
Same

EXERCISES
Same

Aerobics

GOAL
Work for 20 minutes at target heart rate.

EXERCISES
Same

Cool-Down from Aerobics

GOAL
Same

Strength Training

GOAL
Sets: 1. 10 × 60% 1 r.m.
     2. 8 × 70% 1 r.m.
     3. 6 × 80% 1 r.m.

EXERCISES
1 through 5, plus
6. sit-ups (60 ×)
7. back extensions (60 ×)
8. arm curls
9. triceps extensions
10. leg extensions
11. leg curls
12. calf raises

Stretching

GOAL
Perform each exercise 8 times for 40 seconds.

EXERCISES
1 through 4, plus
5. back roll
6. hurdler's stretch

ADVANCED

Flexibility

GOAL
Perform each exercise 9 times for 45 seconds.

EXERCISES
Same

Warm-Up for Aerobics

GOAL
Same

EXERCISES
Same

Aerobics

GOAL
Work for 30 minutes at target heart rate.

EXERCISES
Same

Cool-Down from Aerobics

GOAL
Same

Strength Training

GOAL
Sets: 1. 10 × 50% 1 r.m.
     2. 8 × 60% 1 r.m.
     3. 6 × 70% 1 r.m.
     4. 4 × 80% 1 r.m.

EXERCISES
1 through 12, except for
6. sit-ups (90 ×)
7. back extensions (90 ×)

Stretching

GOAL
Perform each exercise 12 times for 60 seconds.

EXERCISES
1 through 6, plus
7. four-corner neck stretch

Exercise Program for
RACQUETBALL HANDBALL TENNIS SQUASH

Programs for the racquet sports focus on a high degree of muscular and cardiovascular endurance. These sports require only moderate muscular strength in both the upper and lower body. They demand torso strength and stability to control rapid, unplanned changes of direction, which often occur over very short distances. They also demand intense concentration and good depth perception.

BASIC

Flexibility

GOAL
Perform each exercise 3 times for 15 seconds.

EXERCISES
1. neck bend
2. waist stretch
3. triangle
4. fish
5. suspended stretch
6. waist hang

Warm-Up for Aerobics

GOAL
Perform any of these activities for 2 to 5 minutes at minimum resistance, setting, or speed.

EXERCISES
row, or
treadmill, or
rebound

Aerobics

GOAL
Work for 15 minutes at target heart rate.

EXERCISES
row, or
treadmill, or
rebound with hand weights

Cool-Down from Aerobics

GOAL
Gradually reduce intensity of exercise until heart rate drops below 110 beats per minute.

Strength Training

GOAL
Sets: 1. $10 \times 50\%$ 1 r.m.
       2. $10 \times 60\%$ 1 r.m.

EXERCISES
1. flys
2. lat pull-downs
3. triceps extensions
4. arm curls
5. wrist curls
6. hand gripper squeeze
7. leg press

Stretching

GOAL
Perform each exercise 4 times for 20 seconds.

EXERCISES
1. knee tuck and hip twist
2. standing ankle grab
3. cat stretch
4. sit and reach

INTERMEDIATE

Flexibility

GOAL
Perform each exercise 6 times for 30 seconds.

EXERCISES
Same

Warm-Up for Aerobics

GOAL
Same

EXERCISES
Same

Aerobics

GOAL
Work for 30 minutes at target heart rate

EXERCISES
Same

Cool-Down from Aerobics

GOAL
Same

Strength Training

GOAL
Sets: 1. 20 × 60% 1 r.m.
      2. 20 × 70% 1 r.m.

Gradually increase to two complete circuits.

EXERCISES
1 through 7, plus
8. side bends
9. bent-over twist
10. leg curls
11. leg extensions

Stretching

GOAL
Perform each exercise 8 times for 40 seconds.

EXERCISES
1 through 4, plus
5. back roll
6. hurdler's stretch

ADVANCED

Flexibility

GOAL
Perform each exercise 9 times for 45 seconds.

EXERCISES
Same

Warm-Up for Aerobics

GOAL
Same

EXERCISES
Same

Aerobics

GOAL
Work for 40 minutes at target heart rate.

EXERCISES
Same

Cool-Down from Aerobics

GOAL
Same

Strength Training

GOAL
Sets: 1. 20 × 60% 1 r.m.
      2. 20 × 70% 1 r.m.

Gradually increase to three complete circuits.

EXERCISES
1 through 11

Stretching

GOAL
Perform each exercise 12 times for 60 seconds.

EXERCISES
1 through 6, plus
7. four-corner neck stretch

Exercise Program for
RUNNING CYCLING SOCCER SKATING HIKING CROSS-COUNTRY SKIING

These activities require high muscular endurance, medium muscular strength, and very high cardiovascular endurance. The demands on your cardiovascular system are a bit different from those for racquet sports, however. In these activities, you usually cover longer distances, your speed is more constant and slower, and your basic movements are more repetitious and predictable. Long, slow distance training coupled with occasional interval training is ideal for the sports on this list. Focus weight training on your legs and back for both strength and endurance, since performance in these sports puts most of its demands on the legs and back. The upper body muscles need training, too, but not as much, since they are mostly used for rhythm, balance, and coordination. Since these activities take place outdoors, over different kinds of terrain, and for long periods of time, good equipment (shoes, skates, skis, bindings, boots, seat cushions) is essential.

BASIC

Flexibility

GOAL
Perform each exercise
3 times for 15 seconds.

EXERCISES
1. neck bend
2. waist stretch
3. triangle
4. fish
5. suspended stretch
6. waist hang

Warm-Up for Aerobics

GOAL
Perform any of these activities for
2 to 5 minutes at minimum
resistance, setting, or speed.

EXERCISES
treadmill, or
bicycle

Aerobics

GOAL
Work for 20 minutes
at target heart rate.

EXERCISES
treadmill, or
bicycle

Cool-Down from Aerobics

GOAL
Gradually reduce intensity of
exercise until heart rate drops
below 110 beats per minute.

Strength Training

GOAL
Sets: 1. $10 \times 50\%$ 1 r.m.
      2. $10 \times 60\%$ 1 r.m.

EXERCISES
1. bench press
2. upright row
3. leg press
4. calf raises
5. sit-ups ($15 \times$)
6. knee-ups ($15 \times$)

Stretching

GOAL
Perform each exercise
4 times for 20 seconds.

EXERCISES
1. knee tuck and hip twist
2. standing ankle grab
3. cat stretch
4. sit and reach

INTERMEDIATE

Flexibility

GOAL
Perform each exercise
6 times for 30 seconds.

EXERCISES
Same

Warm-Up for Aerobics

GOAL
Same

EXERCISES
Same

Aerobics

GOAL
Work for 40 minutes
at target heart rate.

EXERCISES
Same

Cool-Down from Aerobics

GOAL
Same

Strength Training

GOAL
Sets: 1. 20 × 50% 1 r.m.
     2. 20 × 60% 1 r.m.

Gradually increase to two
complete circuits.

EXERCISES
1 through 4, plus
5. sit-ups (30 ×)
6. knee-ups (30 ×)
7. leg extensions
8. leg curls
9. back extensions (20 ×)

Stretching

GOAL
Perform each exercise
8 times for 40 seconds.

EXERCISES
1 through 4, plus
5. back roll
6. hurdler's stretch

ADVANCED

Flexibility

GOAL
Perform each exercise 9
times for 45 seconds.

EXERCISES
Same

Warm-Up for Aerobics

GOAL
Same

EXERCISES
Same

Aerobics

GOAL
Work for 60 minutes
at target heart rate.

EXERCISES
Same

Cool-Down from Aerobics

GOAL
Same

Strength Training

GOAL
Sets: 1. 20 × 50% 1 r.m.
     2. 15 × 60% 1 r.m.
     3. 10 × 70% 1 r.m.

Gradually increase to three
complete circuits.

EXERCISES
1 through 9, except for
5. sit-ups (60 ×)
6. knee-ups (60 ×)
9. back extensions (40 ×)

Stretching

GOAL
Perform each exercise
12 times for 60 seconds.

EXERCISES
1 through 6, plus
7. four-corner neck stretch

Exercise Program for
SOFTBALL
GOLF
BOWLING
WATER SKIING

These sports require moderate upper body strength, as well as substantial leg and torso tone and control. They also involve twisting the torso, which may predispose it to pulls or strains in the lower back or midsection. These strains usually result from unplanned movements (falls, reaching too far, etc.). All four sports make low demands on muscular endurance and the cardiovascular system. So this training program is geared toward making moderate gains in upper and middle body and leg strength, and in torso stability and flexibility.

BASIC

Flexibility

GOAL
Perform each exercise 3 times for 15 seconds.

EXERCISES
1. neck bend
2. waist stretch
3. triangle
4. fish
5. suspended stretch
6. waist hang

Warm-Up for Aerobics

GOAL
Perform any of these activities for 2 to 5 minutes at minimum resistance, setting, or speed.

EXERCISES
row, or
rebound

Aerobics

GOAL
Work for 15 minutes at target heart rate.

EXERCISES
row, or
rebound with hand weights

Cool-Down from Aerobics

GOAL
Gradually reduce intensity of exercise until heart rate drops below 110 beats per minute.

Strength Training

GOAL
Sets: 1. $10 \times 50\%$ 1 r.m.
      2. $10 \times 60\%$ 1 r.m.

EXERCISES
1. bench press
2. pull-overs
3. squats
4. wrist curls
5. sit-ups ($15 \times$)

Stretching

GOAL
Perform each exercise 4 times for 20 seconds.

EXERCISES
1. knee tuck and hip twist
2. standing ankle grab
3. cat stretch
4. sit and reach

INTERMEDIATE

Flexibility
GOAL
Perform each exercise 6 times
for 30 seconds.

EXERCISES
Same

Warm-Up for Aerobics
GOAL
Same

EXERCISES
Same

Aerobics
GOAL
Work for 20 minutes at target
heart rate.

EXERCISES
Same

Cool-Down from Aerobics
GOAL
Same

Strength Training
GOAL
Sets: 1. $10 \times 50\%$ 1 r.m.
2. $8 \times 60\%$ 1 r.m.
3. $6 \times 70\%$ 1 r.m.

EXERCISES
1 through 4, plus
5. sit-ups ($30 \times$)
6. arm curls
7. triceps extensions
8. bent-over twist
9. hand gripper squeeze

Stretching
GOAL
Perform each exercise 8 times
for 40 seconds.

EXERCISES
1 through 4, plus
5. back roll
6. hurdler's stretch

ADVANCED

Flexibility
GOAL
Perform each exercise 9 times
for 45 seconds.

EXERCISES
Same

Warm-Up for Aerobics
GOAL
Same

EXERCISES
Same

Aerobics
GOAL
Work for 30 minutes at target
heart rate.

EXERCISES
Same

Cool-Down from Aerobics
GOAL
Same

Strength Training
GOAL
Sets: 1. $10 \times 50\%$ 1 r.m.
2. $8 \times 60\%$ 1 r.m.
3. $6 \times 70\%$ 1 r.m.
4. $4 \times 80\%$ 1 r.m.

EXERCISES
1 through 9, except for
5. sit-ups ($60 \times$)

Stretching
GOAL
Perform each exercise 12 times
for 60 seconds.

EXERCISES
1 through 6, plus
7. four-corner neck stretch

Exercise Program for
WATER POLO SWIMMING ROWING

Swimming and rowing activities require maximum muscular endurance, muscular strength, and cardiovascular endurance. All require excellent upper body strength, and water polo additionally requires superior muscular endurance and strength in the legs. Treading water constantly, and then periodically recruiting those muscles to propel the body out of the water to reach high balls, puts an incredible demand on the leg muscles.

BASIC

Flexibility

GOAL
Perform each exercise 3 times for 15 seconds.

EXERCISES
1. neck bend
2. waist stretch
3. triangle
4. fish
5. suspended stretch
6. waist hang

Warm-Up for Aerobics

GOAL
Perform any of these activities for 2 to 5 minutes at minimum resistance, setting, or speed.

EXERCISES
row, or
bicycle

Aerobics

GOAL
Work for 15 minutes at target heart rate.

EXERCISES
row, or
bicycle with hand weights

Cool-Down from Aerobics

GOAL
Gradually reduce intensity of exercise until heart rate drops below 110 beats per minute.

Strength Training

GOAL
Sets: 1. $10 \times 50\%$ 1 r.m.
    2. $8 \times 60\%$ 1 r.m.
    3. $6 \times 70\%$ 1 r.m.
    4. $4 \times 80\%$ 1 r.m.

EXERCISES
1. bench press
2. shoulder press
3. lat pull-downs
4. leg press
5. inner thigh pull
6. outer thigh pull
7. sit-ups ($30 \times$)

Stretching

GOAL
Perform each exercise 4 times for 20 seconds.

EXERCISES
1. knee tuck and hip twist
2. standing ankle grab
3. cat stretch
4. sit and reach

INTERMEDIATE

Flexibility

GOAL
Perform each exercise 6 times
for 30 seconds.

EXERCISES
Same

Warm-Up for Aerobics

GOAL
Same

EXERCISES
Same

Aerobics

GOAL
Work for 30 minutes at target
heart rate.

EXERCISES
Same

Cool-Down from Aerobics

GOAL
Same

Strength Training

GOAL
Sets: Same

Gradually increase to two
complete circuits.

EXERCISES
1 through 6, plus
7. sit-ups (60×)
8. bent-over twist
9. squats
10. pulley row
11. back extensions (30×)

Stretching

GOAL
Perform each exercise 8 times
for 40 seconds.

EXERCISES
1 through 4, plus
5. back roll
6. hurdler's stretch

ADVANCED

Flexibility

GOAL
Perform each exercise 9 times
for 45 seconds.

EXERCISES
Same

Warm-Up for Aerobics

GOAL
Same

EXERCISES
Same

Aerobics

GOAL
Work for 45 minutes at target
heart rate.

EXERCISES
Same

Cool-Down from Aerobics

GOAL
Same

Strength Training

GOAL
Sets: Same

Gradually increase to three
complete circuits.

EXERCISES
1 through 6, plus
7. sit-ups (90×)
8 through 10, plus
11. back extensions (60×)

Stretching

GOAL
Perform each exercise 12 times
for 60 seconds.

EXERCISES
1 through 6, plus
7. four-corner neck stretch

INDEX TO PERSONAL PROGRAM EXERCISES